Cognitive Informatics in Biomedicine and Healthcare

Series Editor

Vimla L. Patel, Center for Cognitive Studies in Medicine and Public Health, New York Academy of Medicine, New York, USA

Enormous advances in information technology have permeated essentially all facets of life. Although these technologies are transforming the workplace as well as leisure time, formidable challenges remain in fostering tools that enhance productivity, are sensitive to work practices, and are intuitive to learn and to use effectively. Informatics is a discipline concerned with the applied and basic science of information, the practices involved in information processing, and the engineering of information systems.

Cognitive Informatics (CI) is the multidisciplinary study of cognition, information and computational sciences. It has been adopted and applied particularly in the fields of biomedicine and health care. The field investigates cognitive aspects of human problem solving and is accordingly closely linked to artificial intelligence (AI) and decision-support systems. It includes all facets of computer applications in biomedicine and health care, including system design and computer-mediated intelligent action. The discipline of CI is strongly grounded in methods and theories derived from cognitive science. It provides a framework for the analysis, modeling and evaluation of complex human performance in technology-mediated settings, thereby contributing to the design, development and safe improvement of information systems for biomedicine and health care.

Despite the significant growth of the field, there have been few systematic reference books or instructional volumes intended for working professionals, scientists or graduate students in both human cognition and biomedical informatics. This series was introduced to meet those needs. Although information technologies are now in widespread use for promoting increased self-reliance in patients, there is often a disparity between the scientific and technological knowledge underlying healthcare practices and the lay beliefs, mental models and cognitive representations of illness and disease. The topics covered in this series also address the key research gaps in biomedical informatics related to the applicability of theories, models and evaluation frameworks of human-computer interaction, human factors and human-centered AI as they apply to health professionals as well as to the lay public.

Kai Zheng · Johanna Westbrook · Vimla L. Patel
Editors

Reengineering Clinical Workflow in the Digital and AI Era

Toward Safer and More Efficient Care

Second Edition

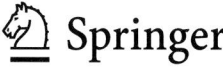 Springer

Editors
Kai Zheng
Department of Informatics
University of California
Irvine, CA, USA

Johanna Westbrook
Australian Institute of Health Innovation
Macquarie University
North Ryde, NSW, Australia

Vimla L. Patel
Center for Cognitive Studies in Medicine
and Public Health
The New York Academy of Medicine
New York, NY, USA

ISSN 2662-7280   ISSN 2662-7299 (electronic)
Cognitive Informatics in Biomedicine and Healthcare
ISBN 978-3-031-82970-3   ISBN 978-3-031-82971-0 (eBook)
https://doi.org/10.1007/978-3-031-82971-0

1st edition: © Springer Nature Switzerland AG 2019
2nd edition: © The Editor(s) (if applicable) and The Author(s), under exclusive license to Springer
Nature Switzerland AG 2025

This Springer imprint is published by the registered company Springer Nature Switzerland AG
The registered company address is: Gewerbestrasse 11, 6330 Cham, Switzerland

If disposing of this product, please recycle the paper.

Edward H. (Ted) Shortliffe

We would like to express our gratitude to him for his lifelong dedication to enhancing clinical practice through the contribution of decades of work on biomedical computing and artificial intelligence. His recognition of the importance of cognitive, social scientific, and educational research has been invaluable in advancing the field of biomedical informatics.

Foreword

Clinical care problems today—inefficiency, errors, applying best evidence.

There is universal recognition that healthcare today is expensive, inefficient and plagued by failure to deliver high quality. Nowhere is this truer than the United States, with its fragmented system of providers and payers and it its singularly huge health expenditures per capita as a proportion of gross domestic product. It is hardly controversial to propose that part of the solution is to improve efficiency through communication and coordination among all the stakeholders.

Current communication and coordination are largely related to financial matters, especially payment to healthcare providers. Where "workflow" is addressed, it is largely administrative in nature (admission, discharge, transfer, referral for clinical procedures, and documentation for billing purposes). Yet the real workflow—moving the patient through the healthcare system to transform the sick patients to healthy ones and keep them that way—what the administrative processes were created for in the first place—often garners less study for process improvement. As a result, clinical workflows take a back seat to administrative ones. By way of illustration, I once worked at a hospital where transfer of a patient from a medical or surgical service to the rehabilitation service required formally discharging the patient, with attendant discharge summary and orders, and then readmitting them, with attendant intake and admission orders—even though the patient might not physically move from one bed to another. The opportunity for degraded continuity of care, such as order transcription errors, was only one of the problems that this process imposed.

In the United States, the Affordable Care Act has led to rapid adoption of electronic health record (EHR) systems, largely commercial products, many of which with serious flaws that had previously impeded their adoption. The unintended consequences of this experience can inform similar efforts in other countries. Nevertheless, EHR adoption has been held out as a way to improve healthcare effectiveness and efficiency through automation of, in part, the communication and coordination related to workflow processes.

It is fair to say that the clinical (previously "medical") informatics research community has been poised to help with information-technology-based workflow for decades, at least since the inception of the Symposium on Computer Applications in Medical Care in 1977 (now renamed as the Annual Symposium of the American Medical Informatics Association). The work presented at that conference alone, over it 40-plus years, comprises many thousands of informatics projects, the majority of which failed to find long-term adoption.

While early evaluation of informatics solutions consisted of demonstrating that programs could run to completion without errors, and could do so faster and more accurately than previous attempts, current evaluations examine issues such as usability and usefulness. Yet even systems that fair well in such assessments find that enthusiasm for their use is underwhelming.

To a large extent, the lack of success of most of these projects has been related to failure to integrate them into healthcare systems and, even where integrated, failure to support workflow processes in natural, intuitive ways. For example, nurses and physicians find work-arounds in using electronic clinician order entry systems to the detriment of patients, while alerts and reminders are overridden more often than not as being inappropriate and bothersome. In my own experience, a tool I developed called the Medline Button, the first version of a class of applications called infobuttons that attempt to anticipate and assist with clinician information needs. The Medline Button executed medical literature searches based on a patient's ICD9 codes in the pre-PubMed era. It was a technical success, making the retrieval of relevant information possible with the touch of a button. However, it was a practical failure because it used data generated at the time of hospital discharge that were no longer relevant during a subsequent hospital admission.

What has largely been missing from efforts to health information technology-based efforts to improve clinical workflow, as evidenced by the Medline Button experience, are studies of cognitive processes of patient care providers and their impact on health care team communication and coordination. In subsequent infobutton research, for example, successful adoption did not occur until I partnered with Vimla Patel, one of this book's editors, and her team of cognitive scientists at McGill University to study clinicians' information needs through formal observational think-aloud studies in actual clinical settings.

Which brings me to the purpose and place of this book. Its reviews, essays, and case studies will collectively raise the reader's awareness of the myriad issues that relate health information technology to clinical workflow, not from the perspective of administrative processes, but based on cognitive processes that such systems are intended to support. Once enlightened with that perspective, the reader should consider the systems present (or needed) in his or her own institution and how they should be studied. Hopefully, some of these readers will be decision-makers at their institutions, who will be able to include cognitive researchers in the task of putting the findings of their research into practice. This book will then be at the right place at the right time to provide insight into the types of tools and evaluation expertise that will be needed to better match workflow systems to intended, rather than unintended, consequences.

Birmingham, AL, USA   James J. Cimino, MD

Contents

Contributors

Joanna Abraham Department of Anesthesiology and Institute for Informatics, School of Medicine, Washington University in St. Louis, St. Louis, MO, USA

Nate Apathy University of Maryland, College Park, MD, USA

Ann M. Bisantz University at Buffalo, Buffalo, NY, USA

Guy André Boy CentraleSupélec (Paris Saclay University), ESTIA Institute of Technology, Bidart, France

Timothy Buchman Emory University, Atlanta, USA

Kenrick Cato School of Nursing, University of Pennsylvania, Philadelphia, PA, USA

Yunan Chen University of California, Irvine, USA

Elizabeth L. Ciemins AMGA, Alexandria, VA, USA

Joanna Clive Centre for Health Systems and Safety Research, Australian Institute of Health Innovation, Faculty of Medicine, Health and Human Sciences, Macquarie University, Sydney, Australia

Enrico Coiera Macquarie University, North Ryde, Australia

William T. M. Dunsmuir Department of Statistics, School of Mathematics and Statistics, University of New South Wales, Sydney, Australia

Patricia C. Dykes Department of Medicine, Division of General Internal Medicine and Primary Care, Brigham and Women's Hospital, Harvard Medical School, Boston, MA, USA

Elizabeth V. Eikey University of California, San Diego, USA

Rollin J. Fairbanks MedStar Health Research Institute, Columbia, MD, USA; Georgetown University School of Medicine, Washington, DC, USA

Paul Fu Jr. City of Hope, Duarte, USA

Aaron Zachary Hettinger MedStar Health Research Institute, Columbia, MD, USA;
Georgetown University School of Medicine, Washington, DC, USA

Cheryl Hiddleson Emory University, Atlanta, USA

Jan Horsky Parexel International, Newton, USA

R. Stanley Hum McGill University, Montreal, Canada

A. Jay Holmgren UC San Francisco, San Francisco, CA, USA

Eugene Y. Kim Department of Emergency Medicine, Columbia University Irving Medical Center, New York, NY, USA

Craig E. Kuziemsky Office of Research Services, MacEwan University, Edmonton, AB, Canada

Holly J. Lanham University of Texas Health Science Center, San Antonio, TX, USA

Ling Li Centre for Health Systems and Safety Research, Australian Institute of Health Innovation, Faculty of Medicine and Health Sciences, Macquarie University, Sydney, Australia

Curt Lindberg Partners in Complexity, Waitsfield, VT, USA

Marcelo Lopetegui HICAPPS SpA, La Reina, Santiago, Chile

Sunny Lou Washington University, St. Louis, MO, USA

Keertana Nambiar Department of Informatics, School of Informatics and Computer Science, University of California, Irvine, CA, USA

Laurie Novak Vanderbilt University Medical Center, Nashville, USA

Mustafa Ozkaynak College of Nursing, University of Colorado-Denver, Denver, USA;
College of Nursing, University of Colorado I Anschutz Medical Campus, Aurora, CO, USA

Vimla L. Patel Cognitive Studies in Medicine and Public Health, The New York Academy of Medicine, New York, NY, USA;
The New York Academy of Medicine, New York, USA

Philip Payne Institute for Informatics, Data Science, and Biostatistics, Washington University in St. Louis, St. Louis, MO, USA

Siddarth Ponnala Saama Technologies, Chennai, India

Magdalena Z. Raban Centre for Health Systems and Safety Research, Australian Institute of Health Innovation, Faculty of Medicine, Health and Human Sciences, Macquarie University, Sydney, Australia

Madhu C. Reddy Department of Informatics, School of Informatics and Computer Science, University of California, Irvine, CA, USA

Sarah Rossetti Department of Biomedical Informatics, School of Nursing, Columbia University, New York City, NY, USA

Emilie M. Roth Roth Cognitive Engineering, Stanford, CA, USA

Kumiko Schnock Department of Medicine, Division of General Internal Medicine and Primary Care, Brigham and Women's Hospital, Harvard Medical School, Boston, MA, USA

Zhe Shan Farmer School of Business, Miami University, Oxford, OH, USA

Bryan Steitz Vanderbilt University, Nashville, TN, USA

Edward H. Suh Department of Emergency Medicine, Columbia University Irving Medical Center, New York, NY, USA

Jennifer Thate Siena College, Albany, NY, USA

Akshay Vankipuram Tempe, Arizona, USA

Jonathan Wald SmarterDx, New York City, USA

Scott R. Walter National Institute for Health and Care Research, Applied Research Collaboration West (NIHR ARC West), University Hospitals Bristol and Weston NHS Foundation Trust, Bristol, UK;
Population Health Sciences, Bristol Medical School, University of Bristol, Bristol, UK;
Centre for Health Systems and Safety Research, Australian Institute of Health Innovation, Faculty of Medicine and Health Sciences, Macquarie University, Sydney, Australia

Nicole E. Werner Departments of Anesthesiology and Biomedical Informatics, School of Medicine, Vanderbilt University, Nashville, USA

Johanna Westbrook Centre for Health Systems and Safety Research, Australian Institute of Health Innovation, Faculty of Medicine, Health and Human Sciences, Macquarie University, Sydney, Australia;
Macquarie University, North Ryde, Australia

Novia Wong Department of Informatics, School of Informatics and Computer Science, University of California, Irvine, CA, USA

Danny T. Y. Wu Department of Biostatistics, Health Informatics, and Data Sciences, University of Cincinnati College of Medicine, Cincinnati, OH, USA

Po-Yin Yen Institute for Informatics, Data Science, and Biostatistics, Washington University School of Medicine in St. Louis, St. Louis, MO, USA;
Goldfarb School of Nursing, Barnes-Jewish College, BJC HealthCare, St. Louis, MO, USA

Sean Yu Regeneron Pharmaceuticals Inc, Tarrytown, NY, USA

Kai Zheng University of California, Irvine, CA, USA

Chapter 1
Clinical Workflow in the Digital and Artificial Intelligence Era

Kai Zheng, Johanna Westbrook, and Vimla L. Patel

1.1   Introduction

Health information technology (IT) in general, electronic health records (EHR) in particular, hold great promise to cross the quality chasm of the healthcare system and to bend the curve of ever-rising costs (). However, health IT implementation projects globally have experienced a wide range of issues, from rollout delays to budget overruns (Kaplan and Harris-Salamone 2009). Successfully deployed systems often fail to generate anticipated results (Black et al. 2011; Kellermann and Jones 2013); some are even associated with unintended adverse consequences (Ash et al. 2007; Campbell et al. 2006; Koppel et al. 2005; Zheng et al. 2016).

In the U.S., for example, over $30 billion were invested in accelerating EHR adoption and promoting its "meaningful use" through the appropriation from the Health Information Technology for Economic and Clinical Health (HITECH) Act 2009 (Blumenthal 2010; Blumenthal and Tavenner 2010). While the program was successful in boosting EHR penetration rates across U.S. hospitals and clinics (ONC 2016), research on the effectiveness of the systems implemented has showed mixed results (Jones et al. 2010; Romano and Stafford 2011). In their Health Affair article entitled "*What it will take to achieve the as-yet-unfulfilled promises of health information technology,*" Kellermann and Jones concluded that despite the widespread adoption of health IT, the quality and efficiency of patient care in the U.S. were only

K. Zheng (✉)
University of California, Irvine, USA
e-mail: kai.zheng@uci.edu

J. Westbrook
Macquarie University, North Ryde, Australia

V. L. Patel
The New York Academy of Medicine, New York, USA

© The Author(s), under exclusive license to Springer Nature Switzerland AG 2025
K. Zheng et al. (eds.), *Reengineering Clinical Workflow in the Digital and AI Era*,
Cognitive Informatics in Biomedicine and Healthcare,
https://doi.org/10.1007/978-3-031-82971-0_1

marginally better; and the annual aggregate expenditures on healthcare continue to soar (Kellermann and Jones 2013).

Disruption to clinical workflow as a result of health IT implementation has been repeatedly shown as a major cause for the under-realized value of health IT. A key issue is that today's health IT systems are often designed to simply mimic existing paper-based forms, and thus provide little support for the cognitive tasks of clinicians or the workflow of the people who must actually use the system (National Research Council 2009). In a systematic review of the health IT evaluation literature, Buntin and colleagues found that a considerable number of studies reported negative or mixed findings, and that "most negative findings within these articles relate to the work-flow implications of implementing health IT, such as order entry, staff interaction, and provider-to-patient communication (Buntin et al. 2011, p. 467)."

"More/New Work" and "Unfavorable Workflow Change" are two workflow disruptions that have been most often discussed in the literature; both are directly attributable to the radical changes to established clinical workflow associated with introduction of health IT (Ash et al. 2007; Campbell et al. 2006; National Research Council 2009; Niazkhani et al. 2009). While some changes are purposefully planned—to reengineer existing processes to take full advantage of new capabilities offered by health IT—some are manifestations of a wide range of problems such as poor software usability, misaligned end-user incentives, rushed implementation processes, and the lack of sociotechnical considerations to effectively integrate software systems into their complex behavioral, organizational, and societal contexts (Ash et al. 2007; Campbell et al. 2006; National Research Council 2009; Niazkhani et al. 2009).

It is therefore critical to develop a comprehensive understanding of the impact of health IT on clinical workflow, in addition to their root causes, mechanisms, and consequences. Unfortunately, studies of these phenomena are still relatively scarce, and available findings are often inconclusive or conflicting (Unertl et al. 2010; Zheng et al. 2010; Carayon and Karsh 2010). Further, a consensus on the research definition of "clinical workflow" remains elusive, especially in the context of assessing workflow changes introduced by health IT (Unertl et al. 2010).

While conceptual models are available, e.g., (Unertl et al. 2010) many challenges remain in the development and application of robust measures of changes to clinical workflow (Zheng et al. 2010). Methods used in existing workflow studies vary to a great extent (Unertl et al. 2010; Zheng et al. 2010, 2011; Carayon and Karsh 2010; Lopetegui et al. 2014). Even among studies using the same method, a considerable degree of discrepancies exists in application of the method and interpretation of study results (Zheng et al. 2011; Lopetegui et al. 2014) For example, time and motion is considered to be the "gold standard" approach for obtaining quantitative assessments of clinical workflow; yet among the time and motion studies published, there has been a large degree of methodological inconsistencies in the design, execution, and results reporting of those studies, such as how inter-observer reliability is assessed and how multitasking is handled (Zheng et al. 2011; Lopetegui et al. 2014). This issue has significant implications for the rigor and generalizability of time and motion studies, diminishing our ability to accumulate knowledge as a field. As commented by

Carayon and Karsh in a comprehensive literature survey report commissioned by the U.S. Agency for Healthcare Research and Quality (AHRQ), the empirical evidence of health IT's impact on clinical workflow has been "anecdotal, insufficiently supported, or otherwise deficient in terms of scientific rigor (Carayon and Karsh 2010, p. 7)."

This book intends to address some of these knowledge gaps by assembling a team of experienced researchers and practitioners who have dedicated their career to studying and improving clinical workflow. Several chapters included in this book are results of a series of research or quality improvement efforts spanning multiple decades; some are syntheses of the research literature since early 1900s, bringing together what we know about clinical workflow, where gaps remain, and how these gaps can be addressed in future research. In this second edition, most chapters have been updated to reflect new developments of the field since the first edition of the book was published in 2019. This second edition also includes several new chapters that provide in-depth discussions on emerging methods for studying clinical workflow and workflow implications when introducing new, artificial intelligence (AI)-enabled health IT applications.

This book is organized into four Sections and 23 Chapters. The first Section, *Clinical Workflow, Health IT, and Artificial Intelligence*, orientates readers to the problem domain, basic concepts (e.g., cognitive behavior, workflow modeling, healthcare AI), and consequences of disrupted workflow due to health IT implementation. Chapter 3 is a new addition in the second edition that specifically looks into the promises and challenges originating from implementing AI-based tools.

The second Section, *the State of the Art of Workflow Research*, summarizes workflow studies conducted in healthcare in the past few decades. Chapter 6 is a new addition in this second edition of the book that reviews the most recent research developments since 2019. We purposefully include in this section workflow research from a non-healthcare domain, aviation, to draw a comparison between how clinical workflow differs from workflows in other industries and how they are conceptualized and studied differently. Section 2 also includes a chapter specifically on multitasking and interruptions, which are two defining characteristics of clinical workflow that have significant efficiency, care quality, and patient safety implications; in addition to chapters that address nursing and patient perspectives, and workflow-related issues during patient handoff and when patients transition from one healthcare setting to another, i.e., workflow at the edges.

Section 3, *Research Methods for Studying Clinical Workflow*, introduces research methodologies that have been commonly used in clinical workflow studies, including work sampling, time and motion, human factors engineering, and emerging methods that leverage sensor technology for automated data collection and real-time workflow assessment. Section 3 also includes a chapter that discusses the unique characteristics of quantitative workflow data and consequently unique challenges to statistically analyzing such data.

Section 4, *Applications and Case Studies*, first presents three large clinical workflow studies supported by the U.S. Agency for Healthcare Research and Quality (AHRQ) that looked into how health IT systems, introduced as part of ambulatory care practice redesign, impact clinical workflow. Section 4 then presents three case studies each focusing on a distinct perspective. These include effort in reengineering clinical workflow to enable a cross-continental collaboration on creating continuously monitored intensive care units, and efforts in enhancing clinical pathways, clinical rounding, and patient handoff communications.

By compiling a collection of high-quality scholarly works that seeks to provide clarity, consistency, and reproducibility in workflow research, we hope to create a repository of knowledge to inform future studies on health IT design, implementation, and evaluation. In addition to a research reader, this book offers pragmatic insights for practitioners in assessing workflow changes in the context of health IT adoption, and in implementing remedial interventions when such strategies are warranted. The book is also designed to present the state of the art on clinical workflow research, providing an excellent reader for graduate students in all clinical disciplines as well as in biomedical and health informatics.

References

The Office of the National Coordinator for Health Information Technology (ONC); Office of the Secretary, United States Department of Health and Human Services (HHS). 2016 Report to Congress on Health IT Progress: Examining the HITECH Era and the Future of Health IT; accessed August 20, 2018, https://dashboard.healthit.gov/report-to-congress/2016-report-con gress-examining-hitech-era-future-health-information-technology.php.

Ash JS, Sittig DF, Poon EG, Guappone K, Campbell E, Dykstra RH. The extent and importance of unintended consequences related to computerized provider order entry. J Am Med Inform Assoc. 2007;14(4):415–23.

Black AD, Car J, Pagliari C, Anandan C, Cresswell K, Bokun T, McKinstry B, Procter R, Majeed A, Sheikh A. The impact of eHealth on the quality and safety of health care: A systematic overview. PLoS Med. 2011;8(1): e1000387.

Blumenthal D. Launching HITECH. N Engl J Med. 2010;362(5):382–5.

Blumenthal D, Tavenner M. The, "meaningful use" regulation for electronic health records. N Engl J Med. 2010;363(6):501–4.

Buntin MB, Burke MF, Hoaglin MC, Blumenthal D. The benefits of health information technology: A review of the recent literature shows predominantly positive results. Health Aff (Millwood). 2011;30(3):464–71.

Campbell EM, Sittig DF, Ash JS, Guappone KP, Dykstra RH. Types of unintended consequences related to computerized provider order entry. J Am Med Inform Assoc. 2006;13(5):547–56.

Carayon P, Karsh B-T. Incorporating health information technology into workflow redesign—summary report. AHRQ Publication No. 10–0098-EF. Rockville, MD: Agency for Healthcare Research and Quality. 2010.

Girosi F, Meili R, Scoville R. Extrapolating evidence of health information technology savings and costs. Santa Monica, CA: RAND Corp.; 2005.

Jones SS, Adams JL, Schneider EC, Ringel JS, McGlynn EA. Electronic health record adoption and quality improvement in US hospitals. Am J Manag Care. 2010;16(12 Suppl HIT):SP64–71.

Kaplan B, Harris-Salamone KD. Health IT success and failure: recommendations from literature and an AMIA workshop. J Am Med Inform Assoc. 2009;16(3):291–9.

Kellermann AL, Jones SS. What it will take to achieve the as-yet-unfulfilled promises of health information technology. Health Aff (Millwood). 2013;32(1):63–8.

Koppel R, Metlay JP, Cohen A, Abaluck B, Localio AR, Kimmel SE, Strom BL. Role of computerized physician order entry systems in facilitating medication errors. JAMA. 2005;293(10):1197–203.

Lopetegui M, Yen PY, Lai A, Jeffries J, Embi P, Payne P. Time motion studies in healthcare: What are we talking about? J Biomed Inform. 2014;49:292–9.

Institute of Medicine (U.S.). Crossing the quality chasm: A new health system for the 21st century. Washington D.C.: National Academy Press; 2001.

National Research Council. Computational technology for effective health care: Immediate steps and strategic directions. Washington D.C.: National Academies Press; 2009.

Niazkhani Z, Pirnejad H, Berg M, Aarts J. The impact of computerized provider order entry systems on inpatient clinical workflow: A literature review. J Am Med Inform Assoc. 2009;16(4):539–49.

Romano MJ, Stafford RS. Electronic health records and clinical decision support systems: Impact on national ambulatory care quality. Arch Intern Med. 2011;171(10):897–903.

Unertl KM, Novak LL, Johnson KB, Lorenzi NM. Traversing the many paths of workflow research: Developing a conceptual framework of workflow terminology through a systematic literature review. J Am Med Inform Assoc. 2010;17(3):265–73.

Zheng K, Haftel HM, Hirschl RB, O'Reilly M, Hanauer DA. Quantifying the impact of health IT implementations on clinical workflow: A new methodological perspective. J Am Med Inform Assoc. 2010;17(4):454–61.

Zheng K, Guo MH, Hanauer DA. Using the time and motion method to study clinical work processes and workflow: Methodological inconsistencies and a call for standardized research. J Am Med Inform Assoc. 2011;18(5):704–10.

Zheng K, Abraham J, Novak LL, Reynolds TL, Gettinger A. A survey of the literature on unintended consequences associated with health information technology: 2014–2015. Yearb Med Inform. 2016;1:13–29.

Part I
Clinical Workflow, Health IT, and Artificial Intelligence

Chapter 2
Cognitive Support for Decisions in the Context of Clinical Workflows

Jan Horsky

Abstract Modern medical care has one of the most complex organizational structures in society, with many non-linear work processes and intricate networks of professional relationships of people who often have interdependent individual and collective responsibilities. Healthcare organizations share many attributes with those in other safety–critical domains that are science-based and information-intensive, and therefore the initiative to improve the quality and safety of care has often been informed by interventions that proved to be effective in those industries. At the same time, many important features of care delivery do not have corresponding examples elsewhere. Researchers analyzing clinical workflows must often do so without the benefit of models that can be readily adapted from other fields, as standard models can describe such extensive and complex work environments only to a limited degree. The ability to reliably assess and model work processes is crucial for developing safe and effective health information technology that needs to be tightly integrated into workflows without adding extraneous complexity and cognitive effort. However, studies have historically investigated primarily the business process of care, and today many workflow analyses show conflicting results and may lack sufficient rigor. Work organization and processes in a socio-natural system that has many non-linear and non-additive functions that characterize healthcare are difficult to model and predict because complex systems are non-reducible to their constituent parts. This chapter discusses several analytic and explanatory frameworks that can guide studies that model workflows and cognitive processes associated with decision making that is often done with incomplete or unreliable information and where goals and priorities often need to be rearranged in response to dynamically changing circumstances. The application of artificial intelligence to the areas of care where they can have a sizeable effect is also reviewed. Patient care can be greatly advanced by the careful harnessing of powerful new forms of information technology into a collaborative environment where complex reasoning and ethics are the exclusive responsibilities of clinicians.

J. Horsky (✉)
Parexel International, Newton, USA
e-mail: horsky@live.com

© The Author(s), under exclusive license to Springer Nature Switzerland AG 2025　　　9
K. Zheng et al. (eds.), *Reengineering Clinical Workflow in the Digital and AI Era*,
Cognitive Informatics in Biomedicine and Healthcare,
https://doi.org/10.1007/978-3-031-82971-0_2

Keywords Clinical workflow · Complex systems · Socio-technical systems · Decision making · Medical cognition · Distributed cognition · Workflow modeling · Cognitive workload · Medical error · Patient safety · Cognitive engineering · Health Information Technology · Artificial Intelligence

2.1 Complex Work Environments

The healthcare industry comprises, at the highest level, a wide array of organizational entities, from small private practices and independent clinics to hospitals and large healthcare delivery networks. Many often work together to provide different or specialized types of care to patients, and each institution also interacts with a multitude of ancillary and support service businesses, insurance and payer companies, public, administrative and regulatory bodies, research centers and academic institutions that jointly form one of the most complex organizational structures in society today (Begun et al. 2003; McDaniel et al. 2013). Modern healthcare has primarily evidence-based character that routinely uses many kinds of medical and information technology that, in turn, shape the work environments where care is delivered. Individuals engaged directly or indirectly in patient care and its administration typically collaborate across professional and institutional boundaries. The quality of their work, level of performance and patient safety are highly dependent on health information technology (HIT) to collect, store, and share information in the complex settings of clinical care.

Decision-making and reasoning of clinicians is as often autonomous as it is contingent on the expertise and decisions made by others at different times and locations. This intricate combination of individual and collective responsibilities, actions and judgements tends to generate many non-linear work processes that account for much of the dynamism and elasticity of both personal and collaborative workflows (Fig. 2.1). Standard workflow models intended to reliably predict outcomes with precision have therefore only limited utility in describing extensive, interconnected processes, especially where dependencies are not always clearly apparent and may change over time.

Many salient characteristics of healthcare work are unique to the domain and do not have good corresponding examples in other industries. Researchers analyzing clinical workflows must often do so without the benefit of models that can be readily adapted from other fields. The primary responsibility of all clinicians is to ensure that patients receive timely, appropriate, and effective care whenever and wherever needed. It means that, in practice, goals, their sequence of completion and plans—the constituent parts of workflow analysis—are quickly reorganized and modified to accommodate emergent events. Interventions that conflict with prior or existing objectives or are outside of normative pathways are sometimes carried out to prevent the exacerbation of minor issues into greater problems. Decisions and actions may be deferred, substituted, or finalized only to a sufficient degree when time or resources are limited, so that tasks with higher priority get completed in full. For example,

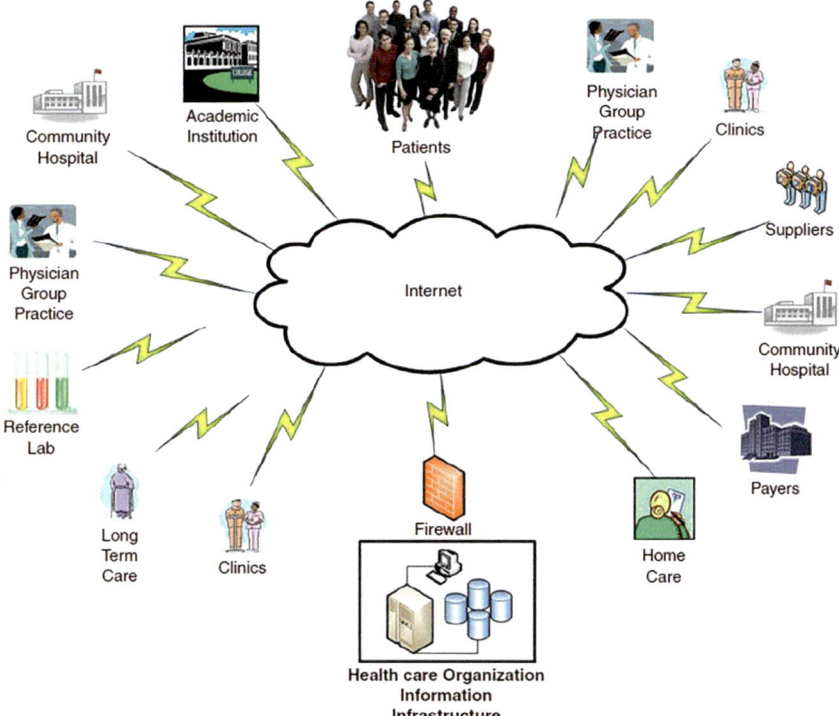

Fig. 2.1 Major organizational components of an integrated. Reprinted from Vogel (2014). Management of information in health care Organizations. Biomedical informatics: Computer applications in health care and biomedicine. E. H. Shortliffe and J. J. Cimino. London, Heidelberg, New York, Dordrecht, Springer: 443–474

planned procedures or evaluations may be postponed or replaced when updated laboratory test results become available, or when new findings require immediate attention. Patients may get treated without delay for acute problems while care for their long-term conditions may be temporarily limited to stabilization or postponed to more opportune time. An important part of improving care quality by making clinical work primarily evidence-based is the reduction of unwarranted variation (Wennberg 2002). At the same time, seeming aberrations and deviations from plans and norms can frequently be considered as necessary corrections to counter evolving risks.

Many public and private organizations have complicated internal structures and employ a large workforce where scientists, researchers, lawyers, professionals and administrative and support personnel collaborate across the boundaries of different expertise and responsibilities. The National Aeronautics and Space Agency (NASA), many national airlines, technology corporations and power-generating companies conduct their work and research in an environment that is science-based, safety–critical and where considerable risks need to be well understood and controlled.

Healthcare organizations share many of these critical attributes and many have therefore informed their effort to increase safety, quality, and effectiveness by considering initiatives successfully implemented in other industries, such as long-term investment in information technology.

There are considerable differences, to be sure, between an engineered system on one hand (the aircraft, engineering), and biological, natural systems (the patient, medical science) on the other. The provision of healthcare has in fact many characteristics that are not typically found in engineered systems and therefore accelerating the uneven pace of progress towards greater effectiveness and safety requires new insights into the specifics and idiosyncrasies of this knowledge and information-intensive domain and its work organization (Durso and Drews 2010). Understanding how health information technology can be best used to advance these goals remains a challenge.

Biomedicine is, in many respects, quite unlike other applied and natural scientific disciplines. One defining but elusive feature of physiologic systems is their remarkable complexity arising from the interaction of a myriad of structural units and regulatory feedback loops that operate over a wide range of temporal and spatial scales, enabling an organism to adapt to environmental stresses (Glass 2001). Medical care and research encompass the properties and behavior of human beings—organisms whose complexity have no counterpart in other sciences. Many properties of natural systems are opaque; for example, important interactions can often be only deduced and in fact may not be fully understood. Individual elements of biological systems occurred without intentional design and are the result of reorganization and evolution in order to adapt to changing environment (Durso and Drews 2010). Medical investigations and discourse therefore includes an aspect of uncertainty that inevitably creates variability among individuals and makes clinical information systematically different from information used in physics, engineering, or even clinical chemistry (Shortliffe and Barnett 2014).

Much of decision making in healthcare involves reasoning with inherently probabilistic information. The level of uncertainty in diagnostic hypotheses or treatment options that clinicians seek to reduce by testing and by gathering data is further affected by information that is often incomplete, dated, or unreliable. For example, observations, laboratory results and narrative reports may not have been completed in time or cannot be obtained when needed, their interpretation could be erroneous and be in apparent conflict (Weber et al. 2017; Smithson 1999). When the history of respiratory problems is not found in the patient record, its lack could be interpreted as an indication of the absence of prior problems by a clinician hypothesizing about the possibility of acute lung disease, even if such assessment occurred but simply was not documented. The value of any patient information rises in the eyes of clinicians when the record is comprehensive: typically, completeness needs to reach 85% or above for the content to be truly useful to clinicians (Yasnoff 2014).

Gathering and reviewing the information that is available adds yet another obstacle that HIT needs to successfully navigate. Somewhat ironically, paucity and excess of information may coincide even in the record of a single patient. Clinicians routinely write assessments, case summaries and test reports and collect laboratory data but individual findings are often meaningful only in the relevant context, either in retrospect, when estimating progress, or relative to other concurrent conditions when considering severity. However, this information may be stored in multiple electronic health record systems (EHR), or in ancillary systems that may or may not be functionally interoperable. Patients treated in different locations receiving specialty care and services may only have portions of their historical data recorded in any one EHR system, and the reviewing clinician may not be aware of critical events described in unconnected sources (Weber et al. 2017). Even information that can be found in a single system may not be easily accessible for appropriate contextual review. Data in different modules and displayed on separate screens complicate their meaningful visual aggregation that a clinician needs to gain specific insights or to compare outcomes over time and across treatments. Poor system design may necessitate repeated searches and navigation through the record to retrieve information that is relevant at the moment, adding time and cognitive burden to already complex medical decisions (Stoller 2013). Narratives in visit and progress notes may also contain repetitive, dated or inaccurate content that occurs as the unintended consequence of too-facile recycling of old text through cut-and-paste functions. This so-called "note bloat" trend inhibits the ongoing questioning and ascertainment process that helps monitor diagnostic accuracy as illnesses evolve over time (Graber et al. 2017).

The complex biomedical science, the pragmatics of making decisions with uncertain or incomplete information, the intricacies of mixed collaborative and individual responsibilities and the dynamics of established and ill-defined goals are all characteristic of a field in which work demands can exceed the bounds of unaided human cognition (Masys 2002). Every year, the volume of new knowledge and revised understanding of established concepts grow rapidly and need to be mastered and applied to practice. It is estimated that while it took 50 years to double the number of medical research publications in 1950, in 1980 it was merely 7 years, only 3.5 years in 2010 and was projected to be just 73 days in 2020 (Challenges and Education 2011). This tremendous wealth of evidence, that continuously expands, can only be channeled to practical use by HIT that is unobtrusively embedded into workflows and effectively supports clinicians in their decision making. It is a crucial component of safe, effective, high-quality care. Success in this endeavor is predicated on our ability to reliably assess and model healthcare work so that new technology can become its integral part without adding yet another layer of complexity.

2.2   The Challenge of Modeling Healthcare Work

Healthcare institutions are paradigmatic examples of complex organizations where clinicians interact with other professionals and with a myriad of information systems and technology in non-linear way, and where work plans often include emergent goals (Martínez-García and Hernández-Lemus 2013). Complex work environments are distinctly different from those that are merely complicated: they are more difficult to analyze, and predictions of future system states are not always reliable. Complicated problems and processes originate from singular causes or from the actions of identifiable agents, and when they combine to create a problem state, the sources can be distinguished and addressed individually. Complex problems, on the other hand, evolve from networks of multiple interacting causes that may not be possible to differentiate and interventions to address them need to consider systems in their entirety. Feedback and circular processes in such systems also modify and intensify the causes so that effects are often disproportional to their origins (Poli 2013).

Healthcare can therefore be characterized as a socio-natural system with many non-linear and non-additive functions that may be opaque and more difficult to understand than within engineered systems, such as those typified by aviation or manufacturing, where nonlinearity is often a sign of malfunction (Durso and Drews 2010). Standard, reusable processes that are known to engender safe practices, and therefore allow for the monitoring of anomalies that may gradually become problems, have more limited use in healthcare. Clinicians may prioritize or trade off a variety of short and longer-term goals to restore a patient to a stable state or to reduce their immediate discomfort. Members of teams regularly help one another without waiting for explicit requests, and engage when anticipating imminent need for extra resources (Rivera-Rodriguez and Karsh 2010). Actions that are planned or in progress are frequently interrupted by personal contact with other clinicians, telephone conversations and pagers or computer-generated alerts. This dynamic is inherent to clinical work and is generally considered to be necessary and adaptive, even as interruptions increase the risk of error (Li et al. 2011).

Clinical objectives that may not be fully formed initially but progress rapidly into to more focused and defined goals as insight is gained may be characterized as emergent (Klein 2009). Emergent properties of systems and processes are difficult to model and predict because complex systems are non-reducible to their constituent parts. In the hypothetico-deductive approach to diagnostic reasoning, for example, data and observations are added to a growing stack of findings, and are used to reformulate or refine the active hypotheses until one reaches a threshold of certainty, when management, disposition or therapeutic decisions can be made (Shortliffe and Blois 2014). Parts of a therapeutic plan that define patient trajectory and workflows affecting multiple clinicians may therefore be only tentative, even in situations when more distant goals are clearly defined. The idea of work that "flows" may be entirely foreign to nurses, for example, whose work is typically irregular, even turbulent, and punctuated by interruptions, handoffs, and patient turnover that drive up cognitive workload (Jennings et al. 2021). Each new observation and information related to them will inform the order of care and the next activity in their mental "stack" of tasks to complete (Ebright et al. 2003). One of the fundamental principles of establishing a productive work environment can be described as "designing out" system barriers by implementing technology that appropriately supports both routine and complex tasks (Ebright 2010).

2.3 Efforts to Improve Safety and Quality Across Industrial Domains

Large companies in the late nineteen eighties started turning their research focus towards cross-functional business processes, and away from studying strictly individual, functional and transactional operations such as procurement, manufacturing, and sales. They defined the concept of a business process as a set of logically related tasks performed to achieve a specific business outcome (Davenport and Short 1990). Their essential insight was that decisions that affect multiple processes at once, either in parallel or as antecedents to events further down the workflow, should be given more weight in the overall analysis than ad-hoc and local decision making.

A similar effort emerged about a decade later in healthcare, spearheaded largely by academic institutions, professional societies and regulatory bodies that aimed to improve quality by modernizing care continuity across primary and specialty practices and by decreasing unwarranted variation (Wennberg 1999). They started creating and disseminating collections of evidence-based recommendations (clinical guidelines) for quality care that outlined clinical goals for a variety of specific conditions and treatments and instructions on how to achieve them. These guidelines today provide the basis for higher-level decision making, somewhat analogous to the multiple-process decisions in other industries, that are often complemented by locally developed clinical protocols that monitor compliance with higher-level guidelines but do not strictly define individual steps in any one process. Each care institution may also create its own clinical pathways, best practices recommendations and structured multidisciplinary plans of care aligned with clinical guidelines. However, there are today no formal industry standards for completing care processes, and clinicians have largely their own ways of interacting with patients and prioritizing tasks as necessary (Karsh 2009).

Healthcare work analyses have historically investigated the business process associated with care or the flow of patients and staff through large hospital buildings rather than the dependencies of clinical decisions. Advancing a planned strategy to improve the effectiveness and safety of care was much less of a motivation than the immediate need to address inefficiencies and disruptions in a reactive way when problems were identified or were introduced by new technologies. For example, there are no standard descriptions of workflow for care processes that would guide decisions about where and how to integrate computer-based decision-support interventions (Shiffman et al. 2004). The interest in analyzing clinical work processes and collaboration developed later, as care teams have grown, and clinicians become more focused and specialized. Currently, workflow studies that were once scarce are done more frequently although their findings are often inconclusive or conflicting (Zheng et al. 2015). Many lack scientific rigor because they describe workflows only indirectly or do not explain conflating or mediating factors such as training and organizational culture within the socio-technical context of HIT implementation and use (Carayon and Karsh 2010).

The term workflow is generally understood, in the context of modeling, to apply to the control dimension of a business process, that is the dependencies among tasks that must be respected during its execution (Delacoras et al. 2000). It is used more broadly in healthcare and its meaning can have local variations. It can describe both individual and group goals and processes, tests and examination a clinician performs during a visit, and also the abstract representation of tasks, information needs, error conditions or the navigation pathways through the screens of a patient records system.

Any workflow model is in its essence a simplified representation of past, actual or future processes that can be described by routing, allocation, and execution components. It may have a narrow focus, such as the support for decision making, but usually has a broader purpose (Reijers 2003). There are several leading frameworks for the study of healthcare processes. Bricon-Souf and colleagues describe a proprietary modeling approach for medical intensive care units that explicitly distinguishes urgency in determining the authorization of a resource to perform a task (Bricon-Souf et al. 1999). The Systems Engineering Initiative for Patient Safety (SEIPS) (Carayon et al. 2006) model is more broadly applicable and defines the work system as an interactive environment that structures workflows, affects the performance of clinicians and therefore indirectly patient outcomes. The authors also proposed the Workflow Elements Model (WEM) (Carayon et al. 2012), a related framework that conceptualizes the activity of individuals and groups working asynchronously as dynamic and temporal characteristics of workflows. System elements, in this view, create a context that constrains or enables workflows that encompass converging and diverging goals. The dynamism of these processes is considered the emergent property of work.

One theoretical perspective on work in healthcare organizations holds that complex social interactions, conflicting objectives, personal preferences and work demands determine how clinicians use information technology and to what effect (Anderson and Aydin 2005). Predictive analyses therefore require robust understanding of organizational dynamics, the skills and performance characteristics of individuals, and the effects that information systems have on coordination and information sharing. Simply modeling the levels of independent variables hypothesized to predict change cannot be productive (Mohr 1982; Markus and Robey 1988). A useful paradigm for situating the description of work processes, pathways and interactions that healthcare workflow studies reference may be found in the work of Holden and Karsh (Holden and Karsh 2009), who have formulated a theoretical model of multilevel work system to understand the behavior of clinicians working with the support of information technology. It was derived in part empirically from HIT evaluation studies and implementation literature, and in part from theories used in communications sciences, psychology, sociology, management, organizational behavior and human factors research. This model, when applied to explain the determinants of technology use behavior, (Smith and Sainfort 1989; Carayon et al. 2003; Klein et al. 1994; House et al. 1995; Klein and Kozlowski 2000) postulates, that physical, cognitive and social-behavioral performance of individuals is affected and constrained by nested structural elements of healthcare organization (Karsh 2009).

The lowest tier of this model describes the integration (or fit) of core constructs, such as clinician-HIT interaction and collaborative and workflow patterns within the constraints and workflow patterns that are active on the levels above. At the top of this four-tier hierarchy is the entire health care industry, where standards, regulations, legislative oversight, social influence and labor force characteristics guide the work of organizations. Below are healthcare institutions of different size, from care delivery networks to private practices, that create administrative structures of their own, formulate policies, norms and best practices, set priorities and provide training, financial resources and expertise appropriate to its constituent work groups and units that are on the next level down. Each organizational setting has its own constraints determined by technological and administrative factors, by its core mission that affects the professional and specialization makeup of the workforce and by the characteristics of the target patient population that collectively contribute to the complexity of workflows and task structure. The work of individuals, at the base tier, is therefore done in an environment responsive to the effects of activities on each higher level that can be disruptive or conducive to attention, situational awareness, decision making, problem solving and cognitive labor. Conduits between and within levels then create a rich and information-intensive context for organizational, patient care and mental workflows (Holden and Karsh 2009).

A compelling viewpoint on the analysis of healthcare work, complementary to the structural dynamism found in other models, is the conceptual lens of the patient trajectory, in which the analytical anchor point is the pathway of an individual patient through the care process. The patient-oriented workflow model (Ozkaynak et al. 2013) references the cognitive, social and work behavior of agents in a complex sociotechnical system (Berg 1999a; Sittig and Singh 2010) where actions are not centered around individuals or groups but rather distributed among roles in the work setting that converge around the care of a specific patient. What partially determines the basic directions and outlines of the care process is a structured sequence of activities, events, and occurrences related to a patient's particular illness trajectory. Workflows therefore align with the way in which an illness typically unfolds, in both sequential and temporal order, and analyses focus on the embedding of illness trajectory within the care process (Reddy et al. 2006). Clinicians planning interventions and tests often need to understand where on the trajectory a patient currently is and where they should be relative to the characteristic unfolding of a disease progression. Their reasoning concerns not only individual data points at the time of decisions, but also patterns and trends over time and their interpretation in the larger context of known outcomes over many patients (Hilligoss and Zheng 2013). Developing these models is methodologically and practically challenging, however, because of the large variability of data types that are meaningful and relevant in each setting, and also due to the lack of a comprehensive and robust conceptual framework that limits their consistent interpretation (Ozkaynak et al. 2013).

The similarly conceptualized multidimensional Triangle Evaluation Model (Ancker et al. 2012) identifies elements of healthcare structure and process that should be assessed concurrently and in the context of quality and safety outcome variables. Its structure-level predictors include HIT characteristics and how clinicians interact with it, organizational setting and a typical patient population at the care institution. These foci align well with the multi-level, dynamic perspective on much of healthcare work. Dynamic workflows that self-adapt to the present situation and evolve at execution time as a function of personal insight pose a challenge to the creation of accurate models. Clinicians often encounter ill-defined and under-specified problems they need to address, and their cognitive task is to determine the form of the solution. Such systems are called "loosely coupled" and it is useful to see dynamic workflows as situated in historical records where tightly-coupled elements provide a bound to loosely-coupled relationships and event sequences that are largely non-deterministic (Covvey et al. 2011). An example of work environment that can be best characterized in such terms is emergency and critical care (Horsky et al. 2015).

2.4   Analyzing Cognitive Process and Collaborative Work

A prominent attribute of clinical work is the presence of both tightly and loosely coupled organizational and work relationships. It is essential that smaller units orga-nize their work autonomously from central control and that individuals have the appropriate level of discretion to make independent decisions in the management of evolving needs in patient care. Typically, clinicians have loosely-coupled interac-tions with policy-setting authorities in administrative and medical oversight roles who monitor institutional guidelines and strategies and regulatory mandates from local and national bodies (the higher tiers of the multi-level model). They are highly trained professionals who collaborate with other experts but retain individual responsibility for decisions (Pinelle and Gutwin 2006). However, multi-disciplinary and special-ized (e.g., surgical) teams often have an ordered structure with tightly-coupled and clearly defined roles and relationships. For example, attending physicians, residents, interns, medical students, nurses and support staff in hospitals have roles delineated in an explicit hierarchy and patient care directives are communicated through verbal and written orders.

A theoretical framework that can be employed to study problem solving and collaborative work in healthcare is Distributed Cognition (DCog), which concep-tualizes human cognition as extended beyond the boundaries of an individual and is manifest in artefacts (physical and electronic), and social and work relationships (Hollan et al. 2000; Hutchins et al. 1991; Hutchins 1995, 2000). Its focus is the representational transformation of information that occurs in external media and are coordinated by human and technological actors (Wright et al. 2000; Furniss and Blandford 2006; Cowley and Vallée-Tourangeau 2017; Horsky et al. 2003). It is perhaps the most clearly articulated, critiqued, commonly used and well known form of exploring how distributed action can be examined as a cognitive process (Perry et al. 2017) The problem structure that DCog can analyze with relatively little difficulty is often defined a-priori: goals are known and defined, changes follow pre-determined processes, and many tasks are repetitive and could be trained. Studies that typically produce clearly identifiable examples of problem solving and cognition distributed over artefacts and collaborators usually involve well-defined activities, explicit boundaries of control and influence, and an environment, where work roles and protocols are pre-set and generally static and constrained, such as ship navigation or the work of pilots.

The tightly-coupled components of healthcare workflows are appropriate objects of such analyses. For example, the patient trajectory workflow model is closely related to that patient's illness trajectory, as clinicians make decisions that follow a specific reasoning process, or an "illness script." It is conceptualized as an internal representation of the pathophysiology, epidemiology, time course, signs and symptoms of a particular illness or a disease and organized as a summary—or mental model—that includes diagnostics and treatment (Custers 2015). Such models are initially acquired through medical training and further developed and internalized by professional experience. They represent knowledge in three broad categories: predisposing conditions (context), pathophysiological insult (causal chain) and clinical consequences (signs and symptoms) (Schmidt and Rikers 2007). Expert clinicians have over time expanded, refined and contextualized this knowledge to form durable mental models in which the presence or absence of significant script characteristics carry certain predictive value for a diagnosis. Their ability to differentiate between illnesses with similar presentations allows them to make more accurate diagnostic and care decisions more quickly.

Clinicians are less likely to associate illnesses with a particular script when they have atypical presentation or when they encounter them infrequently. Their diagnostic reasoning then becomes more laborious and vulnerable to errors, biases and misconceptions (Jones et al. 2014). Uncertainty is inherent to clinical work and its level is associated with diseases that vary greatly in the degree of symptom ambiguity (Leykum et al. 2014). For example, patients who have a more typical progression of an illness can be more reliably and predictably treated according to existing standards of care than others, for whom population-derived guidelines are a poor fit and who require more personalized care. The downside is that outcomes dependent on individual characteristics or manifestations that may be unknowable are far less certain.

The DCog framework is less effective for the analysis of loosely-coupled structures that have dynamic workflows and emergent goals. Uncertainty takes many forms in health care (Plsek and Greenhalgh 2001) and derives from three main sources: the complexity of the system itself, the unpredictable trajectories of some illnesses, and the limits of current medical knowledge (Han et al. 2011). It has been conceptualized as a multidimensional phenomenon with theoretically distinct constructs that are potentially measurable and related to different outcomes, mechanisms of action and management strategies (Gerrity et al. 1990). For example, a measure developed to study clinical reasoning strategies during patient visits includes an assessment of uncertainty that refers to how well the limitations of available information are recognized and explained and how solutions are planned to adjust to the current situation (Weir et al. 2012). A study of clinical reasoning and communication in an emergency department examined the amount of detail conveyed in narrative accounts of care during handoffs as an approximation of the uncertainty level (Horsky et al. 2015). However, uncertainty of diagnostic and treatment decisions within complex systems is often irreducible and its measurement and management challenging. It is the product of non-linear dynamics and the information needed to reduce this type of uncertainty may not exist (Lanham et al. 2014). Application of the DCog approach in settings, where shifting problem space and specific, local solutions are central to the performance of both individual actors and the entire system therefore remains problematic.

There are several published reports on DCog analyses that have come close in their application to highly dynamic and loosely structured settings (Hazlehurst et al. 2008, 2007; Holder 1999) although the problems described have been carefully "bounded" to create a simplified problem space that does not account for the layers of setting context (Cowley and Vallée-Tourangeau 2017). Many other studies, however, have used DCog as a methodological and explanatory framework or were designed to extend its methodology (Horsky et al. 2003; Kaufman et al. 2003, 2009; Furniss et al. 2016a; Sedig et al. 2015; Grundgeiger et al. 2010; Cohen et al. 2006; Xiao 2005; Nemeth et al. 2004; Berg 1999b; Zhang 2002; Zhang and Norman 1994; Horsky 2008) Importantly, the DCog framework allows researchers to identify and discuss the difference between tightly and loosely coupled system analysis of activity systems in terms of their informational content and problem solving activities (Cowley and Vallée-Tourangeau 2017).

Healthcare that is highly specialized and where teams of clinicians and experts are involved in the treatment of one patient requires a high level of coordination. It means that all parties need to understand the position of their collaborators in the shared problem space, and how their mental models and work progress align, in order to reduce diagnostic or therapeutic uncertainty and to resolve ill-structured problems. Situation Awareness (SA) and decision-making also become distributed and an emergent property of a collaborative system: they represent something that resides in the interaction between agents of the system rather than separately in the minds of individuals (Salmon 2009). Analyses then need to pay attention to how agents are made aware of ongoing but problem-unrelated situation monitoring in order to self-organize (Perry et al. 2017).

2.5 Cognitive Load

There are natural limits to the span and effectiveness of attention, perception, recognition and recall memory, learning, problem solving, reasoning and decision making that bound their application primarily to the core purpose of clinical work—pursuing medical goals. These resource are simultaneously needed for interaction with technology, organization and work coordination.(25) Situation Awareness relates to the dynamic and transient state of a mental model which is produced by an ongoing process of information gathering and interpretation (Hendy 1995) It is a construct that can be thought of as an internal mental model of the current state of an individual's environment, or the perception of the elements in the environment within time and space confines, the comprehension of their meaning and the projection of their status in the near future (Mica 1988). SA is one component of dynamic, distributed decision making, along with task, system and individual factors. It changes as the environment changes in response to decisions and actions of individuals or due to automated technology interventions (Wright et al. 2004) Dynamic systems are therefore extremely demanding on human cognitive resources. Mental workload increases along with system complexity while situation awareness is more difficult to maintain.

Even in routine medical care, cognitive workload is immense. Family physicians, for example, have to perceive, process, integrate and make decision on four to five problems in one visit (Beasley et al. 2004). They need to identify and diagnose each problem and plan testing and treatment. The complexity of decisions further rises with the number of comorbidities and concurrent problems that may interact or have causal relationships and when indicated treatment options may be in conflict. The burden on primary care clinicians in terms of coordination, information gathering, cognitive workload and decision-making is compounded not only by frequent interruptions and multiple parallel tasks but also by incomplete information; it is estimated that physicians have about eight unanswered questions for every ten ambulatory visits (Bates et al. 2003).

Research in cognitive psychology offers ample evidence of the detrimental effect of interruptions on human cognition (Altmann and Trafton 2007), and reports from healthcare studies show, that interruptions and distractions contribute to medical error (Ashcroft et al. 2005) and may increase the risk to patient safety during certain types of clinical tasks (Li et al. 2011). Sophisticated and robust information technology and evidence-based clinical decision support (CDS) are therefore essential tools. Any concerted effort aimed at the reduction of errors and increase in care quality needs to consider alleviating the cognitive burden of clinicians as one of its primary objectives of safe, high-performance care.

2.6   Effects of Technology on Work Organization

Newly implemented information technology invariably changes established processes, from documentation to decision making and coordination. Personal and team workflows are often significantly affected, requiring clinicians to change long-standing and familiar practices and to adopt new ones. Many often express a range of personal viewpoints on the benefits and hazards of new work organization and how it may affect the quality of care or safety. While the utility of work reorganization may be perceived very differently by individuals, evidence from research shows a net increase in patient safety over time that can be attributed to the use of advanced information systems. Many patient injuries still occur every year but severe harm arises from relatively few initial causes, including hospital-acquired infections, adverse drug events, surgical injuries, deep venous thromboses and pulmonary emboli, falls and pressure ulcers that account for most of the adverse events in hospitals (Bates and Sheikh 2015). However, it is the quality of HIT design, advanced functions and rigorous implementation that seems to lead to real gains in safety and efficiency. The emphasis on technological and design quality and extensive functionality is crucial, however: basic EHRs with limited functions are less likely to have a significant positive effect. For example, a review of randomized clinical trials evaluating order entry and decision support interventions reported that only three out of ten studies showed measurable decrease of unsafe prescribing and only a half reduced medication errors (Lainer et al. 2013). At the same time, only about a half of US hospitals use EHRs with integrated advanced decision support and other functions known to reduce error, in what appears to be an emerging digital divide in the use of technology (Adler-Milstein et al. 2017). On the plus side, there seems to be a real, long-term progressive trend in both technology adoption and its quality.

Large and comprehensive HIT systems have many components that need to retain largely immutable design structures in order to keep the software reliable and compatible with legacy iterations, and to have the ability to maintain and develop it even as individual implementations are adapted to function according to local requirements. Dynamic work systems, however, have unique constraints where any single technology may have distinctly different effects than anticipated (Zheng et al. 2015). The shared responsibility of all key stakeholders in the multilevel work system described earlier, (Holden and Karsh 2009) such as vendors, care providers, healthcare organizations, information technology departments and public and private agencies, is to monitor and manage the safety of HIT and to guide their efforts towards resolving their often conflicting priorities and requirements (Singh and Sittig 2016) For example, vendors and developers should provide health systems with guidance on decisions regarding configuration (e.g., changing default settings of medication administration times to better match local workflows), customization and optimizing usability while clinician must be responsible for learning how to use the EHR safely (Sittig et al. 2017) Technology that can effectively meet the work demands of complex socio-technical systems requires the active participation and expertise of all involved parties from inception to implementation.

Clinicians have the most direct experience with long-term and frequent use of HIT that affords them a unique insight into its effects on their work, positive or otherwise, and therefore can report the perceived advantages and flaws to engineers and designers. At the same time, skilled professionals in general have only limited ability to describe and explain how they perform complex tasks and reasoning. They may not have the right vocabulary to convey to non-medical professionals how they arrive at care decisions or to articulate how technology may best support them. Understanding how HIT can best support them is not as simple as asking what they want, an all too common approach (Andre and Wickens 1995). Clinician-oriented approaches can capture the effect of technology on specific and diverse individual roles and their work. However, designers, implementers and workflow engineers should not fall into the "one size fits all" fallacy as validation of the design in practice requires thorough experimental testing based on well-defined performance criteria and rich, nuanced understanding of healthcare work (Karsh et al. 2010). Established methods such cognitive analysis (Bisantz et al. xxxx; Hettinger et al. 2017; Roth and Bisantz 2013; Vicente 1999; Schraagen et al. 2000), workflow and task analysis and human-centered design evaluations have consistently generated useful guidance to HIT designers (Roth et al. 2002; Zhang et al. 2014; Lowry 2014; Schumacher and Lowry 2010). Biomedical science and clinical work are uniquely complex but not impenetrable to researchers from outside of the domain, even as it is a highly intricate and structured process of problem discovery and clarification in the context of unbounded complexity (Carroll 1997).

Findings that are developed from the results of studies in biomedical informatics, usability, workflow and cognitive engineering fields need to be reformulated again by researchers into models that can best inform the work of technology designers and engineers. A workshop about the usability of medication-alerting clinical decision support and its evaluation outlined how this transfer of knowledge into practical design guidance may take place (Marcilly et al. 2016) Participants preferred design principles in the form of checklists and guidelines for design and procurement of software and hardware, and needed help in interpreting and understanding critiques of prototypes that clinicians provided as a part of user-centered cyclical evaluation. An important component of specific advisories was their justification in terms of potential harm if they were to be ignored, evidence of poor and better outcomes from prior studies and visual examples such as prototypes, wireframes and screenshots illustrating alternatives that are more optimal or less for function. Maintaining the research-to-practice continuum of discovery transfer effectively ensures that evidence-based design can make HIT better cognitive and interactive tools in clinical work.

2.7 Integrating New Knowledge into Care

Understanding how disease variants, the genetic makeup of patients and their unique physiological and lifestyle differences may alter the effectiveness of treatments outlined in guidelines is essential to make precision medicine a widely used approach to care. The expansion of genetic testing, advances in drug development and in information technology over the last several decades have created favorable conditions for its more consistent practice, as better genomic and phenomic analytic methods and sophisticated technology have become available. The term, sometimes also called personalized medicine, generally refers to the increasing specificity and accuracy of characterizing the state of patient health, and then selecting the most effective treatment option. Patients admitted to medical centers equipped with the necessary facilities may receive genotyping analyses that become an integral part of the patient record, that also includes data from tests, procedures and findings from history taking or physical examination entered by clinicians (Collen et al. 2015) The process may create well-organized arrays of new knowledge that is poised to inform multiple decisions along the care trajectory, from precise diagnosis to better treatment options more directly related to the distinct health characteristics of a single individual. For example, the knowledge of genetic variations and their effects on disease risk or on drug response would guide clinicians in prescribing safer and more effective medication therapy while also considering the effects of prior and concurrent treatments, comorbidities, and patient preferences.

A design initiative central to the goals of precision medicine is the ability to deliver decision support in forms that reduce high cognitive burden of complex decisions. It means, in broad terms, that decision support systems align the type, form and content of each alert or advisory with the decision it is intended to inform, and deliver it at the precise point of workflow where it can have the strongest effect on prescribing, test ordering and other clinical behavior (Horsky et al. 2012) A recent study that closely analyzed decision making during medication ordering, and the effect of CDS alerts on the reasoning of clinicians, showed that they conceptualized patient risk as a complex set of interdependent tradeoffs specific to individual patients (Horsky et al. 2017) The clinicians showed a strong tendency not to follow automated advice they considered to have low clinical value. In their own words, the value of an intervention (medication interaction and allergy alerts, in this study) was largely in its relevance to the patient they were treating. The specific clinical context in which they evaluated the specificity and appropriateness of given advice included comorbidities, prior drug tolerance and other illness-related factors, and, importantly, the proportion and significance of known, uncertain and absent information. Many clinicians felt that the content of an alert and the logic of its triggering algorithm need to meet a high threshold of veracity, primarily by considering patient-specific and knowledge-based information, to become a trusted and reliable tool. In turn, high reliability would cultivate higher confidence in CDS accuracy over time and increase its use.

The effort to expand the use of precision medicine has benefited from the convergence of two recent trends. Machine-learning studies can analyze vast repositories of clinical and research data to produce current, curated and evidence-based knowledge. Care recommendations can therefore be formulated with insights from the analyses of millions of patient lives and decades of recorded clinical history. The other necessary component is the ability of sophisticated CDS to contextualize this knowledge in real time with individual patient data, such as up-to-date labs, known allergies, pharmacotherapy, and increasingly more often, genetic information. Clinicians then can make decisions guided by evidence that is made specific to the patient they are treating.

Delivering focused and contextualized advice effectively into clinical workflows is an ongoing challenge for researchers and technology makers. Large volumes of genomic data that need to be curated, stored and then analyzed together with clinical care data immensely increase the need for robust HIT infrastructure and computing power (West et al. 2006). The input of more information that needs to be considered, however, cannot result in the net increase in clinician workload due to more interactions with HIT and further diversion of attention away from medical reasoning (Woods et al. 2001). Minimally intrusive forms of CDS can be developed with the help of cognitive engineering and workflow analyses that can identify links between cognitive tasks and specific design features that best support them (Hettinger et al. 2017). Excellent human–computer interaction and usability characteristics are as essential to HIT, as is its functionality, because systems need to attenuate the ever escalating cognitive burden. However, there may be only infrequent opportunities to substantially improve existing systems that are in constant use. Healthcare institutions may choose to redesign HIT systems and associated workflows perhaps only at a time of large-scale EHR transitions or upgrades (Beuscart-Zéphir et al. 2010).

The long-term objective of HIT design is to make systems adaptive to the dynamics of healthcare work, anticipate possible errors and allow corrective actions before an adverse event results (Horsky et al. 2005). Cognitive engineering can make socio-technical systems less prone to errors that emerge as the product of human interaction with technology. Complex systems need to be studied as a single unit of analysis with full consideration of use context and organizational constraints, which is not an easy endeavor, however (Carayon et al. 2013). For example, a common occurrence that often points to poorly designed system functions or errors in process design are recurring and frequent workarounds that clinicians use to circumvent unresponsive or irrelevant states during interactions. Inferior workflow fit will force potentially unsafe workarounds that may defeat built-in safety features, yet there is currently no clear way to distinguish theoretically between maladaptive workarounds and those that are necessary to allow flexibility in atypical situations, where goals are shifted or supplanted but otherwise would be discouraged during routine situations (Patterson 2018). Processes and factors that affect latent safety problems in complex, dynamic socio-technical systems such as cognitive workload, situation awareness, coordination and other measured constructs often require labor-intensive assessment studies that institutions may not be able to carry out to a sufficient degree or repeat after reorganizations and new technology additions.

Unobtrusive methods that may help in the assessment of large systems include simplified data collection using sensor-based technology (SBT). They allow cost and time effective measurement of physical, physiological, cognitive, and behavioral processes at the individual (e.g., mental workload, stress), team (e.g., cohesion, communication, team composition) and system level (e.g., workflow) (Hughes et al. 2018). Such methods may combine radio frequency identification (RFID) tags and physiological monitoring systems into a complementary approach that can identify or infer workflows and higher-level events. For example, a group of researchers combined RFID tag workflow monitoring in one study with ethnographic observations, augmenting data collection with multidimensional activity information that allowed observers to focus on cognitive details rather than simply annotating movement activities (Vankipuram et al. 2011).

Objective assessment of technical and teamwork skills or the tracking and monitoring of clinicians and patient engagement can be in some cases conducted with relatively few resources. Real-time data from sensors and other signals can be triangulated and correlated to provide contextual information (Alemdar and Ersoy 2010). Researchers in another study characterized the interactions of clinicians gathering information for hospital rounds discussions and patient-case presentations in the EHR by applying process-mining methods to system event logs. They triangulated quantitative findings with patient chart review and qualitative data to find that interactive behavior was associated with workflow routines, patient case complexity and variant screen sequence patterns (Furniss et al. 2016b).

Cognitive engineers and others whose work concerns the understanding of complex collaborative processes must address the challenge of gathering empirical evidence and facilitating critical contributions of emergent constructs, mental models and distributed knowledge into analyses. Human-centered technology is a design concept that is essential to building healthcare workplaces that are conducive to information and collaboration-intensive work and allow clinicians to focus their reasoning more directly on patient care (Morrow and Fiore 2013).

2.8   Artificial Intelligence as an Agent in Patient Care Workflows

Machine learning, natural language processing, deep neural networks and other algorithms with autonomous learning have decades-long history of use in healthcare and medical research, from interpreting large volumes of data and clinical notes to assess risk and to predict patient outcomes to early detection of abnormalities in images. These and other advanced computational techniques, commonly referred to as artificial intelligence (AI), have been at the forefront of public and professional attention in the last few years. Researchers have been using this powerful tool to gain new insights into disease progression or to compare patient outcomes between different standards of care and patient populations, among other investigations. The role of AI in direct patient care is being explored at a fast pace today, as many stakeholders in healthcare delivery are asking questions about its optimal use and implementation. For example, early investigations have shown that AI algorithms that analyze radiographic images with excellent results seem to be difficult to integrate into the workflows of radiologists (Blezek et al. 2021). Similarly, vascular surgeons are exploring whether AI can determine and recommend optimal statin treatment based on individual patient risk factors, enhancement of intraoperative fluoroscopy and ultrasound imaging that would demonstrate its usefulness within surgical workflows (Dossabhoy et al. 2023).

Recent comments by clinical leaders at the American Medical Association show that one of their priorities for the application of AI, and where they envision the technology having a sizeable effect, is in improving the work conditions of medical professionals, and, by extension, the quality of care. Excessive work hours, high cognitive load and physician burnout, one of the leading contributors to medical error, is a problem that AI interventions seem to be able to address most directly by their capacity to alleviate much of repetitive and time consuming work by the automation of routine tasks and "intelligent augmentation" of care documentation and administration (Nundy and Hodgkins 2018; Ratwani et al. 2019). The everyday grind of repetitive and laborious tasks is a good candidate for optimization by intelligent agents that tirelessly evaluate, adjust to changes and adapt their interventions in real time as conditions demand. For example, AI can scan written notes for incomplete or potentially erroneous information and suggest corrections. The effect of more complete and accurate data on decision making at later points in patient care could be a significant reduction of uncertainty. Free-text entries can be, at the same time, reformulated and entered into structured fields for machine processing. Dynamic, intelligent scheduling of patient flow and the balancing of staff or resources allocation that is responsive to quickly changing conditions seems to be a good fit for AI automation that has proven its immense strength in controlling self-optimizing workflows in many industries. Patient care can be greatly advanced by the careful harnessing of powerful new forms of HIT into a collaborative environment where human rapport, ethics, and complex reasoning will stay the exclusive domain of healthcare professionals (Jennings et al. 2021).

Acknowledgements The manuscript draft has benefited from conversations with Dr. Vimla Patel.

References

Adler-Milstein J, Holmgren AJ, Kralovec P, Worzala C, Searcy T, Patel V. Electronic health record adoption in US hospitals: The emergence of a digital "advanced use" divide. J Am Med Inform Assoc. 2017;24(6):1142–8.

Alemdar H, Ersoy C. Wireless sensor networks for healthcare: A survey. Comput Netw. 2010;54(15):2688–710.

Altmann EM, Trafton JG. Timecourse of recovery from task interruption: data and a model. Psychon Bull Rev. 2007;14(6):1079–84.

Ancker JS, Kern L, Abramson E, Kaushal R. The Triangle Model for evaluating the effect of health information technology on healthcare quality and safety. J Am Med Inform Assoc. 2012;19(1):61–5.

Anderson JG, Aydin CE. Evaluating the organizational impact of healthcare information systems. 2nd ed. Hannah KJ, Ball MJ, editors. New York, NY: Springer; 2005; xv, p. 344

Andre AD, Wickens CD. When Users Want What's not Best for Them. Ergon Des: Q Hum Factors Appl. 1995;3(4):10–4.

Ashcroft DM, Quinlan P, Blenkinsopp A. Prospective study of the incidence, nature and causes of dispensing errors in community pharmacies. Pharmacoepidemiol Drug Saf. 2005;14(5):327–32.

Bates DW, Ebell M, Gotlieb E, Zapp J, Mullins HC. A proposal for electronic medical records in U.S. primary care. Journal of the American Medical Informatics Association. 2003; 10(1):1–10.

Bates DW, Sheikh A. The role and importance of cognitive studies in patient safety. BMJ Qual Saf. 2015;24(7):414–6.

Beasley JW, Hankey TH, Erickson R, Stange KC, Mundt M, Elliott M, et al. How Many Problems Do Family Physicians Manage at Each Encounter? A WReN Study. The Annals of Family Medicine. 2004;2(5):405–10.

Begun JW, Zimmerman B, Dooley KJ. Health Care Organizations as Complex Adaptive Systems. In: Mick SS, Wyttenbach ME, editors. Advances in Health Care Organization Theory. San Francisco: Jossey-Bass; 2003. p. 253–88.

Berg M. Patient care information systems and health care work: A sociotechnical approach. Int J Med Informatics. 1999a;55(2):87–101.

Berg M. Accumulating and Coordinating: Occasions for Information Technologies in Medical Work. Comput Support Coop Work. 1999b;8(4):373–401.

Beuscart-Zéphir M-C, Pelayo S, Bernonville S. Example of a Human Factors Engineering approach to a medication administration work system: Potential impact on patient safety. Int J Med Informatics. 2010;79(4):e43–57.

Bisantz AM, Burns CM, Fairbanks RJ. Cognitive Systems Engineering in Health Care 2015.

Blezek DJ, Olson-Williams L, Missert A, Korfiatis P. AI Integration in the Clinical Workflow. J Digit Imaging. 2021;34(6):1435–46.

Bricon-Souf N, Renard JM, Beuscart R. Dynamic workflow model for complex activity in intensive care unit. Int J Med Inform. 1999;53(2–3):143–50.

Carayon P, Schoofs Hundt A, Karsh BT, Gurses AP, Alvarado CJ, Smith M, et al. Work system design for patient safety: The SEIPS model. Quality & Safety in Healthcare. 2006; 15(Suppl 1):i50–8.

Carayon P, Karsh B-T. Incorporating Health Information Technology Into Workflow Redesign--Summary Report. Rockville, MD: Agency for Healthcare Research and Quality, (Prepared by the Center for Quality and Productivity Improvement UoWM, under Contract No. HHSA 290–2008–10036C; 2010. Report No.: AHRQ Publication No. 10–0098-EF.

Carayon P, Cartmill R, Hoonakker P, Schoofs Hundt A, Karsh B-T, Krueger GP, et al. Human factors analysis of workflow in health information technology implementation. In: Carayon P, editor. Handbook of human factors and ergonomics in health care and patient safety. Human factors and ergonomics. 2nd ed. Boca Raton, FL: CRC Press; 2012; p. xxvii, p. 848

Carayon P, Wetterneck TB, Rivera-Rodriguez AJ, Hundt AS, Hoonakker P, Holden R, et al. Human factors systems approach to healthcare quality and patient safety. Appl Ergon. 2013.

Carayon P, Alvarado CJ, Brennan PF, Gurses AP, Hundt AS, Karsh B-T, et al. Work system and patient safety. Proceedings of human factors in organizational design and management-VII; October 1–2; Aache, Germany 2003; p. 58–588.

Carroll JM. Human-computer interaction: Psychology as a science of design. Annu Rev Psychol. 1997;48(1):61–83.

Challenges DP, Education OFM. Trans Am Clin Climatol Assoc. 2011;122:48–58.

Cohen T, Blatter B, Almeida C, Shortliffe EH, Patel VL. A cognitive blueprint of collaboration in context: Distributed cognition in the psychiatric emergency department. Artif Intell Med. 2006; 37(2):73–83.

Collen MF, Greenes RA. Medical Informatics: Past and Future. In: Collen MF, Ball MJ, editors. The History of Medical Informatics in the United States. London: Springer, London; 2015. p. 725–48.

Covvey HD, Cowan DD, Alencar P, Malyk W, So J, Henriques D, et al. Model human behavior: don't constrain it! In: Borycki E, editor. International perspectives in health informatics. Studies in health technology and informatics. Amsterdam ; Fairfax, VA: IOS Press; 2011; xvi, p. 431

Cowley SJ, Vallée-Tourangeau F. Cognition beyond the brain: Computation, interactivity and human artifice 2017.

Custers EJ. Thirty years of illness scripts: Theoretical origins and practical applications. Med Teach. 2015;37(5):457–62.

Davenport TH, Short JE. The new industrial engineering: Information technology and business process redesign. Sloan Management Review. 1990;31(4):11–27.

Delacoras C, Klein M. A knowledge-based approach for designing robust business practices. In: Desel J, Oberweis A, editors. Van der Aalst WMP. Business process management. Lecture notes in computer science. Berlin: Springer-Verlag; 2000. p. 50–65.

Dossabhoy SS, Ho VT, Ross EG, Rodriguez F, Arya S. Artificial intelligence in clinical workflow processes in vascular surgery and beyond. Semin Vasc Surg. 2023;36(3):401–12.

Durso FT, Drews FA. Health Care, Aviation, and Ecosystems: A Socio-Natural Systems Perspective. Curr Dir Psychol Sci. 2010;19(2):71–5.

Ebright PR, Patterson ES, Chalko BA, Render ML. Understanding the complexity of registered nurse work in acute care settings. J Nurs Adm. 2003; 33(12):630–8.

Ebright P. The Complex Work of RNs: Implications for Healthy Work Environments. Online J. Issues Nurs. 2010; 15.

Furniss D, Blandford A. Understanding emergency medical dispatch in terms of distributed cognition: a case study. Ergonomics. 2006;49(12–13):1174–203.

Furniss SK, Burton MM, Larson DW, Kaufman DR. Modeling Patient-Centered Cognitive Work for High-Value Care Goals. Proceedings of the international symposium on human factors and ergonomics in health care. 2016a;5(1):112–9.

Furniss SK, Burton MM, Grando A, Larson DW, Kaufman DR. Integrating process mining and cognitive analysis to study EHR workflow. AMIA Annu Symp Proc. 2016b;2016:580–9.

Gerrity MS, DeVellis RF, Earp JA. Physicians' reactions to uncertainty in patient care. A new measure and new insights. Med Care. 1990; 28(8):724–36.

Glass L. Synchronization and rhythmic processes in physiology. Nature. 2001;410(6825):277–84.

Graber ML, Byrne C, Johnston D. The impact of electronic health records on diagnosis. dx. 2017; 0(0).

Grundgeiger T, Sanderson P, MacDougall HG, Venkatesh B. Interruption management in the intensive care unit: predicting resumption times and assessing distributed support. J Exp Psychol Appl. 2010;16(4):317–34.

Han PK, Klein WM, Arora NK. Varieties of uncertainty in health care: A conceptual taxonomy. Med Decis Making. 2011;31(6):828–38.

Hazlehurst B, McMullen CK, Gorman PN. Distributed cognition in the heart room: How situation awareness arises from coordinated communications during cardiac surgery. J Biomed Inform. 2007;40(5):539–51.

Hazlehurst B, Gorman PN, McMullen CK. Distributed cognition: An alternative model of cognition for medical informatics. Int J Med Informatics. 2008;77(4):226–34.

Hendy KC. Situation awareness and workload: Birds of a feather? AGARD AMP Symposium on Situational Awareness: Limitations and Enhancements in the Aviation Environment; 24–28 April. Brussels: Belgium; 1995.

Hettinger AZ, Roth EM, Bisantz AM. Cognitive engineering and health informatics: Applications and intersections. Journal of Biomedical Informatics. 2017; 67(Supplement C):21–33.

Hilligoss B, Zheng K. Chart biopsy: an emerging medical practice enabled by electronic health records and its impacts on emergency department-inpatient admission handoffs. J Am Med Inform Assoc. 2013;20(2):260–7.

Holden RJ, Karsh B-T. A Theoretical Model of Health Information Technology Usage Behaviour with Implications for Patient Safety. 28.1 (2009): 21–38. Web. Behaviour & Information Technology. 2009; 28(1):21–38.

Holder BE. Cognition in flight: Understanding cockpits as cognitive systems [Ph.D.]. San Diego, CA: University of California, San Diego; 1999.

Hollan J, Hutchins E, Kirsh D. Distributed cognition: Toward a new foundation for human-computer interaction research. ACM Transcations Comput-Hum Interact. 2000;7(2):174–96.

Horsky J. Distributed Cognitive Resources: A Framework for the Analysis of Human Interaction with Complex Health Information Technology. Saarbrücken, Germany: VDM Verlag; 2008.

Horsky J, Kaufman DR, Oppenheim MI, Patel VL. A framework for analyzing the cognitive complexity of computer-assisted clinical ordering. J Biomed Inform. 2003;36(1–2):4–22.

Horsky J, Zhang J, Patel VL. To err is not entirely human: complex systems and user cognition. J Biomed Inform. 2005;38(4):264–6.

Horsky J, Schiff GD, Johnston D, Mercincavage L, Bell D, Middleton B. Interface design principles for usable decision support: A targeted review of best practices for clinical prescribing interventions. J Biomed Inform. 2012;45(6):1202–16.

Horsky J, Suh EH, Sayan O, Patel V. Uncertainty, case complexity and the content of verbal handoffs at the emergency department. AMIA Annu Symp Proc. 2015;2015:630–9.

Horsky J, Aarts J, Verheul L, Seger DL, van der Sijs H, Bates DW. Clinical reasoning in the context of active decision support during medication prescribing. Int J Med Informatics. 2017;97:1–11.

House R, Rousseau DM, Thomas-Hunt M. The meso paradigm: a framework for the integration of micro and macro organizational behavior. Research in Organizational Behavior. 1995;17:71–114.

Hughes AM, Zajac S, Razjouyan J, Ahmed R. Sensor based assessment for learning and care quality: The new frontier. AMIA Annual Fall Symposium; San Francisco, CA 2018. p. 118–20.

Hutchins E. The social organization of distributed cognition. In: Resnick LB, Levine JM, editors. Perspectives on socially shared cognition. Washington, DC: American Psychological Association; 1991. p. 283–307.

Hutchins E. The cognitive consequences of patterns of information flow. Intellectica. 2000;30:53–74.

Hutchins E. Cognition in the wild. Cambridge, MA: MIT Press; 1995 1995. xviii, 381 p p.

Jennings BM. Workflow, Turbulence, and Cognitive Complexity. In: Baernholdt M, Boyle DK, editors. Nurses Contributions to Quality Health Outcomes. Cham: Springer International Publishing; 2021. p. 85–107.

Jones B, Brzezinski WA, Estrada CA, Rodriguez M, Kraemer RR. A 22-year-old woman with abdominal pain. J Gen Intern Med. 2014;29(7):1074–8.

Karsh B-T. Clinical practice improvement and redesign: How change in workflow can be supported by clinical decision support. Rockville, MD: Agency for Healthcare Research and Quality; 2009 June. Contract No.: AHRQ Publication No. 09–0054-EF.

Karsh B-T, Weinger MB, Abbott PA, Wears RL. Health information technology: Fallacies and sober realities. J Am Med Inform Assoc. 2010;17(6):617–23.

Kaufman DR, Patel VL, Hilliman C, Morin PC, Pevzner J, Weinstock RS, et al. Usability in the real world: Assessing medical information technologies in patients' homes. J Biomed Inform. 2003;36(1–2):45–60.

Kaufman DR, Pevzner J, Rodriguez M, Cimino JJ, Ebner S, Fields L, et al. Understanding workflow in telehealth video visits: Observations from the IDEATel project. J Biomed Inform. 2009;42(4):581–92.

Klein GA. Streetlights and Shadows: Searching for the Keys to Adaptive Decision Making. London, UK: MIT Press; 2009.

Klein KJ, Danserau F, Hall RJ. Levels issues in theory development, data collection, and analysis. Acad Manag Rev. 1994;24:243–8.

Klein KJ, Kozlowski SWJ. Multilevel theory, research, and methods in organizations : foundations, extensions, and new directions. San Francisco: Jossey-Bass; 2000; xxix, p. 605.

Lainer M, Mann E, Sonnichsen A. Information technology interventions to improve medication safety in primary care: a systematic review. Int J Qual Health Care. 2013;25(5):590–8.

Lanham HJ, Sittig DF, Leykum LK, Parchman ML, Pugh JA, McDaniel RR. Understanding differences in electronic health record (EHR) use: linking individual physicians' perceptions of uncertainty and EHR use patterns in ambulatory care. J Am Med Inform Assoc. 2014;21(1):73–81.

Leykum LK, Lanham HJ, Pugh JA, Parchman M, Anderson RA, Crabtree BF, et al. Manifestations and implications of uncertainty for improving healthcare systems: an analysis of observational and interventional studies grounded in complexity science. Implementation Science : IS. 2014;9:165.

Li SYW, Magrabi F, Coiera E. A systematic review of the psychological literature on interruption and its patient safety implications. J Am Med Inform Assoc. 2011;19(1):6–12.

Lowry S. Integrating electronic health records into clinical workflow: an application of human factors modeling methods to ambulatory care. 2014.

Marcilly R, Monkman H, Villumsen S, Kaufman D, Beuscart-Zephir M-C. How to present evidence-based usability design principles dedicated to medication-related alerting systems to designers and evaluators? results from a workshop. Stud Health Technol Inform. 2016;228:609–13.

Markus ML, Robey D. Information technology and organizational change: Causal structure in theory and research. Manage Sci. 1988;34:583–98.

Martínez-García M, Hernández-Lemus E. Health systems as complex systems. Am J Oper Res. 2013;3(1A):113–26.

Masys DR. Effects of current and future information technologies on the health care workforce. Health Aff (Millwood). 2002;21(5):33–41.

McDaniel RR, Driebe DJ, Lanham HJ. Health care organizations as complex systems: new perspectives on design and management. Adv Health Care Manag. 2013;15:3.

Mica RE. Design and evaluation for situation awareness enhancement. Proceedings of the human factors society annual meeting. 1988;32(2):97–101.

Mohr LB. Explaining organizational behavior. 1st ed. San Francisco: Jossey-Bass; 1982. xv, 260 p. p.

Morrow PB, Fiore SM. Team Cognition: Coordination across Individuals and Machines. In: Lee JD, Kirlik A, editors. The Oxford Handbook of Cognitive Engineering. Oxford Library of Psychology. New York: Oxford University Press; 2013.

Nemeth CP, Cook RI, O'Connor M, Klock PA. Using cognitive artifacts to understand distributed cognition. IEEE Trans Syst Man Cybern. 2004;34(6):726–35.

Nundy S, Hodgkins ML. Health Affairs Blog [Internet]: Health Affairs. 2018. [cited 2024].

Ozkaynak M, Flatley Brennan P, Hanauer DA, Johnson S, Aarts J, Zheng K, et al. Patient-centered care requires a patient-oriented workflow model. J Am Med Inform Assoc. 2013;20(e1):e14–6.

Patterson ES. Workarounds to intended use of health information technology: a narrative review of the human factors engineering literature. Hum Factors. 2018;60(3):281–92.

Perry M. Socially Distributed Cognition in Loosely Coupled Systems. In: Cowley SJ, Vallée-Tourangeau F, editors. Cognition Beyond the Brain: Computation, Interactivity and Human Artifice. Cham: Springer International Publishing; 2017. p. 19–41.

Pinelle D, Gutwin C. Loose coupling and healthcare organizations: deployment strategies for groupware. Comput Supported Coop Work. 2006;15(5–6):537–72.

Plsek PE, Greenhalgh T. Complexity science: The challenge of complexity in health care. Br Med J. 2001;323(7313):625–8.

Poli R. A Note on the difference between complicated and complex social systems. CADMUS [Internet]. 2013 [cited 2017; 2(1):pp. 142–7 pp. Available from: http://cadmusjournal.org.

Ratwani RM, Reider J, Singh H. A decade of health information technology usability challenges and the path forward. JAMA. 2019;321(8):743–4.

Reddy M, Dourish P, Pratt W. Temporality in medical work: time also matters. Comput Support Coop Work. 2006;15(1):29–53.

Reijers HA. Workflow Modeling. In: Reijers HA, editor. Design and Control of Workflow Processes: Business Process Management for the Service Industry. Berlin, Heidelberg: Springer Berlin Heidelberg; 2003. pp. 31–59.

Rivera-Rodriguez AJ, Karsh B-T. Interruptions and distractions in healthcare: review and reappraisal. Qual Saf Health Care. 2010;19(4):304–12.

Roth EM, Bisantz AM. Cognitive Work Analysis. In: Lee JD, Kirlik A, editors. The Oxford Handbook of Cognitive Engineering. Oxford Library of Psychology. New York: Oxford University Press; 2013.

Roth EM, Patterson ES, Mumaw RJ. Cogntitive engineering: Issues in user-centered system design. In: Marciniak JJ, editor. Encyclopedia of software engineering. Wiley-Interscience. New York: John Wiley & Sons; 2002.

Salmon PM. Distributed situation awareness: Theory, measurement and application to teamwork. Farnham, England ; Burlington, VT: Ashgate; 2009. xx, p. 246.

Schmidt HG, Rikers RM. How expertise develops in medicine: Knowledge encapsulation and illness script formation. Med Educ. 2007;41(12):1133–9.

Schraagen JM, Chipman SF, Shalin VL, editors. Cognitive task analysis. Mahwah, NJ: Lawrence Erlbaum Associates, Inc.; 2000.

Schumacher RM, Lowry SZ. NIST Guide to the Processes Approach for Improving the Usability of Electronic Health Records. Washington, D.C.: National Institute of Standards and Technology; 2010. Report No.: NISTIR 7741.

Sedig K, Parsons P, Naimi A, Willoughby K. Reconsidering healthcare evidence as dynamic and distributed: the role of information and cognition. Int J Evid Based Healthc. 2015;13(2):43–51.

Shiffman R, Michel G, Essaihi A, Thornquist E. Bridging the guideline implementation gap: A systematic, document-centered approach to guideline implementation. J Am Med Inform Assoc. 2004;11:418–26.

Shortliffe EH, Barnett GO. Biomedical Data: Their Acquisition, Storage, and Use. In: Shortliffe EH, Cimino JJ, editors. Biomedical informatics: Computer applications in health care and biomedicine. Fourth edition ed. London 2014. p. 39–66.

Shortliffe EH, Blois MS. Biomedical Informatics: The Science and the Pragmatics. In: Shortliffe EH, Cimino JJ, editors. Biomedical informatics: Computer applications in health care and biomedicine. Fourth edition ed. London: Springer; 2014; pp. 3–38.

Singh H, Sittig DF. Measuring and improving patient safety through health information technology: The Health IT Safety Framework. BMJ Qual Saf. 2016;25(4):226–32.

Sittig DF, Belmont E, Singh H. Improving the safety of health information technology requires shared responsibility: It is time we all step up. Healthcare. 2017.

Sittig DF, Singh H. A new sociotechnical model for studying health information technology in complex adaptive healthcare systems. Qual Saf Health Care. 2010;19(Suppl 3):i68-74.

Smith MJ, Sainfort F. Balance theory of job design for stress reduction. Int J Ind Ergon. 1989;4:67–79.

Smithson M. Conflict aversion: preference for ambiguity vs conflict in sources and evidence. Organ Behav Hum Decis Process. 1999;79(3):179–98.

Stoller JK. Electronic siloing: an unintended consequence of the electronic health record. Cleve Clin J Med. 2013;80(7):406–9.

Vankipuram M, Kahol K, Cohen T, Patel VL. Toward automated workflow analysis and visualization in clinical environments. J Biomed Inform. 2011;44(3):432–40.

Vicente KJ. Cognitive work analysis: Toward safe, productive & healthy computer-based work. Mahwah, NJ: Lawrence Erlbaum Associates, Inc.; 1999. xix, p. 392

Weber GM, Adams WG, Bernstam EV, Bickel JP, Fox KP, Marsolo K, et al. Biases introduced by filtering electronic health records for patients with "complete data." J Am Med Inform Assoc. 2017;24(6):1134–41.

Weir C, Drews FA, Leecaster MK, Barrus RJ, Hellewell JL, Nebeker JR. The orderly and effective visit: impact of the electronic health record on modes of cognitive control. AMIA Annu Symp Proc. 2012;2012:979–87.

Wennberg JE. Unwarranted variations in healthcare delivery: Implications for academic medical centres. Br Med J. 2002; 325(7370):961–4.

Wennberg JE. Understanding geographic variations in health care delivery.[comment]. New England Journal of Medicine. 1999; 340(1):52–3.

West M, Ginsburg GS, Huang AT, Nevins JR. Embracing the complexity of genomic data for personalized medicine. Genome Res. 2006;16(5):559–66.

Woods DD, Patterson ES. How Unexpected Events Produce An Escalation Of Cognitive And Coordinative Demands. In: Hancock PA, Desmond PA, editors. Stress workload and fatigue. Hillsday, NJ: Lawrence Erlbaum Associates; 2001. p. 2290–304.

Wright PC, Fields RE, Harrison MD. Analyzing human-computer interaction as distributed cognition: The resources model. Hum-Comput Interact. 2000;15(1):1–41.

Wright MC, Taekman JM, Endsley MR. Objective measures of situation awareness in a simulated medical environment. Qual Saf Health Care. 2004;13(Suppl 1):i65-71.

Xiao Y. Artifacts and collaborative work in healthcare: Methodological, theoretical, and technological implications of the tangible. J Biomed Inform. 2005;38(1):26–33.

Yasnoff WA. Health Information Infrastructure. In: Shortliffe EH, Cimino JJ, editors. Biomedical informatics: Computer applications in health care and biomedicine. Fourth edition. / edited by Edward H. Shortliffe, James J. Cimino. ed. London 2014.

Zhang J. Representations of health concepts: A cognitive perspective. J Biomed Inform. 2002;35(1):17–24.

Zhang J, Norman DA. Representations in distributed cognitive tasks. Cogn Sci. 1994;18(1):87–122.

Zhang J. Better EHR. Houston, TX: National Center for Cognitive Informatics & Decision Making in Healthcare; 2014.

Zheng K, Ciemins EL, Lanham HJ, Lindberg C. Examining the Relationship Between Health IT and Ambulatory Care Workflow Redesign. Rockville, MD: Agency for Healthcare Research and Quality, 2902010–0019I-1 BCuCN; 2015 July. Report No.: AHRQ Publication No. 15–0058-EF Contract No.: AHRQ Publication No. 15–0058-EF.

Chapter 3
Transforming Clinical Workflows with Artificial Intelligence (AI)-Based Technologies

Paul Fu Jr.

3.1 Introduction

Artificial Intelligence (AI), especially the circa 2023 breakthroughs in generative AI performance, has been rapidly transforming the entire healthcare sector, bringing about efficiencies and capabilities that were unimaginable just a few years ago. Relative to other innovative technologies, AI has the potential to be more disruptive across the spectrum of clinical workflows. From managing messaging in baskets, to improving diagnostic test accuracy, personalizing treatment plans, and providing population level health insights, AI is positioned to revolutionize the way healthcare providers work and how patients receive care.

All AI technologies are based on machine learning, the concept of which was first theorized by McCulloch and Pitts (1943) and implemented in 1957 with the development of the "Perceptron" by Rosenblatt (1958). Although there was great promise, the capabilities of early machine learning were limited because of insufficient computational power and a lack of available data in the suitable digital formats, and the interest subsequently waned. Two factors led to the re-emergence of the interest shortly before the turn of the 21st Century: a tipping point in microchip transistor density that allowed for much greater computational power with manageable power demands and the digitization and electronic exchange of large datasets prompted by major advances in networking and interoperability.

At the core, healthcare AI utilizes complex algorithms and software to emulate human cognition in the analysis, interpretation, and comprehension of complicated medical and healthcare data. Although there is currently a very high level of excitement about AI, in fact, machine-learning tools in varied forms have been in production and in the marketplace for decades, helping to improve clinical workflows across the

P. Fu Jr. (✉)
City of Hope, Duarte, USA
e-mail: pafu@coh.org

spectrum of care delivery through automation of repetitive analytical tasks, personalization of data analysis and presentation, and improving precision and accuracy. For example, predictive analytics uses a combination of very large datasets, statistical algorithms, and machine learning in order to make a probabilistic assessment of a future state such as risk of uncontrolled diabetes in 12 months in a diabetes management program (Khalilnejad et al., 2024), forecasting disease outbreak surges (Comito and Pizzuti, 2022), or prediction of 3-month mortality in patients with metastatic solid tumors (Zachariah et al., 2022).

AI-based diagnostic tools are also employed at the point of care to improve diagnostic accuracy and provide critical real-time information to clinicians. Using digitally captured fundoscopic images, AI algorithms perform acceptably to screen for diabetic retinopathy regardless of whether images are analyzed on a server or workstation, on a hand-held fundus camera with embedded software, or on a smartphone-based application (Joseph et al., 2024; Hasan and Siddiqui, 2023). Machine learning has been applied near-real-time to improve image quality for breast ultrasound, digital mammography, and MRI with downstream improvements in interpretation accuracy and tumor grading as well as reducing inter- and intra-observer variability (Coffey et al., 2024; Shamir et al., 2024). Deep learning shows additional promise in identifying cancer in more complex 3-dimensional models derived from 2-dimensional images (Bi et al., 2019). Improvements in diagnostic accuracy will yield better risk stratification and targeted management.

Genomic data is derived using molecular techniques such as next-generation sequencing (NGS) to articulate the genetic makeup of tumors and includes the identification of genetic mutations, alterations, and expression patterns that can enables precision medicine. AI algorithms are frequently used to facilitate the analysis of the enormous datasets generated by NGS, including detecting single nucleotide polymorphisms (SNPs) and structural variations or helping to distinguish between true variants and sequencing errors (Cosgun and Oh, 2020; Danis et al., 2021; Choon et al., 2024).

3.2   Defining Basic AI Technologies

Figure 3.1 exhibits an overview of key AI technologies. The definition of each of them is presented below.

Artificial Intelligence (AI) is the set of computer science methods and tools that enable machines to perceive their environment in the form of data, and then use learning to iteratively provide a desired result (Russell and Norvig, 2021).

Machine Learning (ML) is a method that teaches computers to learn from and make decisions based on data. Early machine learning applications sifted through large datasets to analyze relationships, such as between prevention health interventions and disease treatments, to identify interventions that would improve patient outcomes or identify those at risk of developing a condition.

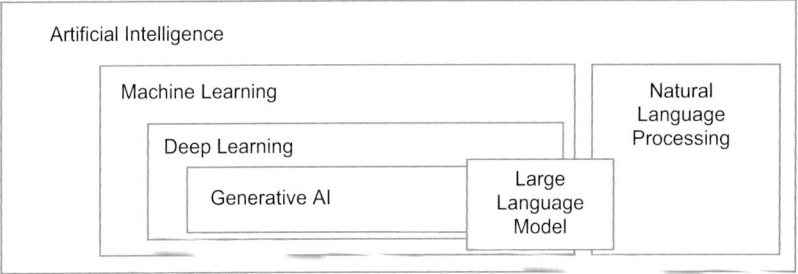

Fig. 3.1 Overview of key AI technologies

Deep Learning is a subset of ML that uses neural networks with multiple layers (i.e., "deep") of computation to analyze complex data. In healthcare, deep learning is commonly used for radiographic image analysis, such as detecting abnormalities in mammography (Hanis et al., 2022) and MRI imaging (Mazurowski et al., 2019).

Neural networks are the foundation of deep learning that recognize patterns by mimicking human decision making using a combination of nodes and layers. Nodes are analogous to neurons in that they are the core processing unit that receive different data inputs and perform tasks based upon in which layer the node resides, leading to an output. Layers consist of multiple nodes and are the highest-level building blocks for neural networks.

There are three types of layers in a neural network: input layer, hidden layer(s), and output layer. Layers are stacked and the output from each node of one layer is sent to each node of the subsequent layer. The input layer uses nodes to represent the distinct features of the initial dataset and passes this categorization to the first hidden layer. Hidden layers are where all computations are performed. The outputs from preceding layer nodes are weighted and summed, and then an adjustment is applied using a bias constant. The bias is to ensure a threshold or baseline result. The adjusted result is then passed through an activation function that performs matrix multiplication between the inputs and weights and outputs a non-linear transformation of the data.

```
activation function: sum(inputs * weights) + bias = output
```

Each hidden layer typically contains only one activation function, essentially looking at one aspect or recognizing one feature of the input data. Adding additional hidden layers allows for analysis of additional aspects or features of the input data and as the outputs from each node pass to each node of the subsequent hidden layer, it becomes possible to compound the learning and recognize more complex specific features layer by layer. The greater the number of hidden layers, the "deeper" the learning. The final output layer transforms the result of data processing into an expected output and there is one output layer node for each output variable.

The stacked layers are critical to the ability for neural networks to recognize patterns and structures within different data types (images, alphanumeric, numeric). Traditional machine-learning models require manual extraction of features, or an individually measurable characteristic. Neural networks automate this identification and extraction process by simultaneously using multiple data inputs, stacking hidden layers, each looking for a specific feature, and then integrating the outputs much more quickly and accurately than if a similar analysis were to be performed in series.

"Training" a neural network refers to an iterative process where the input weights are optimized to get to the expected output. This allows the neural network to adapt to new, previously unseen data variations, such as applying a common AI tool to patients with different phenotypes. Once appropriately trained, neural networks can process new data at quickly, compactly, and scalably, allowing for real-time decision support within a clinical workflow.

Traditional machine-learning algorithms classify input data based upon what they have learned. Traditional neural networks analyze input data to produce a statistically likely output based upon existing classifications. Generative AI models such as Generative Adversarial Networks (GANs) and Generative Pre-trained Transformer (GPT) take a different approach: they create completely new images, texts, or data that mimic the original datasets. Training involves the model learning the statistical properties, patterns, and structures within the training set. During training, the model self-adjusts parameters to minimize the difference between the output data that the model generates and the source data. In healthcare, this could mean generating synthetic medical data for research without exposing patient data.

Natural Language Processing (NLP) focuses on the interaction between computers and human language (either written or spoken) with the goal of making sense of language in a way that is meaningful and useful and that can be acted upon. The two foundations of NLP are syntax (the arrangement of words in such a manner as to make sense to the reader or listener) and semantics (i.e., the meaning of the words). Syntactic algorithms are used to compare and align natural language input with coded grammatical rules. Tokenization divides text into sentence tokens and then sentence tokens are divided into word tokens. Part-of-speech tagging then takes each word token and identifies its part, such as noun, verb, or adjective, or grammatical category. Lemmatization and stemming are a text normalizing processes that take a word token and break it down into a common base form. This allows different word tokens to be associated with each other. While lemmatization uses a vocabulary and morphological analysis of the word token and part-of-speech tag to identify the base form, stemming takes a more direct approach and truncates the end of the word token. Semantic algorithms subsequently use that base form data to provide an interpretation of the meaning of the original natural language. Named Entity Recognition (NER) detects and categorizes key pieces of information (i.e., named entities) such as names, locations, organizations, events, and time codes. Identifying the key semantic elements of a sentence allows for a quantitative understanding of the general knowledge contained within the original text. This fully parsed set of data can then be used by sentiment analysis algorithms that can determine the emotional state or sentiment behind the original text, typically classifying as positive, negative, or neutral. Together, these processing steps allow the NLP model to accurately extract information from documents as well as sort and categorize the documents themselves. Challenges in NLP are often related to cultural variations or colloquialisms that impact the ability to understand context appropriately.

Large language models (LLM) sit at the intersection of deep learning and NLP, enabled through the current generations of specialized processors that allow for training on very large repositories of text data. NLP methods are used to break down textual data with the largest models containing billions of parameters (or weights). Generative AI transformer models, such as GPT or Bidirectional Encoder Representations from Transformers (BERT) can weigh the importance of different words in a sentence, helping with the NLP context challenge. These models are also designed for highly paralleled computation, which makes training on large datasets feasible. While extremely versatile, the complexity of LLMs results in challenges around understanding and reducing bias in training data.

3.3 Reengineering Clinical Workflows to Accommodate AI

IT implementation projects have a high failure or incompletion (overbudget, delayed, unmet objectives) rate ranging from 52% (Bloch et al., 2012) to 65% (Johnson and Mulder, 2020) or 75% (Wu and Misra, 2023) depending on project scope and complexity. Implementation projects for health IT (HIT) are no different (Wears and Misra, 2005). Studies of unsuccessful implementations of HIT have looked at poor technology design, poor adoption, and various socio-organizational factors that contribute to a technology–workflow mismatch (Yen et al., 2017; Kaplan 2001). With this perspective, it is critical that the introduction of AI into the clinical setting is met with re-engineered workflows that recognize the transformative nature of AI.

3.3.1 Conceptual Frameworks

Sittig and Singh (2010) defined a model for use in identifying and addressing socio-technical challenges involved with the full cycle of HIT implementation. This model differs from traditional HIT evaluation approaches that look at the ternary success measures of on-budget, on-time, and goals-achieved, and recognizes the inherent difficulty of recomposing those gross measures to reflect implementation in a complex adaptive system. The socio-technical model looks at the HIT intervention through 8 dimensions: (1) hardware and software computing infrastructure, (2) clinical content, (3) human–computer interface, (4) people, (5) workflow and communication, (6) internal organizational policies, procedures, and culture, (7) external rules, regulations, and pressures, and (8) system measurement and monitoring. In this framework, the eight components are interacting and interdependent and do not stand alone (Sittig and Singh, 2010).

AHRQ defines workflow as "the sequence of physical and mental tasks performed by various people within and between work environments" (AHRQ, 2024) However, Unertl et al. (2010) conducted a literature review that revealed significant variability in the definition of the term 'workflow' as well as in methods to study workflow and subsequently proposed a conceptual framework for conducting workflow research.

Under this framework (exhibited in Fig. 3.2), clinical workflows refer to the entire breadth of activities or actions that are performed by users within the healthcare setting in order to deliver service to patients and consumers. The performance of actions in contemporary healthcare workflows is often enabled partially or completely by HIT, such as the electronic health record (EHR). Modernizing these workflows with the advancement of HIT can lead to significant improvements in patient care and operational efficiencies.

What defines an optimal workflow can be highly subjective as clinical workflows must balance clinician efficiency and experience, patient outcomes and experience, patient safety, and enhance the overall quality of care as well as reflect the contextual needs of the organization and its staff. The two conceptual models are complementary; however, both were designed for a pre-AI HIT landscape and the role-breaking nature of advanced AI provides a challenge to appropriately define and optimize AI-embedded clinical workflows depending on where the human is in the loop.

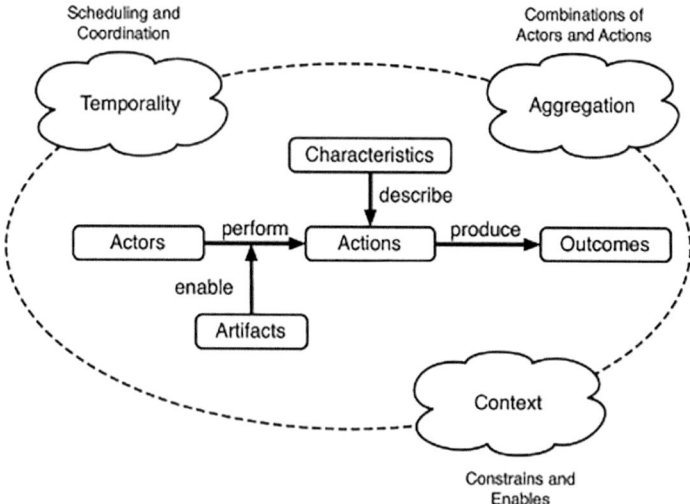

Fig. 3.2 Conceptual framework for workflow research. *Source* Unertl et al. (2010). Unertl KM, Novak LL, Johnson KB, Lorenzi NM. Traversing the many paths of workflow research: developing a conceptual framework of workflow terminology through a systematic literature review. J Am Med Inform Assoc. 2010;17(3):265–73. https://www.ncbi.nlm.nih.gov/pmc/articles/PMC2995718/figure/fig3/

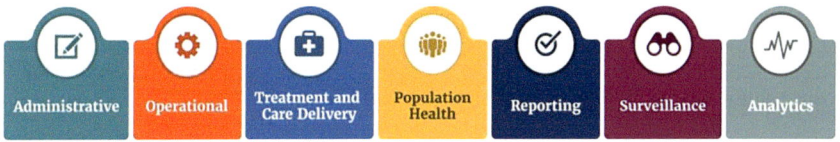

Fig. 3.3 Health care automation domains. *Source* Zayas-Cabán et al. (2022). Public domain

3.3.2 Healthcare Domains and Automation Opportunities

Opportunities for workflow automation are typically found in workflows with low process complexity, frequent and consistent task repetition, and well-defined rules and processes that use well-structured data. Workflow automation becomes far more difficult when there are complex processes that involve the use of multiple data points for decision making (Zayas-Cabán et al., 2021).

What makes AI different from other HIT innovations is the fact that it is not a monolithic product, but a technology stack that can be applied narrowly or broadly across healthcare domains. In fact, depending on the context, a single AI-based tool, such as a specialty-trained LLM, can be simultaneously used both narrowly **AND** broadly by different users for different use cases, and that flexibility can be multiplied within and across domains, flexing to meet organizational and individual needs. Shown in Fig. 3.3, the U.S. Office of the National Coordinator for Health Information Technology (ONC) proposed a set of healthcare domains that could be used to frame national priorities to accelerate workflow automation (Zayas-Cabán et al., 2022).

3.3.3 Principles of Designing AI-Driven Workflows

Basic principles for designing AI-driven healthcare workflows are no different than those that guide the implementation of non-AI tools and are noted elsewhere in this book. In general, it is ill-advised to add any technology to an existing ineffi-cient process without sufficient redesign so that it does not simply becomes a faster (decreased cycle time) inefficient process. Similarly, the use of any HIT should be focused on an outcome that supports one or more of the Institute of Medicine's Six Aims for Improvement: Safe, Timely, Effective, Efficient, Equitable, and Patient-Centered care (STEEEP). However, AI requires some additional considerations (Table 3.1).

Identify Capacity to Support AI-Driven Workflow Augmentation

Based on key informant interviews, literature reviews, and a multidisciplinary expert workshop, ONC proposed a set of considerations (Fig. 3.4) to assist stakeholders in

Table 3.1 Key questions for designing AI-driven workflows

1. Identify capacity to support AI-driven workflow augmentation
    a. Is there a sufficiently robust dataset to support the AI-based technology?
    b. Do users trust the technology?
2. Identify desired level of shared decision making
    a. Is the current workflow well-understood?
    b. What are the opportunities as a result of AI adoption?
    c. What level of AI autonomy is desired and/or acceptable?
3. Identify the level of role displacement based upon the level of tool autonomy
    a. Which actions will be redefined?
    b. Which actors will be eliminated?
    c. Which sources and messages will be modified?

the work to make healthcare more efficient through adoption of workflow automation solutions (Zayas-Cabán et al., 2022).

Understanding the workflows of opportunity and setting the goal of automation to add value are baseline considerations for any process improvement project. In the context of AI, these considerations are inextricably tied to the others. There must be a sufficiently large high-quality dataset available to develop or train AI models. Concomitantly, unlike process automations of which the beginning and end states are visible and verifiable, there must be trust in the development of AI, as much of the inner workings of AI algorithms such as LLMs are transformer models that are completely opaque, and it is not possible to consistently reproduce the same result given the way how such models work.

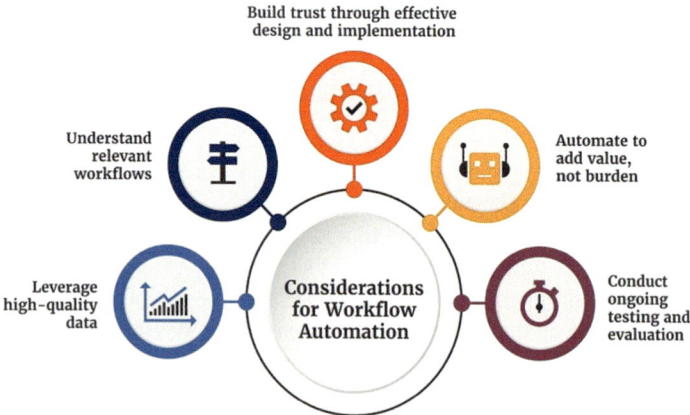

Fig. 3.4 Considerations for healthcare workflow automation. *Source* Zayas-Cabán et al. (2022). Public domain

Identify the Desired Level of Shared Decision Making

A thorough understanding of existing workflow processes, as well as identification of opportunities for improvement, are the first steps towards effectively incorporating new AI-based tools. As an example, clinician burnout is a significant issue, and dissatisfaction with EHR use and the amount of time spent on clerical and repetitive tasks has been reported to be a risk factor (Shanafelt et al., 2016; Melnick et al., 2019). In-basket message volume and delivery timing have also been reported to delay the opening of time-sensitive EHR alert messages (Cutrona, 2017). Therefore, an opportunity to alleviate the cognitive burden could lie in leveraging AI to off-load or simplify in-basket message replies and improve alerting for critical abnormal value reports. Once such opportunities are identified, the next step is to choose the desired level of human involvement relative to the output and the risks and benefits.

In Human-in-the-Loop (HITL) models, the AI system is integrated into an existing clinical workflow, where a human user reviews and approves all AI proposed actions. For example, this might be used in radiology image interpretation workflow where AI suggests likely diagnoses based on image analysis concurrent with a radiologist performing a manual interpretation; the interpreting radiologist subsequently must confirm or reject the AI recommendation. The benefit of presumed higher accuracy and lower error risk is countered by the addition of an extra step to the clinical workflow.

In Human-on-the-Loop (HOTL) models, the AI system completely supplants portions of the existing clinical workflow, and the human user adds supervision and monitoring tasks to allow for timely intervention if system performance deviates from the expected outcome. An example is remote patient monitoring systems that use AI to track vital signs and alert staff when abnormal data is detected. This allows for efficient and highly scalable monitoring, as the capacity of automated range monitoring greatly exceeds human capacity, but the effectiveness relies heavily on model precision and the responsiveness of human supervisors to alerts. This is typically the "sweet spot" for balancing efficiency gains with risk mitigation.

In Human-out-of-the-Loop (HOOTL) models, the workflow is completely displaced by the AI system, which functions completely autonomously without human intervention. Any risk or safety monitoring requires a completely new user workflow to be developed. An example is an automated medication dispensing system which uses a combination of robotics and AI to select, package, label, and prepare medications for distribution. HOOTL models represent the highest efficiency gain as all repeatable tasks are fully automated, but concomitantly carry the highest potential risk without appropriate model and performance supervision.

Table 3.2 lists more examples of HITL, HOTL, and HOOTL according to ONC's healthcare domains.

In addition to the level of AI system autonomy (i.e., HITL, HOTL, HOOTL), the concept of shared decision making is another important construct to frame the use of any AI tool to address a workflow improvement opportunity. For example, Elwyn et al. (2012) introduced a three-step model for collaborative decision making with patients. In this model (Fig. 3.5), Choice Talk ensures that patients understand the

Table 3.2 Examples of HITL, HOTL, and HOOTL

Domain	Clinical workflow examples	HITL	HOTL	HOOTL
Administrative	Patient scheduling and registration; billing claims processing	Pre-processing of claims by extracting required data	Automated infusion bed scheduling	
	Care documentation	Documentation suggestions	Chart summarization	
Operational	pharmacy management	Pharmacogenomic drug interaction checking		Automated dispensing cabinets
	Bed management	Readmission risk prediction	Patient discharge forecasting	
	Staff resourcing	Staff level/demand forecasting	Automated staff scheduling	
	Demand management			
Treatment and care delivery	assessment	Genomic analysis	AI-based decision support	
	Diagnosis	Rare disease diagnosis assistance; Imaging tagging	Imaging analysis	Automated diabetic retinopathy screening
	Treatment planning	Personalized treatment plans	Clinical trial matching	
	Treatment	Surgical planning (e.g., 3d modeling)	Robotic surgery	
	Monitoring		Early warning/clinical deterioration prediction	Remote patient monitoring; critical event notification and intervention
	Follow-up	Monitoring medication adherence		
	Patient education	Medication and appointment reminders; treatment summarization	Chatbots	Generation of language and literacy level appropriate patient health information
Population health		Point-of-care preventive health recommendations	Care coordination	Screening reminders

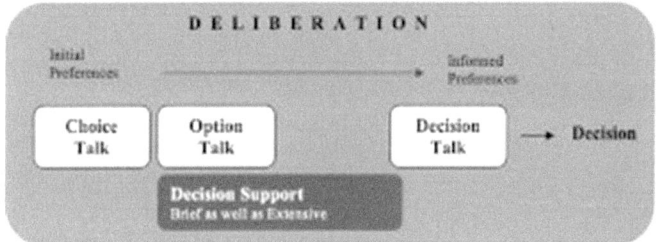

Fig. 3.5 Elwyn shared decision-making model (distributed under creative commons license). *Source* https://www.ncbi.nlm.nih.gov/pmc/articles/PMC3445676/figure/Fig1/

options available to them for care; Option Talk provides detailed information related to those options; and Decision Talk facilitates the decision making based upon patient preferences. This model can be adapted for use with HITL and HOTL AI tools with the user taking the place of the patient. The AI model takes the role of the clinician and provides the decision support (HITL) or a decision recommendation (HOTL) that supports decision making.

Identify the Level of Workflow Role Displacement

The conceptual framework developed by Unertl et al. (2010) describes five entities that are involved in the workflow process: actor, artifact, actions, characteristics (that describe actions), and outcomes. Traditional HIT systems are generally artifacts that enable the actor's decision-making process. However, AI-based tools have the ability serving as artifact (HITL), actor + artifact + recommended action (HOTL), or actor + artifact + action + outcome (HOOTL). Similarly, there is compression of social-technical dimensions as certain AI tools (such as LLM combined with a chat interface) are inherently multi-dimensional and combine computing infrastructure, clinical content, user interface, and workflow and communication dimensions.

Many healthcare workflows are inherently non-linear and the staff performing those workflows often have a high level of expertise and specialization. However, those same individuals frequently have high levels of autonomy, tribal behaviors, and variable personal styles of working (Westbrook et al., 2009). With many of these individuals working in collaborative teams to provide care to patients, it represents a remarkable challenge to data/information transfer and communication.

Berlo's Source-Message-Channel-Receiver (SMCR) model of communication is a linear model where the source of communication determines a message and its success can be impacted by communication skills, attitudes, knowledge level, and

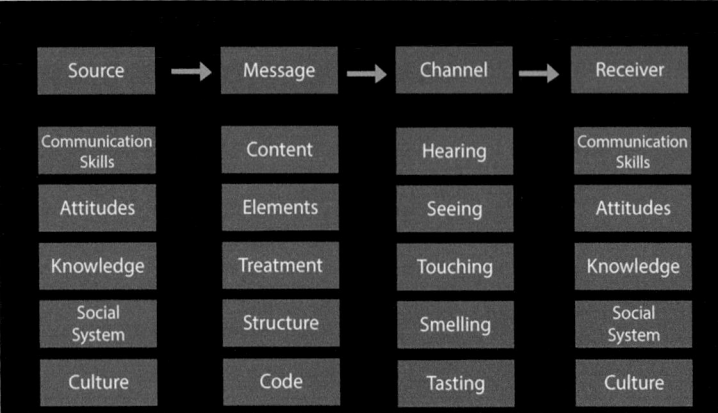

Fig. 3.6 Berlo's (1960) Source-message-channel-receiver model of communication. (Used under creative commons license. The top row represents the core elements of the model and the rows beneath the process flow represent the key characteristics of each model element. https://www.researchgate.net/figure/Berlos-1960-Source-Message-Channel-Rec eiver-Model-of-Communication-Developed-from_fig1_331435468)

position within a social-cultural system (Berlo, 1960). It is similar to the social-technical model in that it defines a mode of communications where success is dependent upon factors that may not be directly related to the actual message being communicated. At a high level, the source encodes a message, sends it via a channel, which then decodes the message for the receiver (Fig. 3.6).

Where there is a 1:1:1:1 relationship between source:message:channel:receiver, automation solution is usually straightforward and the benefits are easy to quantify. A simplistic example is a laboratory instrument resulting a single test result, encoding it as an Health Level 7 (HL7) message, and sending it through the data network to the EHR HL7 interface listener. If one of the relationships changes to many, then the complexity begins to increase but is still manageable. For example, a 1:1:1:many relationship can be seen with a single email message with multiple recipients. Once two or more of the relationships change to many:many, the complexity can become overwhelming rapidly, and many of the challenges in healthcare are related to the issue of managing too many messages and information overload. AI tools can be used to simplify many:many relationships back to 1:many or even 1:1, such as using generative AI to summarize large numbers of messages into a single message, or facilitate the personalization of messages to multiple recipients.

3.3.4 AI Tool Development Lifecycle

There are several distinct stages in the development lifecycle of an AI-based tool (Samala, 2024). **Discover** represents the initial research and ideation phase and

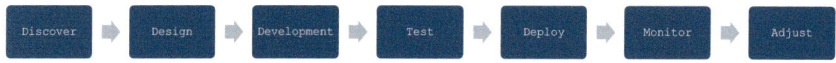

Fig. 3.7   Development lifecycle of AI

often uses formal methods such as design thinking to identify needs and develop functional and non-functional requirements (Parizi, 2022). The **Design** phase takes these requirements and converts them into conceptual designs and plans, which are then used during the **Development** phase to prototype and iterate until there is a testable minimum viable product, or a basic version of the tool that has enough features to be used by testers to provide feedback for refinement. The **Test** phase involves aggregating an appropriately representative training dataset for training an AI model. Once the model has been trained, a validation dataset is used to tune the model's parameters. Finally, a test dataset is used to evaluate the performance of the final model. Validation and test datasets are often referred to as "holdout" datasets because they are not used during initial training and thus provide an unbiased evaluation of model performance using unseen data. Implementation of the tool into workflow occurs in the **Deploy** phase. Once deployed, performance and effectiveness are **Monitor**ed and depending on the type of AI, the underlying models may be continuously **Adjust**ed to improve performance (Fig. 3.7).

3.3.5   *Challenges and Considerations*

While many clinical decision-support (CDS) systems have been shown to improve quality and efficiency in lab or single-site settings, most have struggled to show efficacy when implemented more broadly (Sittig, 2008; Chaudry, 2006). The ability for an HIT tool to generalize effectively is critical because while clinical workflows may share high-level commonalities across institutions and care delivery settings, their characteristics often vary widely based on role definitions, clinical staffing models, organizational culture, and geography. Traditional CDS tools work in collaboration with human experts through HITL or HOOTL models, supporting clinicians in health or disease management intervention though integration into existing clinical workflows. Advances in AI-based CDS have the potential of changing this dynamic by directly affecting health and wellness, and thus forcing the development of entirely new clinical workflows that completely take the human out of the loop.

Trust in AI

As AI systems become increasingly autonomous, it is essential that the output of these systems can be trusted, especially as humans move on the loop and out of the loop. However, many AI systems are "black boxes" where the inner workings are opaque to end users. All systems output a numeric value. In some instances, those values are displayed directly to the end user, such as a sepsis risk score, while others use that score to trigger subsequent actions, such as an alert that prompts the ordering of a sepsis order set. Trust begins with a recognition by the end user that the needs and requirements that drove the model development are sufficiently aligned or similar to the destination organization where the model is to be deployed and that the datasets and algorithms do not foster inequity.

As an example, City of Hope, a dedicated cancer center in Duarte, CA, deployed a third-party machine learning-based early sepsis detection system in 2018 that presented a numerical risk score in an inpatient list summary report. While the vendor-supplied sensitivity and specificity data suggested an acceptable data-clinical status correlation, in clinical practice, the risk score was quickly noted as impractical as it was flagging most inpatients as high risk. A root cause analysis suggested that the general inpatient population that the vendor used to create the training and validation datasets was not sufficiently similar to the oncology post-bone marrow transplant patients that represent the bulk of the inpatient population at City of Hope. While further tuning of the vendor model did decrease false negative flagging, the initial poor performance led to a general abandonment of the system by the clinical staff due to a lack of confidence. A subsequent foray using a home-grown sepsis risk score model that was trained on ten years of City of Hope oncology inpatient data was far more successful.

As illustrated by the example, the complexity of the healthcare socio-technical system makes it unlikely to have a single source of data sufficiently broad to train an AI model (Wu, 2022). For example, differences in data definitions, coding definitions, and population demographics may result in a model trained using data from one setting not applicable in another (Vollmer, 2020; Larson, 2024). The large volume of data required to train AI models also raises challenge to bias assessment. Differences in data collected (or not collected) for training datasets can lead to amplification of bias in vulnerable populations such as those characterized by age, gender, race, geography, or economic status, and can result in unwittingly suboptimal decision support or actions (Johnson, 2020).

In addition to issues arising from training data, AI systems must be sufficiently **transparent** so that human users can interact with these systems to provide effective oversight (Endsley, 2017). Traditional neural network models can support this level of transparency but may require a data scientist to fully understand the parameters and weighting. As AI systems advance in complexity, it will become increasingly difficult for humans to be trained to maintain an accurate mental model of how they work in real-time, as tools such as generative AI, by their very nature, are designed to learn over time (USAF, 2019). **Explainability**, or the retrospective provision of information about why and how (logic, process, reasoning, variables) a specific decision was made or action taken, is increasingly required for these more complex AI tools.

Recognition of Workflow Complexity

Suboptimal adoption of AI-based tools is often not due to poor algorithmic performance, but rather a lack of understanding of how to effectively integrate such tools into clinical workflow to support the significant complexity of the modern healthcare workplace (Yang, 2019; Jaspers 2011). Kawamoto (2005) conducted a systematic review of trials to identify CDS success factors and noted four features that were consistently correlated with successful implementations: (1) automatic as part of workflow, (2) support at the time and point of care for decision making, (3) actionable recommendations, and (4) computer involvement. While this review predated the general prevalence of EHRs (hence obviating the need to call out computer involvement), the first three continue to be highly relevant almost two decades later for contemporary HITL and HOTL AI tools.

Personnel time required for implementation of AI-based tools must also be taken into consideration as it is often the largest resource required (Sendak, 2020). Where the tool focuses on a single individual, such as supporting an HITL or HOTL radiologist diagnostic process, the time demand impact is often low and limited to a single (1:1:1:1) or small group of users (1:1:1:many). However, when a single tool provides information to many members of a multidisciplinary care teams, such as patients who are candidates for early discharge, the aggregate amount of personnel time required to appropriately validate the implementation increases significantly.

New Challenges with Generative AI

Concomitant with the rapid evolution of AI in the recent decade, there has been a significant growth in AI tools brought to the healthcare market (Muehlematter, 2021). The FDA tripled the number of approved AI-enabled medical devices between 2019 and 2023 (FDA, 2024). There are many more commercially available healthcare AI tools that are not subject to FDA approval as they are not considered to be medical devices (Fig. 3.8).

Historically, AI-based systems used in healthcare have utilized traditional machine-learning techniques with focused integration to match the HITL or HOTL workflow. Models are discrete, logic is transparent, outputs can be reproduced, and results can be easily explained. The cognitive burden on end users is the same as with any other discrete data point that requires interpretation. However, the rapid development of generative AI and LLM models, and their integration into tools that support the entire spectrum of healthcare activities and services, pose a challenge to existing approaches towards the identification and mitigation of unintended consequences.

As opposed to traditional AI models, the technical and logical architectures of generative AI and LLM are not discrete outside of parameter configuration and weighting; and explainability can be challenging due to model complexity. Every LLM model has output differences that are the product of the billions of parameters used and then filtered by what the model developers deem to be the optimal approach

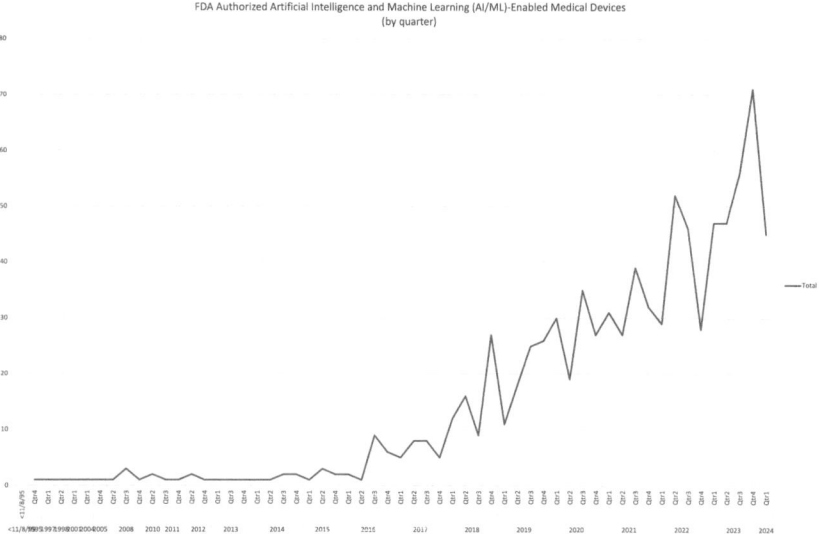

Fig. 3.8 FDA approvals of AI-enabled medical devices by quarter (1995–2024)

towards delivering the output. Advanced AI tools can use multiple LLMs to cross-check and validate results in order to minimize hallucinations and other factitious outputs. However, healthcare organizations utilizing these tools must make the effort to ensure that they understand a model's inherent strengths and weakness and the fit with the proposed use case, and also train the clinical workforce to ask the right question (prompt engineering, or how to design the inputs to produce the optimal output), critically evaluate the output to ensure that it is the right answer, and provide the right level of model supervision depending on if the workflow is HITL, HOTL, or HOOTL.

Many commercial products leverage the same few generative AI LLM models through application programming interfaces (APIs) and are distinguishing their offerings by pre-model prompt engineering and post-model user interface design. Most organizations are skilled at evaluating product design and usability but now must also develop core competencies in evaluating how commercial tools interact with AI LLMs in the background.

Data Privacy and the Development of Large Clinical Datasets

Vendors and software developers frequently partner with healthcare delivery systems in order to create training and test datasets to enhance AI model development. These arrangements are typically contractual and explicitly define model intellectual property rights, data privacy protections, data reuse allowances, and data ownership. For traditional AI tools, there is the theoretical possibility for a healthcare system to revoke those permissions and require the removal of the contributed data from future training and test datasets. Traditional AI models can be subsequently retrained and tuned on the redacted datasets and the difference in output can be measured and reproduced. This is no longer the case with generative AI and LLMs, as contributed data is simply part of a very large training dataset that is used to train the model but does not directly affect the output and is not weighted directly.

Increasingly, the need to collect more specialized and deeper datasets is prompting developers to partner using a "freemium" model where healthcare organizations are given free or low-cost access to the tool in exchange for de-identified patient data that will then be used to continue to refine the AI model. It will be important for healthcare organizations to review such partnerships closely to ensure that data considered to be organizational intellectual property, such as clinical trials data, or data that has the potential of "fingerprinting" patients, such as genomic variant testing, is appropriately safeguarded.

3.4 Conclusion

While AI has been part of the HIT ecosystem for several decades and used in human in the loop and human on the loop clinical workflows, only recently has the technology advanced to the point where it can now be considered for human out of the loop scenarios. As such, there is a pressing need to develop appropriate transparency, explainability, and supervision measures, and to balance the reliance on emerging AI tools and ensuring system reliability with workflow efficiency and effectiveness gains.

A key consideration when adopting AI tools in healthcare is to understand the underlying reason to deploy the tool in clinical workflow: Is it to decrease burnout by off-loading low-yield cognitive work? Is it to improve quality of care through human-AI synergy? Is it to improve efficiency? Answering this question allows the design of the right level of integration of AI into the clinical workflow. For example, do end users need to review and approve all proposed actions (HITL) or their involvement is only needed for supervision and monitoring (HOTL)? If the process is completely automated (HOOTL), what is the impact on the workforce, and does it change our traditional communications model where some or all the components of the sender-message-channel-receiver flow can be combined? How should clinical workflow be altered in order to accommodate different models of AI tool interaction?

In many ways, with respect to healthcare AI, the genie is out of the lamp. Governmental agencies are now rushing to develop regulations to ensure its safe use. The European AI Act (2024) is a legal framework enacted to support the development of trustworthy AI, as well as establishing the governance and enforcement rules. Using a risk-based approach, it specifies how developers must support transparency and accountability for AI systems. However, advancing technology will continue to outstrip regulatory bodies and healthcare organizations must develop a strategy to adapt to ever-evolving AI-driven solutions.

References

Agency for healthcare research and quality. What is workflow? 21 February 2020. https://digital. ahrq.gov/health-it-tools-and-resources/evaluation-resources/workflow-assessment-health-it-toolkit/workflow. Accessed 2 June 2024.

Berlo DK. The process of communication. New York: Holt, Rinehart and Winston; 1960.

Bi WL, Hosny A, Schabath MB, Giger ML, Birkbak NJ, Mehrtash A, Allison T, Arnaout O, Abbosh C, Dunn IF, Mak RH, Tamimi RM, Tempany CM, Swanton C, Hoffmann U, Schwartz LH, Gillies RJ, Huang RY, Aerts HJWL. Artificial intelligence in cancer imaging: clinical challenges and applications. CA Cancer J Clin. 2019; 69(2):127–57. https://doi.org/10.3322/caac.21552. Epub 2019 Feb 5. PMID: 30720861; PMCID: PMC6403009.

Bloch M, Blumberg S, Laartz J. Delivering large-scale IT projects on time, on budget, and on value. McKinsey. www.mckinsey.com. Published 1 Oct 2012. https://www.mckinsey.com/capabilit ies/mckinsey-digital/our-insights/delivering-large-scale-it-projects-on-time-on-budget-and-on-value/. Accessed 18 May 2024.

Chaudhry B, Wang J, Wu S, Maglione M, Mojica W, Roth E, Morton SC, Shekelle PG. Systematic review: impact of health information technology on quality, efficiency, and costs of medical care. Ann Intern Med. 2006;144(10):742–52. https://doi.org/10.7326/0003-4819-144-10-200 605160-00125. Epub 2006 Apr 11 PMID: 16702590.

Choon YW, Choon YF, Nasarudin NA, Al Jasmi F, Remli MA, Alkayali MH, Mohamad MS. Artificial intelligence and database for NGS-based diagnosis in rare disease. Front Genet. 2024;25(14):1258083. https://doi.org/10.3389/fgene.2023.1258083.PMID:38371307;PMCID: PMC10870236.

Coffey K, Aukland B, Amir T, Sevilimedu V, Saphier NB, Mango VL. Artificial intelligence decision support for triple-negative breast cancers on ultrasound. J Breast Imaging. 2024;6(1):33–44. https://doi.org/10.1093/jbi/wbad080. PMID: 38243859.

Comito C, Pizzuti C. Artificial intelligence for forecasting and diagnosing COVID-19 pandemic: a focused review. Artif Intell Med. 2022;128:102286. https://doi.org/10.1016/j.artmed.2022. 102286. Epub 2022 Mar 28. PMID: 35534142; PMCID: PMC8958821.

Cosgun E, Oh M. Exploring the consistency of the quality scores with machine learning for next-generation sequencing experiments. Biomed Res Int. 2020;25(2020):8531502. https://doi.org/ 10.1155/2020/8531502.PMID:32219145;PMCID:PMC7061114.

Cutrona SL, Fouayzi H, Burns L, Sadasivam RS, Mazor KM, Gurwitz JH, Garber L, Sundaresan D, Houston TK, Field TS. Primary care providers' opening of time-sensitive alerts sent to commer-cial electronic health record InBaskets. J Gen Intern Med. 2017;32(11):1210–19. https://doi.org/ 10.1007/s11606-017-4146-3. Epub 2017 Aug 14. PMID: 28808942; PMCID: PMC5653559.

Danis D, Jacobsen JOB, Carmody LC, Gargano MA, McMurry JA, Hegde A, Haendel MA, Valentini G, Smedley D, Robinson PN. Interpretable prioritization of splice variants in diagnostic next-generation sequencing. Am J Hum Genet. 2021;108(9):1564–77. https://doi.org/10.1016/j.ajhg. 2021.06.014. Epub 2021 Jul 21. Erratum in: Am J Hum Genet. 2021 Nov 4;108(11):2205. PMID: 34289339; PMCID: PMC8456162.

Elwyn G, Frosch D, Thomson R, Joseph-Williams N, Lloyd A, Kinnersley P, Cording E, Tomson D, Dodd C, Rollnick S, Edwards A, Barry M. Shared decision making: a model for clinical practice. J Gen Intern Med. 2012;27(10):1361–7. https://doi.org/10.1007/s11606-012-2077-6. Epub 2012 May 23. PMID: 22618581; PMCID: PMC3445676.

Endsley MR. From here to autonomy. Hum Factors. 2017;59(1):5–27. https://doi.org/10.1177/001 8720816681350. Epub 2016 Dec 15 PMID: 28146676.

Food and Drug Administration. Artificial intelligence and machine learning (AI/ML)-enabled medical devices. FDA. Published online May 13, 2024. https://www.fda.gov/medical-devices/ software-medical-device-samd/artificial-intelligence-and-machine-learning-aiml-enabled-med ical-devices#:~:text=With%20this%20update%2C%20the%20FDA. Accessed June 7, 2024.

Hanis TM, Islam MA, Musa KI. Diagnostic accuracy of machine learning models on mammography in breast cancer classification: a meta-analysis. Diagnostics (Basel). 2022;12(7):1643. https://doi.org/10.3390/diagnostics12071643.PMID:35885548;PMCID:PMC9320089.

Hasan SU, Siddiqui MAR. Diagnostic accuracy of smartphone-based artificial intelligence systems for detecting diabetic retinopathy: a systematic review and meta-analysis. Diabetes Res Clin Pract. 2023;205: 110943. https://doi.org/10.1016/j.diabres.2023.110943. Epub 2023 Oct 5 PMID: 37805002.

Jaspers MW, Smeulers M, Vermeulen H, Peute LW. Effects of clinical decision-support systems on practitioner performance and patient outcomes: a synthesis of high-quality systematic review findings. J Am Med Inform Assoc. 20111;18(3):327–34. https://doi.org/10.1136/amiajnl-2011-000094. Epub 2011 Mar 21. PMID: 21422100; PMCID: PMC3078663.

Johnson J, Mulder, H. Endless modernization: how infinite flow keeps software fresh. Theh Standish Group. https://www.researchgate.net/profile/Hans-Mulder-2/publication/348849361_Endless_Modernization_How_Infinite_Flow_Keeps_Software_Fresh/links/60132878299bf1b 33e30c29e/Endless-Modernization-How-Infinite-Flow-Keeps-Software-Fresh.pdf. Published 2020. Accessed 18 May 2024.

Joseph S, Selvaraj J, Mani I, Kumaragurupari T, Shang X, Mudgil P, Ravilla T, He M. Diagnostic accuracy of artificial intelligence-based automated diabetic retinopathy screening in real-world settings: a systematic review and meta-analysis. Am J Ophthalmol. 2024;263:214–230. https://doi.org/10.1016/j.ajo.2024.02.012. Epub ahead of print. PMID: 38438095.

Kaplan B. Evaluating informatics applications–some alternative approaches: theory, social interactionism, and call for methodological pluralism. Int J Med Inform. 2001;64(1):39–56. https://doi.org/10.1016/s1386-5056(01)00184 8. PMID: 11673101.

Kawamoto K, Houlihan CA, Balas EA, Lobach DF. Improving clinical practice using clinical decision support systems: a systematic review of trials to identify features critical to success. BMJ. 2005;330(7494):765. https://doi.org/10.1136/bmj.38398.500764.8F. Epub 2005 Mar 14. PMID: 15767266; PMCID: PMC555881.

Khalilnejad A, Sun RT, Kompala T, Painter S, James R, Wang Y. Proactive identification of patients with diabetes at risk of uncontrolled outcomes during a diabetes management program: conceptualization and development study using machine learning. JMIR Form Res. 2024;26(8): e54373. https://doi.org/10.2196/54373.PMID:38669074;PMCID:PMC11087850.

Larson DB, Doo FX, Allen B Jr, Mongan J, Flanders AE, Wald C. Proceedings from the 2022 ACR-RSNA workshop on safety, effectiveness, reliability, and transparency in AI. J Am Coll Radiol. 2024;S1546–1440(24)00137–6. https://doi.org/10.1016/j.jacr.2024.01.024. Epub ahead of print. PMID: 38354844.

Mazurowski MA, Buda M, Saha A, Bashir MR. Deep learning in radiology: an overview of the concepts and a survey of the state of the art with focus on MRI. J Magn Reson Imaging. 2019;49(4):939–954. https://doi.org/10.1002/jmri.26534. Epub 2018 Dec 21. PMID: 30575178; PMCID: PMC6483404.

McCulloch W, Pitts W. A logical calculus of ideas immanent in nervous activity. Bull Math Biophys. 1943;5(4):115–33. https://doi.org/10.1007/BF02478259.

Melnick ER, Dyrbye LN, Sinsky CA, Trockel M, West CP, Nedelec L, Tutty MA, Shanafelt T. The association between perceived electronic health record usability and professional burnout among US physicians. Mayo Clin Proc. 2020;95(3):476–87. https://doi.org/10.1016/j.mayocp.2019.09.024. Epub 2019 Nov 14 PMID: 31735343.

Muehlematter UJ, Daniore P, Vokinger KN. Approval of artificial intelligence and machine learning-based medical devices in the USA and Europe (2015–20): a comparative analysis. Lancet Digit Health. 2021;3(3):e195–203. https://doi.org/10.1016/S2589-7500(20)30292-2. Epub 2021 Jan 18 PMID: 33478929.

Parizi R, Prestes M, Marczak S, Conte T. How has design thinking being used and integrated into software development activities? a systematic mapping. J Syst Softw. 2022;187:111217. https://doi.org/10.1016/j.jss.2022.111217.

Rosenblatt F. The perceptron: a probabilistic model for information storage and organization in the brain. Psychol Rev. 1958;65(6):386–408. https://doi.org/10.1037/h0042519.

Russell SJ, Norvig P. Artificial intelligence: a modern approach, 4th ed. Pearson; 2021. p. 4. https://doi.org/10.1109/MSP.2017.2765202.

Samala RK, Drukker K, Shukla-Dave A, Chan HP, Sahiner B, Petrick N, Greenspan H, Mahmood U, Summers RM, Tourassi G, Deserno TM, Regge D, Näppi JJ, Yoshida H, Huo Z, Chen Q, Vergara D, Cha KH, Mazurchuk R, Grizzard KT, Huisman H, Morra L, Suzuki K, Armato SG 3rd, Hadjiiski L. AI and machine learning in medical imaging: key points from development to translation. BJR Artif Intell. 2024;1(1):ubae006. https://doi.org/10.1093/bjrai/ubae006. PMID: 38828430; PMCID: PMC11140849.

Sendak MP, Ratliff W, Sarro D, Alderton E, Futoma J, Gao M, Nichols M, Revoir M, Yashar F, Miller C, Kester K, Sandhu S, Corey K, Brajer N, Tan C, Lin A, Brown T, Engelbosch S, Anstrom K, Elish MC, Heller K, Donohoe R, Theiling J, Poon E, Balu S, Bedoya A, O'Brien C. Real-world integration of a sepsis deep learning technology into routine clinical care: implementation study. JMIR Med Inform. 2020;8(7): e15182. https://doi.org/10.2196/15182.PMID:32673244; PMCID:PMC7391165.

Shamir SB, Sasson AL, Margolies LR, Mendelson DS. New frontiers in breast cancer imaging: the rise of AI. Bioengineering (Basel). 2024;11(5):451. https://doi.org/10.3390/bioengineering11050451.PMID:38790318;PMCID:PMC11117903.

Shanafelt TD, Dyrbye LN, Sinsky C, Hasan O, Satele D, Sloan J, West CP. Relationship between clerical burden and characteristics of the electronic environment with physician burnout and professional satisfaction. Mayo Clin Proc. 2016;91(7):836–48. https://doi.org/10.1016/j.mayocp.2016.05.007. Epub 2016 Jun 27 PMID: 27313121.

Sittig DF, Singh H. A new sociotechnical model for studying health information technology in complex adaptive healthcare systems. Qual Saf Health Care. 2010;19 Suppl 3(Suppl 3):i68–74. https://doi.org/10.1136/qshc.2010.042085. PMID: 20959322; PMCID: PMC3120130.

Sittig DF, Wright A, Osheroff JA, Middleton B, Teich JM, Ash JS, Campbell E, Bates DW. Grand challenges in clinical decision support. J Biomed Inform. 2008;41(2):387–92. https://doi.org/10.1016/j.jbi.2007.09.003. Epub 2007 Sep 21. PMID: 18029232; PMCID: PMC2660274.

Unertl KM, Novak LL, Johnson KB, Lorenzi NM. Traversing the many paths of workflow research: developing a conceptual framework of workflow terminology through a systematic literature review. J Am Med Inform Assoc. 2010;17(3):265–73. https://doi.org/10.1136/jamia.2010.004333. PMID: 20442143; PMCID: PMC2995718.

US Department of the Air Force. Unmanned Aircraft Systems Flight Plan 2009–2047. 2009. p. 41. http://www.govexec.com/pdfs/072309kp1.pdf. Accessed 24 May 2024.

US Department of the Air Force. Autonomous horizons: the way forward. Washington, DC: Office of the U.S. Air Force Chief Scientist; 2019. https://apps.dtic.mil/sti/citations/AD1157410. Accessed 15 June 2024.

Vollmer S, Mateen BA, Bohner G, Király FJ, Ghani R, Jonsson P et al. Machine learning and artificial intelligence research for patient benefit: 20 critical questions on transparency, replicability, ethics, and effectiveness. BMJ 2020;368:l6927. https://doi.org/10.1136/bmj.l6927.

Wears RL, Berg M. Computer technology and clinical work: still waiting for Godot. JAMA. 2005;293(10):1261–3. https://doi.org/10.1001/jama.293.10.1261.

Westbrook J, Braithwaite J, Gibson K, et al. Use of information and communication technologies to support effective work practice innovation in the health sector: a multi-site study. BMC Health Serv Res. 2009;9:201. https://doi.org/10.1186/1472-6963-9-201.

Wu T, Misra RB. Why big projects fail—and how to give yours a better chance of success. Harvard Business Review. Published November 3, 2023. https://hbr.org/2023/11/why-big-projects-fail-and-how-to-give-yours-a-better-chance-of-success. Accessed May 18 2024.

Wu DTY, Barrick L, Ozkaynak M, Blondon K, Zheng K. Principles for designing and developing a workflow monitoring tool to enable and enhance clinical workflow automation. Appl Clin Inform. 2022;13(1):132–138. https://doi.org/10.1055/s-0041-1741480. Epub 2022 Jan 19. PMID: 35045584; PMCID: PMC8769810.

Yang Q, Steinfeld A, Zimmerman J. Unre-markable AI: fitting intelligent decision support into critical, clinical decision-making processes. In: Proceedings of the 2019 CHI conference on human factors in computing systems; May 4–9. Glasgow, Scotland UK. ACM, New York, NY, USA; 2019. p. 11. https://doi.org/10.1145/3290605.3300468.

Yen PY, McAlearney AS, Sieck CJ, Hefner JL, Huerta TR. Health information technology (HIT) adaptation: refocusing on the journey to successful HIT implementation. JMIR Med Inform. 2017;5(3): e28. https://doi.org/10.2196/medinform.7476.PMID:28882812;PMCID: PMC5608986.

Zachariah FJ, Rossi LA, Roberts LM, Bosserman LD. Prospective comparison of medical oncologists and a machine learning model to predict 3 month mortality in patients with metastatic solid tumors. JAMA Netw Open. 2022;5(5): e2214514. https://doi.org/10.1001/jamanetworko pen.2022.14514.PMID:35639380;PMCID:PMC9157269.

Zayas-Cabán T, Okubo TH, Posnack S. Priorities to accelerate workflow automation in health care. J Am Med Inform Assoc. 2022;30(1):195–201. https://doi.org/10.1093/jamia/ocac197.PMID: 36259967;PMCID:PMC9748536.

Zayas-Cabán T, Haque SN, Kemper N. Identifying opportunities for workflow automation in health care: lessons learned from other industries. Appl Clin Inform. 2021;12(3):686–697. https://doi. org/10.1055/s-0041-1731744. Epub 2021 Jul 28. PMID: 34320683; PMCID: PMC8318703.

Chapter 4
Unintended Adverse Consequences of Health IT Implementation: Workflow Issues and Their Cascading Effects

Elizabeth V. Eikey, Yunan Chen, and Kai Zheng

Abstract The implementation of health information technology (IT) in clinical settings can introduce adverse effects to workflow, such as new or increased work, interruptions and distractions, delays or inefficiencies, duplicated work practices, and changed or disrupted communication. These adverse effects, if not managed properly, can result in increased clinician cognitive load and escalated patient safety risks. In this chapter, we summarize the literature on unintended adverse consequences of health IT related to clinical workflow with updates based on the rapid changes in technology during and beyond COVID-19. Based on prior research, we categorize these effects as primary and secondary unintended consequences to conceptualize the workflow issues and their cascading effects. By considering workflow issues as primary consequences and beginning to unpack the complex relationship between these issues and their impact on clinical work, we can better anticipate and address the adverse effects associated with health IT implementation.

Keywords Health information technology (health IT) · Workflow · Unintended consequences · Adverse effects · Workarounds · Healthcare · Clinicians · Patients

4.1 Introduction

Health information technology (IT) has great promise as a means to improve quality of care and patient safety. However, the introduction of health IT can impact healthcare practices in ways that are not by design, leading to unintended consequences. The term "unintended consequences" refers to unforeseen or unpredicted results to a

E. V. Eikey (✉)
University of California, San Diego, USA
e-mail: eeikey@health.ucsd.edu

Y. Chen · K. Zheng
University of California, Irvine, USA

© The Author(s), under exclusive license to Springer Nature Switzerland AG 2025
K. Zheng et al. (eds.), *Reengineering Clinical Workflow in the Digital and AI Era*,
Cognitive Informatics in Biomedicine and Healthcare,
https://doi.org/10.1007/978-3-031-82971-0_4

specific action (Campbell et al. 2006). However, some scholars emphasize an important discernment between unintended and unanticipated consequences. As discussed by Tingvold et al. (2023) *"unintended consequences are not necessarily unexpected and surprising and therefore must be distinguished from unanticipated and unforeseen consequences."* Thus, there are three "types" of consequences: intended or planned consequences, unintended or unplanned but not unanticipated consequences, and unintended (unplanned) and unanticipated consequences (Tingvold et al. 2023). Unintended consequences—whether unforeseen or not—can be positive, negative, or neutral. In this chapter, we focus on unintended consequences that are found to have a detrimental effect. This is not to say that there are no unintended or unanticipated positive effects associated with health IT implementation; within this chapter we simply choose to focus on one aspect that has been more commonly studied.

To date, a considerable body of health IT evaluation research has been devoted to understanding the unintended consequences that it introduces. While many papers have reviewed the relevant literature (Zadeh and Tremblay 2016; Harrington et al. 2011; Marcilly et al. 2015; Kim et al. 2017; Maslove et al. 2011; Menachemi and Collum 2011; Salahuddin et al. 2016; Niazkhani et al. 2009; Gephart et al. 2015; Bloomrosen et al. 2011; Pirnejad et al. 2010; Voshall et al. 2013; Vanderhook and Abraham 2017; Kuziemsky et al. 2016), the purpose of this chapter is to discuss the unintended consequences in the context of clinical *workflow*. Workflow is a core component of clinical practice because it encompasses all the activities and processes through which patient care is delivered. According to the U.S. Department of Health and Human Services (Information and Technology: What is Workflow. 2017), workflow can broadly be defined as *"the sequence of physical and mental tasks performed by various people within and between work environments. It can occur at several levels (one person, between people, across organizations) and can occur sequentially or simultaneously."* While health IT often focused on technologies embedded directly within clinical settings, the lines between clinical and consumer tools are becoming increasingly blurred. Health IT with the potential to impact workflow include but are not limited to:

- **Electronic health record (EHR) systems:** digital records of patients' health information, including medical history, diagnoses, medications, treatment plans, immunization dates, allergies, radiology images, and laboratory test results.
- **Health information exchange (HIE) platforms:** systems that facilitate the secure exchange of patient information among different healthcare providers and systems to support coordinated care.
- **Clinical decision-support systems (CDSS):** software tools that assist healthcare professionals in making clinical decisions by providing relevant information, alerts, and recommendations based on patient data.
- **Legacy systems:** older information systems that may still be in use within healthcare organizations, contributing to challenges in data integration and interoperability.
- **Telehealth and telemedicine platforms (hereby referred to as telehealth):** technologies enabling remote consultations and healthcare services delivery,

often involving videoconferencing and digital communication tools (can be synchronous or asynchronous).

- **Apps, wearable devices and remote patient monitoring tools:** devices that patients use to collect and share health data—either digitally or in person—such as fitness trackers and smartwatches; some data can be automatically sent to providers for monitoring.
- **Specialized healthcare applications:** software applications used for specific purposes, such as radiology information systems, laboratory information systems, and pharmacy management systems.
- **Artificial intelligence (AI):** the application of advanced computational algorithms and machine learning techniques to analyze and interpret complex medical data for tasks such as diagnostic support, predictive analytics, natural language processing, and personalized treatment recommendations.
- **Extended reality (XR) systems (e.g., virtual reality [VR], augmented reality [AR], and mixed reality [MR]):** an umbrella term that encompasses various immersive technologies, including VR, AR, and MR, that offer innovative solutions for spine medicine, surgery, consultation, therapy, education, and rehabilitation.

The surge in healthcare technology since 2020 has rapidly reshaped medical services, with innovations accelerating the adoption of health IT in response to the COVID-19 pandemic. Since 2020, clinical workflow has evolved driven by a convergence of new technologies, innovative service delivery models, and significant demographic shifts. Cutting-edge technologies such as AI (Alowais et al. 2023) and XR (Morimoto et al. 2022) have not only introduced novel tools for healthcare professionals but also ushered in unprecedented changes to traditional clinical processes. Additionally, the widespread adoption of telehealth, particularly in response to the COVID-19 pandemic, has redefined healthcare delivery, emphasizing remote interactions and virtual consultations (Anderson et al. 2022; Shaver 2022). Technologies that blur the lines between the clinical and consumer space, such as mobile apps, have created opportunities and challenges around large amounts of patient-generated data. Demographic changes, notably the increased care needs of older adults (Fulmer et al. 2021), have prompted a demand for more coordinated and adaptable healthcare practices. This confluence of factors has reshaped clinical workflow and necessitated a dynamic approach to health information technology integration, emphasizing the need for an in-depth exploration of the unintended consequences of health IT arising from these multifaceted changes.

Understanding workflow in clinical settings is essential to designing and deploying usable health IT: "*A critically important component of an organization's preparation for an HIT implementation is a thorough review of its workflow processes, procedures, and role assignments; yet the complexity of the healthcare workflow makes it resistant to many conventional workflow modeling and automation approaches*" (Bloomrosen et al. 2011) (page 88). Without carefully engineered integration with clinical workflow, health IT systems will not be embraced by end users and they may cause unintended negative consequences that adversely impact quality and safety of patient care (Sheehan and Bakken 2012; Zheng et al. 2020).

The term unintended consequences in the context of health IT became popularized in the early to mid 2000s by researchers studying the effects of patient care information systems (Paper et al. 2004) and computerized prescriber order entry (CPOE) (Ash et al. 2006). However, the recognition that health IT implementation could bring with unintended effects was not new, which had been reported in the literature even earlier (e.g., Goldstein et al. 2002). Often unintended adverse consequences (UACs) is the most commonly used term in the literature to emphasize the detrimental impact of unintended consequences such as more/new work for clinicians and disrupted/altered communication patterns (Campbell et al. 2006; Zheng et al. 2010a; Cresswell et al. 2017).

While many researchers use the term unintended consequences to refer broadly to unplanned effects related to workflow as a result of health IT implementation (Nanji et al. 2014; Horsky et al. 2006; Harrison et al. 2007; Gephart et al. 2016; Wu et al. 2013; Sergeeva et al. 2016), some researchers call these impacts (Zheng et al. 2010a; Wu et al. 2013; Vishwanath et al. 2010), effects (Vishwanath et al. 2010), residual consequences (Nanji et al. 2014), or simply problems (Horsky et al. 2006). For example, Vishwanath et al. (2010) did not explicitly discuss unintended consequences but talked in depth about the impact of EHR use on outpatient workflows. Wu et al. (2013), on the other hand, used the term unintended consequences, but they also repeatedly referred to these issues simply as impacts. The varied terminology use suggests a broad interest among the health IT research community in studying unintended consequences. However, it also means that it is difficult to synthesize this body of research because of the lack of consensus on how such issues should be defined and described.

This chapter briefly summarizes the extant literature on how health IT implementation may unintendedly introduce adverse consequences to clinical workflow, with the following two goals. First, we attempt to characterize the chain of impact by distinguishing primary unintended consequences that lead to changes in workflow, from secondary unintended consequences that originate from the workflow alterations. Second, we attempt to provide a discussion on the causes of, and some proposed solutions, for these workflow-related UACs. State-of-the-art and emergent health technologies are also discussed, particularly as health IT has evolved during and beyond COVID-19.

4.2   Characterizing Unintended Consequences

Understanding health IT's impact on workflow can be challenging due in part to the fact that workflow encompasses all activities around clinical care. The introduction of health IT is often associated with direct changes in established workflow such as new types of work and new task interdependencies, which has been widely noted in literature (Campbell et al. 2006; Gephart et al. 2015; Kuziemsky et al. 2016).

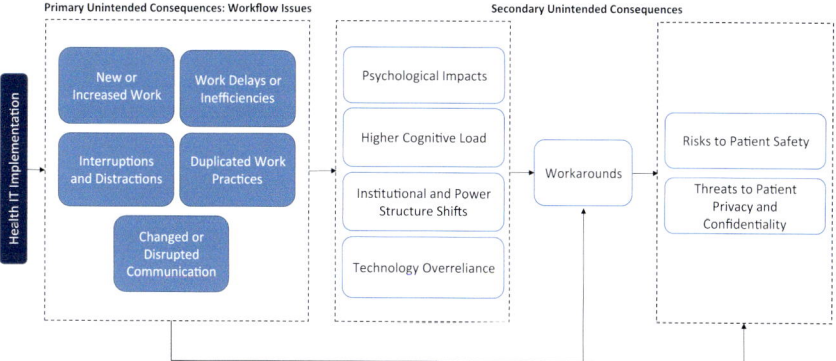

Fig. 4.1 Primary and secondary unintended adverse consequences of health IT

We refer to these as primary unintended consequences. In addition, there are other indirect impacts that occur as a result of these primary consequences. For example, some studies (although varying in their methodological approaches) have found that clinicians may adopt unsafe workarounds in response to disrupted and fragmented workflow, which can lead to an increase in errors resulting in patient safety threats (Ash et al. 2004; Yen et al. 2016; Coiera 2015). This cascading effect, from workflow consequences to other secondary impact, is illustrated in Fig. 4.1.

4.2.1 Workflow Issues as Primary Unintended Consequences

In many cases, unintended consequences of health IT implementation directly affect the work practices of both clinicians (e.g., physicians, nurses, pharmacists) and non-clinical staff (e.g., medical billing and coders, receptionists, and IT staff); even though the former is far more frequently studied. Unintended consequences to clinicians' workflow include new or increased workload (Campbell et al. 2006; Morimoto et al. 2022; Gephart et al. 2016; Hooff and Hafkamp 2017; Addab et al. 2022; Alipour and Hayavi-Haghighi 2021; Austin et al. 2021; Graham et al. 2020; Torous et al. 2021; Powell and Alexander 2021; Schriger et al. 2022; Triberti et al. 2020; Food and Drug Administration 2023) delayed work or time inefficiencies (Zadeh and Tremblay 2016; Zheng et al. 2010a; Horsky et al. 2006; Addab et al. 2022; Alipour and Hayavi-Haghighi 2021; Triberti et al. 2020; Ramaiah et al. 2012; Jeffery Reeves et al. 2021; Kemp et al. 2021; Khoshrounejad et al. 2021); interruptions or distractions (Zheng et al. 2010a; Nanji et al. 2014; Wu et al. 2013; Sergeeva et al. 2016; Lawrence et al. 2023; León et al. 2022); duplicated work practices (Campbell et al. 2006; Nanji et al. 2014; Horsky et al. 2006; Gephart et al. 2016; Cifuentes et al. 2015; Steinkamp et al. 2022) and changed or disrupted communication (Campbell et al. 2006; Wu et al. 2013; Schriger et al. 2022; Triberti et al. 2020; Kemp et al. 2021; Khoshrounejad et al. 2021; Jonasdottir et al. 2022; Baniasadi et al. 2020).

New or increased work: health IT can create new types of work or alter the nature of existing work that may lead to increased workload. For instance, an early study found that use of a CPOE system required added steps in order to get to the "patient overview" as compared to the work practices before the CPOE implementation (Campbell et al. 2006). Further, healthcare providers' workload may increase when they are forced to enter new types of information into computerized systems that were not previously required (Campbell et al. 2006; Gephart et al. 2016) and respond to computer-generated alerts that may not contain relevant or helpful information (Campbell et al. 2006). Workload increases often affect nurses (Gephart et al. 2016; Hooff and Hafkamp 2017), and studies have also found that physicians' administrative workload may also increase due to health IT use (Hooff and Hafkamp 2017).

The surge in patient-generated health data, facilitated through apps or specialty software, has demonstrated significant impacts on clinical workflow. The need for interaction between patients and providers within and outside of these digital environments introduces workflow challenges and necessitates manual processes, further straining healthcare professionals (Austin et al. 2021). For instance, Austin et al. (2021) reported that in 94% of the relevant case studies the utilization of specialized apps or software was needed, often because of the lack of the integration with existing healthcare IT such as the EHR. Attendant workflow is particularly burdensome, as patient-generated health data needs to be manually entered into the EHR.

Remote patient monitoring tools can also increase workload as patients generate data outside of the clinical setting for providers to oversee. The need to review and interpret the continuous stream of data generated by remote monitoring devices can create an additional burden on clinicians' time. In a qualitative review study of acute care, Thomas et al. (2021) reported that while remote patient monitoring has a number of benefits, these vary across contexts, and the additional workload can have trickle down negative impacts, such as slow response times and low adherence, particularly when remote monitoring is poorly integrated into existing clinical workflows. Similarly, as digital mental health interventions (DMHIs) and mental health apps become integral to psychiatric care, clinicians face the need to manage patient-generated health data and adapt to non-traditional workflows (Graham et al. 2020; Torous et al. 2021). These tools could include consumer apps and remote monitoring (e.g., technologies that utilize digital phenotyping). Despite the interest in DMHIs, Torous et al. (2021) report that workflow considerations are underexplored yet critical for successful implementation.

With the adoption of telehealth, accelerated by the COVID-19 pandemic, introduces complexities such as scheduling and documenting virtual appointments, with challenges including internet and connectivity issues that can further add to providers' workloads (Powell and Alexander 2021). One study found that telehealth required increased planning and preparation by clinicians (Schriger et al. 2022). Another found that telehealth added new responsibilities for critical access hospital staff, such as nurses, administrative support staff, ward clerks, and medical assistants (Haque et al. 2021). Compliance with regulatory requirements and navigating reimbursement procedures for telehealth services can introduce administrative complexities.

Clinicians may need to allocate additional time to ensure adherence to regulations and proper billing practices.

Additionally, the integration of XR in healthcare can also increase workloads (Morimoto et al. 2022). While promising for improved interventions, XR requires additional work to make adjustments for each user as well as ongoing technical support, such as in the operative environment (Food and Drug Administration 2023). While AI has the potential to streamline workflows in some cases, increased workloads are also possible with the inclusion of AI to support diagnoses and treatment, especially as clinicians may become mediators between AI and patients to review, approve, refine, and explain the AI's conclusions and recommendations (Triberti et al. 2020).

Interruptions and distractions: As a result of added or more fragmented work, health IT may interrupt clinicians' work processes or distract them from performing their clinical tasks. These disruptions may originate from computerized clinical systems (e.g., EHR and CPOE) due to poorly designed alerts and more rigid structured data entry requirements. The fact that with the introduction of health IT, clinicians must use a computer to complete certain tasks may also disrupt their usual workflow. For instance, clinicians may need to spend more time and exert more energy to find a nearby computer workstation to enter patient information (Zheng et al. 2010a), which is an added step not part of the paper-based workflows. Sometimes, computer-based automation may also result in distractions. For example, in the case of pharmacy workflow, a study found that pharmacy staff were disrupted by the need to restock prescriptions that patients never picked up because of an auto-filling feature added to their IT system (Nanji et al. 2014). Interruptions are also found due to the rapid increase of use of mobile devices in clinical settings. While mobile devices improve access to information and response time (Wu et al. 2013; Sergeeva et al. 2016), they can also become a salient source of disruptions. For instance, the "in the moment" communication afforded by mobile platforms causes frequent interruptions (e.g., imagine a clinician's phone going off every few minutes) (Wu et al. 2013) and disrupts collaborative work practices (Sergeeva et al. 2016). With growing popularity of remote monitoring and patient-generated data, providers face new challenges. The constant stream of data generated by remote patient monitoring devices requires clinicians to regularly review and interpret the information, adding to their workload and potentially causing interruptions during their routine tasks (Lawrence et al. 2023; León et al. 2022). Alerts and notifications from remote patient monitoring devices, indicating changes in a patient's condition, may demand immediate attention from clinicians, causing additional interruptions and diverting focus from other tasks.

Work delays or inefficiencies: Along these same lines, sometimes the introduction of new health IT creates delays in work and decreases time efficiency. For instance, Campbell et al. (2006) reported that CPOE systems could slow the process of clinical documentation and ordering. Similarly, in the context of pharmacy workflow, Zadeh and Tremblay (2016) conducted a literature review on studies of e-prescribing systems from 2008 to 2014 and found that 38% of the studies reported reduced pharmacy workflow efficiency as a result of unintended consequences. Further, inefficiencies are not only found internally within a clinical space; in fact, breakdowns of IT-based external interactions with insurance companies, laboratories, pharmacies, etc., may also cause work delays (Ramaiah et al. 2012). While there are discrepancies between some qualitative and quantitative studies with respect to how health IT impacts workflow efficiency, these may be due to how workflow is defined and measured. For example, Zheng et al. (2010a) reported that many time and motion studies had found the impact on workflow efficiency to be negligible; whereas qualitative studies had found consistent perceptions of decreased efficiency. They explained that this discrepancy may be due to the "design of the time and motion studies, which is focused on measuring clinicians' 'time expenditures' among different clinical activities rather than inspecting clinical 'workflow' from the true 'flow of the work' perspective". Therefore, they developed a set of new methods (e.g., workflow fragmentation assessments, pattern recognition, and data visualization) to assess workflow efficiency, and found that the implementation of a CPOE system caused a higher frequency of task switching and more fragmented workflow. This work suggests that analyses merely focusing on time utilization may not be adequate to capture workflow inefficiencies.

Recent technologies, such as the widespread adoption of telehealth, have introduced both transformative benefits and challenges to clinical workflows, particularly in the realm of work delays and inefficiencies (Jeffery Reeves et al. 2021). While telehealth, accelerated by the COVID-19 pandemic, has become a vital mode of healthcare delivery, most clinics have not been restructured their workflow for telehealth in a way that streamlines healthcare delivery (Jeffery Reeves et al. 2021). Technical issues such as poor internet connectivity, audio or video problems, and glitches in telehealth platforms can also cause delays (e.g., clinicians and patients may experience difficulties in establishing a stable connection) (Kemp et al. 2021; Khoshrounejad et al. 2021). As previously mentioned, there is a lack of integration between telehealth and EHR systems, which in addition to added work, can cause inefficiencies in providing healthcare (Alipour and Hayavi-Haghighi 2021). With AI, delays in healthcare delivery may result from the lack of information about how the AI arrives at the recommendations and decision paralysis, as AI becomes part of the decision-making process (Triberti et al. 2020). Delays can also be caused by XR as it requires setup time (e.g., (Addab et al. 2022)), which may not always be possible with time sensitive care needs.

Duplicated work practices: Another major unintended consequence related to clinical workflow is duplicated work practices. Sometimes health IT requires clinicians to enter redundant information (Gephart et al. 2016; Cifuentes et al. 2015; Steinkamp et al. 2022) or copy data from paper forms into the system (Horsky et al. 2006). For instance, Cifuentes et al. (2015) reported that clinicians often needed to double-enter their work into multiple computerized systems that were not interconnected. In other cases, health IT causes duplicated results, such as with the case of medications. For example, in Campbell et al.'s (2006) early work, they found that emergency orders were often duplicated because they were entered into the CPOE system and then phoned in to ensure efficiency. Similarly, Nanji et al. (2014) found that medication prescriptions were being dually transmitted—once through fax and once through the e-prescribing system—which often resulted in the same medications being filled more than once for each patient.

Another related issue is duplicated documentation. In a study quantifying duplicated notes in the EHR, Steinkamp et al. (2022) found an increase in duplication from 2015 to 2020 from 33.0% to 54.2%, of which over half came from text written by the same author. This significantly increases the burden on clinicians; from their corpus, they translate this into clinicians' workload stating that "*the median record length was 4,285 words; therefore, 10 records is 42,850 words, which is 81 standard single-spaced pages of 500 words each. Thus, a physician seeing 10 patients in a day would be responsible for reviewing at least 85 pages of single-spaced text across 691 notes. The duplicated half of the content not only provides no new information, but also increases the time required for the reading clinician attempting to discern which information is accurate and timely vs false or irrelevant*" (page 8).

Changed or disrupted communication: Communication is critical to clinical work and workflow, which may be altered or disrupted as the result of health IT use. CPOE systems, for example, may inhibit interpersonal communication because ordering information is now conveyed through electronic means that eliminates face-to-face interactions, during which important miscommunication and omissions may be discovered (Campbell et al. 2006). Similarly, Wu et al. (2013) conducted a study on the use of electronic communication tools, particularly smartphones, in clinical settings, and found that they could cause a decrease in verbal communication and negatively impact the relationships among clinicians. Thus, instead of promoting effective communication among healthcare providers and staff, health IT systems often provide only an illusion of communication whereby it is assumed the intended recipient will view and act upon the information entered into the system, which however may not always be the case in reality (Campbell et al. 2006).

Despite its benefits and reported satisfaction, telehealth has also been found to alter communication between patients and clinicians, given the technological medium in which synchronous (e.g., video and audio chatting) and asynchronous (e.g., messages) conversations take place (Kemp et al. 2021; Khoshrounejad et al. 2021; Jonasdottir et al. 2022). For example, two different scoping reviews (Khoshrounejad et al. 2021; Jonasdottir et al. 2022) reported changes in patient–provider communication as a challenge in telehealth due to factors such as loss of personal connection and limited non-verbal cues (Schriger et al. 2022). The shift from traditional in-person care to telehealth requires adjustments in communication and coordination, and the asynchronous nature of some telehealth communications, such as messaging or email consultations, may lead to delays in response times, impacting the timely exchange of information.

Similarly, XR, such as VR, can negatively impact communication and the patient–provider relationship due to diminished face-to-face interactions (Baniasadi et al. 2020). The use of AI in healthcare can also potentially reduce communication between patients and clinicians, as clinicians rely more on the technology, which in turn can impact rapport building, leading to potential issues of trust. Critical patient information may be lost when trying to make it fit within the constraints of AI's capability. Additionally, AI may become another factor that complicates the decision-making process and therefore, alters existing communication practices between clinicians who need to act on timely recommendations (Triberti et al. 2020).

4.2.2 Secondary Unintended Consequences Resulting from Workflow Issues

As a result of the workflow issues, clinicians often face secondary consequences, such as psychological impacts, higher cognitive load, shifts in institutional and power structure, and overreliance on technology. When clinicians are overburdened or upset, they may resort to workarounds in an attempt to ease these secondary consequences. These workarounds, and the workarounds that directly result from the workflow issues, can negatively impact patient safety and privacy.

Adverse Effects on Clinicians

Workflow issues that result from health IT adoption can affect clinicians in many unintended and negative ways, including detrimental psychological impacts such as provoking negative emotions (Campbell et al. 2006; Sittig et al. 2005) and burnout (Ye 2021), increased task fragmentation (Zheng et al. 2010a; Yen et al. 2016; Moy et al. 2023), increased cognitive burden (Moy et al. 2023), changed institutional and power structure (Campbell et al. 2006; Haque et al. 2021), and an overreliance on technology (Campbell et al. 2006; Quinn et al. 2021; Younis et al. 2024). As healthcare providers try to learn a new technologies and contest with changes to their work processes, they may experience guilt, annoyance, sadness, hostility, and disgust (Sittig et al. 2005). These unexpected and negative emotions often occur due to disruptions to clinical workflow and negative feedback from the system (Sittig et al. 2005). Not only are these negative feelings unpleasant for clinicians, but they may also make it difficult for clinicians to attend to complex clinical tasks (Campbell et al. 2006; Sittig et al. 2005). Addressing clinician burnout is increasingly crucial, and studies have shown that health IT can contribute to burnout through disturbed workflows (Ye 2021; Wu et al. 2021). This is particularly true when it comes to issues with patient-generated health data and integration with the EHR (Ye 2021).

Changes and disruptions to established workflow can also result in task fragmentation reflected as higher frequencies of task switching and multitasking (Zheng et al. 2010a; Yen et al. 2016; Moy et al. 2023) This can be disruptive to clinicians' work and are often associated with increased cognitive load and unnecessary physical activities (Yen et al. 2016; Laxmisan et al. 2007; Zheng et al. 2010b). For example, frequent login and logout actions, interruptive alerts, irrelevant reminders, and abrupt phone calls can all lead to more fragmented workflows and higher chance for errors (Yen et al. 2016; Coiera 2015). Within the EHR specifically, providers and nurses perceive increased cognitive burden due to inability to offload tasks, lack of cognitive aids, mismatch of clinical mental models, lack of agency and information overload (Moy et al. 2023).

By requiring added work and altering the ownership of certain clinical activities and tasks, health IT can impact individuals' roles and responsibilities in an organization (Hooff and Hafkamp 2017), leading toward changes to institutional and power structure (Campbell et al. 2006; Haque et al. 2021). For instance, CPOE systems redistribute work through role-based authorization, which rigidly controls who can do what (Campbell et al. 2006). Further, role misfits could occur where individuals experience reduced autonomy (Hooff and Hafkamp 2017). An example is that after the implementation of a new EHR system, nurses must wait for an official order from a physician placed through the system in order to remove a patient's IV, which could be independently performed by nurses in the past (Hooff and Hafkamp 2017). This change shifts the power structure and could create resentment between different types of medical professionals (Campbell et al. 2006).

As clinicians become accustomed to health IT, they may also develop an over-reliance on technology (Campbell et al. 2006; Shepard 2017; Haque et al. 2021; Quinn et al. 2021; Younis et al. 2024)) or certain clinical tasks simply could no longer be accomplished without technology. With newer health IT like AI, this is an increasing concern. This can be problematic when technology fails or is incorrect. It is inevitable that health IT will experience downtimes, both planned and unplanned (Shepard 2017; Kashiwagi et al. 2017). In the event of a system failure or mistakes, clinicians may no longer have the relevant information or knowledge to perform a task, which they relied on health IT to provide (Campbell et al. 2006). This can result in delayed care and/or increased patient safety risks (Campbell et al. 2006; Kashiwagi et al. 2017; Larsen et al. 2018).

Workarounds

Workarounds are mitigating strategies commonly employed by clinicians to overcome barriers to their work introduced by a variety of factors, including primary unintended consequences and their secondary effects. Workarounds can be individual, managerial, or artifact-based, depending on who initiates the workaround and how it is enacted. Common examples of workarounds include using paper and other software systems as intermediaries (Cresswell et al. 2017; Menon et al. 2016; Boonstra et al. 2021), staying logged into the system under a coworker's credential to save time (Ser et al. 2014) or sharing login details (Boonstra et al. 2021), copy-pasting (Boonstra et al. 2021), using separate text fields (Boonstra et al. 2021), and ignoring popups (Boonstra et al. 2021). In the context of test result management, Menon et al. (Menon et al. 2016) found that among the primary care clinicians studied who used workarounds, 70% reported using paper-based methods and 22% reported using a combination of paper and computer-based approaches. These workarounds persist as patient-generated health data and AI become more commonplace in healthcare settings. In terms of XR and telehealth, when encountering issues, clinicians may resort to using personal devices or unsanctioned technologies as workarounds.

Sometimes workarounds can become a routine practice to address workflow issues (Salahuddin et al. 2016). For instance, to combat inefficiencies and to facilitate care coordination, clinicians may write down patient information on a piece of paper (Menon et al. 2016; Boonstra et al. 2021), take photos of the screen of a computer workstation (Eikey et al. 2015), or use applications such as Microsoft Word or Excel (Boonstra et al. 2021). Generally, workarounds are aimed at alleviating secondary consequences that emerge as a result of workflow issues, rather than addressing the underlying workflow issues directly. For example, changes to work processes due to IT use may increase the cognitive load of clinicians, requiring them to use paper-based methods as a memory aid (Menon et al. 2016).

Many researchers have studied workarounds as part of the attempt to better understand disruptions to clinical workflow (Voshall et al. 2013; Cresswell et al. 2017; Ramaiah et al. 2012; Menon et al. 2016; Blijleven et al. 2017). Workarounds are an important phenomenon in this context, as they often signal unaddressed workflow issues. Some workarounds, e.g., those circumventing IT-enforced documentation, privacy/security, legal requirements or patient safety protocols, may also lead to additional adverse consequences (Fulmer et al. 2021; Vishwanath et al. 2010) (Blijleven et al. 2017), while others may be associated with benefits (Blijleven et al. 2017; Tucker et al. 2019). In recent years, researchers have expanded the scope of work on the impact of workarounds beyond quality of care and patient safety to include data quality, privacy and security, workload, laws and regulations, and financial aspects (Blijleven et al. 2017). While workarounds are often informal practices to mitigate workflow issues, they can also become formal organizational mandates when a direct solution is not readily available (Cresswell et al. 2017).

Risks to Patient Safety

The most concerning adverse impact as a result of workflow issues and/or unsafe workarounds is added risks to patient safety (Zheng et al. 2020; Cresswell et al. 2017; Gephart et al. 2016; Menon et al. 2016). Disruptions to workflow can increase the likelihood of errors, leading toward serious adverse events (Campbell et al. 2006; Pirnejad et al. 2010; Voshall et al. 2013; Cresswell et al. 2017; Nanji et al. 2014; Horsky et al. 2006; Ash et al. 2004; Menon et al. 2016). Poor usability of health IT also contributes to the problem. For example, due to poorly designed software user interface, it may become much easier for clinicians to select the wrong option or input an order for the wrong patient (Ash et al. 2004; Schiff et al. 2016). Schiff et al. (2016) provided an overview of common design problems of CPOE, including an illustration of how the overwhelming number of acetaminophen choices displayed on a computer screen could facilitate new types of errors. In addition, health IT requires complete and structured data, which can also cause cognitive overload that makes clinicians more susceptible to making mistakes (Ash et al. 2004; Yen et al. 2016; Coiera 2015; Chao 2016). Apps, remote monitoring devices, wearables, XR, and AI have introduced more data that need to be documented and interpreted, which can also contribute to overload.

Threats to Patient Privacy and Confidentiality

Lastly, workflow issues and unsafe workarounds can adversely affect patient privacy and confidentiality. Particularly, the use of workarounds such as paper notes, screenshots, and photos to improve memory and efficiency can threaten patient privacy and confidentiality by recording and transferring sensitive patient information in an unsecure manner. Similarly, the use of unapproved systems, devices, and software also compromise patient privacy, as their data are likely not protected in the same way as they are in approved systems. Although there are often privacy policies and security measures in place in clinical environments, clinicians may work around them when they deem these policies and measures inhibit their work practices (Eikey et al. 2015; Murphy and Reddy 2014; Chen and Xu 2013).

4.3 Causes and Solutions of Workflow Issues

We now shift the focus to the causes of workflow issues and briefly discuss some solutions that have been proposed in the literature. Most commonly, workflow issues occur when there is poor alignment between work practices and health IT design (Campbell et al. 2006; Horsky et al. 2006; Gephart et al. 2016). Health IT tends to rigidly model workflow according to organizational policies and regulatory requirements, which may not necessarily reflect the reality of day-to-day clinical practice (Campbell et al. 2006). Nuanced, non-linear, complex, and sometimes invisible processes are not easily incorporated in IT design. Health IT also tends to neglect the varied nature of workflow needs; that is, the work practices around the same task may be very different depending on an individual's role, the patient's conditions, etc. (Campbell et al. 2006) Health IT changes work practices; and work practices and social systems around health IT impact how they are used (Harrison et al. 2007).

Affordances of newly introduced technologies may also result in workflow issues. In some cases, barriers to workflow are introduced intentionally for valid reasons; for example, authentication requirements and automatic system timeouts (Eikey et al. 2015; Murphy and Reddy 2014; Chen and Xu 2013) are "limitations" designed purposefully to protect data security and patient privacy, even though they may cause undesirable delays and workflow disruptions. In addition, sometimes the affordances of technology adapted for clinical settings make them prone to disrupt workflow. For instance, smartphones could easily become a source of workflow interruption because of their ability to allow healthcare professionals to contact each other "in the moment" (Wu et al. 2013). Similarly, despite benefits, a study showed that use of iPods in the operating room can be distracting because they are by design fun and entertaining; they allow healthcare providers to do personal activities that may divert their attention from clinical work (Sergeeva et al. 2016).

Additionally, workflow issues may stem from a lack of standardization across different healthcare organizations, such as hospitals, specialty clinics, laboratories, pharmacies, and insurance companies (Ramaiah et al. 2012). While health IT at one site may be well-integrated with the local work practices, clinicians' and staff's work may be negatively impacted when there are barriers to effectively communicating with other entities through health IT. Unfortunately, while significant advancements of health information exchange have been made in recent years, the interoperability between different health IT systems remains poor, which could cause delays and disruptions (Ramaiah et al. 2012).

Throughout the literature, there are numerous proposed solutions to preventing and improving workflow issues and mitigating their unintended adverse effects. First, it has been repeatedly shown that developing a thorough understanding of workflow in clinical settings, both before and after health IT implementation, is critical (Campbell et al. 2006; Gephart et al. 2016). This requires health IT designers and implementers to shift their focus from "anticipated" use to actual use (Harrison et al. 2007), and consider multiple perspectives when designing and evaluating systems (Wu et al. 2013). Some researchers have also argued for the importance of considering the sociotechnical integration of health IT with its use context. For instance, Harrison et al. (2007) developed the Interactive Sociotechnical Analysis (ISTA) framework as a means to better understand healthcare organizations as a sociotechnical system and "stop viewing HIT innovations as things, but instead treat them as elements within unfolding processes of sociotechnical interaction" (page 543).

Constantly gathering feedback from frontline clinicians and staff is also crucial to identify unintended workflow issues and making necessary health IT or organizational changes (Campbell et al. 2006). Such feedback should be taken seriously, and timely incorporated into redesign to customize health IT to better fit end users' workflow (Gephart et al. 2016). As part of this feedback, workarounds also need to be transparent. By tracking workarounds and making them more visible, we can determine if there is solid rationale justifying their use, and if actions should be taken to formalize them as part of organization processes (Cresswell et al. 2017) or to mitigate their risks (Cresswell et al. 2017). The design of IT systems is not stagnant and thus, we must iteratively make design revisions as we discover more about clinical workflow and how it is affected by the use of health IT (Campbell et al. 2006).

4.4   Future Work

Designing a health IT system that is perfectly aligned with clinical workflow is very challenging. This is particularly true for *unanticipated unintended* workflow disruptions which, by definition, cannot be easily anticipated by software designers and implementers. That said, developing a thorough understanding of the clinical work and clinical workflow in the setting where the system will be deployed is possible, and can help to mitigate undesirable effects (Harrison et al. 2007). Then, post-implementation, we need close collaboration between system designers, developers, implementers, clinician champions, and all other end users to monitor adoption and appropriation, and make necessary changes to the system or use additional training to improve workflow and ease secondary consequences. Systems must also be flexible enough to be quickly adapted, capable of incorporating feedback and suggestions. That is, all health IT systems must be treated as a constant "work in progress" in order to maximize their benefits while minimizing potential harm to clinicians, staff, and patients.

Further, it should be acknowledged that the radical workflow change as a result of health IT adoption is inevitable. In the last few years alone, the use of new technologies such as telehealth has increased exponentially. New, IT-enabled processes necessitate new care models and new workflow patterns. However, as demonstrated in the literature, many workflow disruptions associated with health IT implementation could have been avoided; and some of the adverse effects are due to the lack of communication with clinicians and staff on change management and on setting up the right expectations. Thus, we need to develop ways to ease end users' negative emotions, reduce their cognitive load, alleviate concerns about power and role changes, and ensure they do not become over-reliant on technology. Additionally, we need to pay particular attention to unsafe workarounds and their potential detrimental effects on patient safety and privacy and confidentiality.

Addressing these challenges demands a concerted effort to streamline data entry processes, enhance interoperability, and leverage technology to minimize duplicated work, optimizing the overall efficiency and integrity of healthcare workflows. This chapter represents a step toward understanding and unpacking the relationship between what we have termed as primary and secondary unintended consequences. However, in studying unintended consequences of health IT related to workflow, we have to take a holistic approach that addresses systems, users, managerial issues, and the context; and consider the secondary or indirect effects resulting from primary workflow changes. We hope this chapter sparks more research on the different categories of unintended consequences, as well as the causal and perhaps even cyclical connections between them.

While there are many benefits to health IT, there are also challenges that need to be addressed. As the health IT landscape continually evolves, understanding and planning for the integration and impact of new technologies are critical. It is important to note that while this chapter specifically focuses on unintended adverse consequences and their cascading effects in the context of workflow, technologies in healthcare can have far-reaching impacts. Although outside of the scope of this work, it is necessary to more broadly investigate unintended consequences outside of workflow (e.g., Federspiel et al., 2023) by taking a systems approach.

References

Addab S, Hamdy R, Le May S, Thorstad K, Tsimicalis A. The use of virtual reality during medical procedures in a pediatric orthopedic setting: A mixed-methods pilot feasibility study. Paediatr Neonatal Pain. 2022;6:1–15. https://doi.org/10.1002/pne2.12078.

Alipour J, Hayavi-Haghighi MH. Opportunities and challenges of telehealth in disease management during COVID-19 pandemic: a scoping review. Appl Clin Inform. 2021;12:864–76. https://doi.org/10.1055/s-0041-1735181.

Alowais SA, Alghamdi SS, Alsuhebany N, Alqahtani T, Alshaya AI, Almohareb SN, Aldairem A, Alrashed M, Bin Saleh K, Badreldin HA, Al Yami MS, Al Harbi S, Albekairy AM. Revolutionizing healthcare: the role of artificial intelligence in clinical practice. BMC Med Educ. 2023;23:1–15. https://doi.org/10.1186/s12909-023-04698-z.

Anderson JTL, Bouchacourt LM, Sussman KL, Bright LF, Wilcox GB. Telehealth adoption during the COVID-19 pandemic: A social media textual and network analysis. Digit Heal. 2022;8. https://doi.org/10.1177/20552076221090041

Ash J, Berg M, Coiera E. Some unintended consequences of information technology in health care: the nature of patient care information system-related errors. JAMIA. 2004;11:104–12. https://doi.org/10.1197/jamia.M1471.Medical.

Ash JS, Sittig DF, Campbell E, Guappone K, Dykstra RH. An unintended consequence of CPOE implementation: shifts in power, control, and autonomy. AMIA Annu Symp Proc. 2006;2006:11–5. 86321[pii]

Austin E, Lee JR, Amtmann D, Bloch R, Lawrence SO, McCall D, Munson S, Lavallee DC. Use of patient-generated health data across healthcare settings: Implications for health systems. JAMIA Open. 2021;3:70–6. https://doi.org/10.1093/JAMIAOPEN/OOZ065.

Baniasadi T, Ayyoubzadeh SM, Mohammadzadeh N. Challenges and practical considerations in applying virtual reality in medical education and treatment. Oman Med J. 2020;35:1–10. https://doi.org/10.5001/omj.2020.43.

Blijleven V, Koelemeijer K, Jaspers M. Exploring Workarounds Related to Electronic Health Record System Usage: A Study Protocol. JMIR Res Protoc. 2017;6: e72. https://doi.org/10.2196/resprot.6766.

Bloomrosen M, Starren J, Lorenzi NM, Ash JS, Patel VL, Shortliffe EH. Anticipating and addressing the unintended consequences of health IT and policy: A report from the AMIA 2009 Health Policy Meeting. J Am Med Informatics Assoc. 2011;18:82–90. https://doi.org/10.1136/jamia.2010.007567.

Boonstra A, Jonker TL, van Offenbeek MAG, Vos JFJ. Persisting workarounds in Electronic Health Record System use: types, risks and benefits. BMC Med Inform Decis Mak. 2021;21:1–14. https://doi.org/10.1186/s12911-021-01548-0.

Campbell EM, Sittig DF, Ash JS, Guappone KP, Dykstra RH. Types of unintended consequences related to computerized provider order entry. J Am Med Informatics Assoc. 2006;13:547–56. https://doi.org/10.1197/jamia.M2042.Introduction.

Chao CA. The impact of electronic health records on collaborative work routines: A narrative network analysis. Int J Med Inform. 2016;94:100–11. https://doi.org/10.1016/j.ijmedinf.2016.06.019.

Chen Y, Xu H. Privacy management in dynamic groups: understanding information privacy in medical practices. CSCW. 2013;2013:541–52.

Cifuentes M, Davis M, Fernald D, Gunn R, Dickinson P, Cohen DJ. Electronic health record challenges, workarounds, and solutions observed in practices integrating behavioral health and primary care. J Am Board Fam Med. 2015;28:S63–72. https://doi.org/10.3122/jabfm.2015.S1.150133.

Coiera E. Technology, cognition and error. BMJ Qual Saf. 2015;24:417–22. https://doi.org/10.1136/bmjqs-2014-003484.

Cresswell KM, Mozaffar H, Lee L, Williams R, Sheikh A. Workarounds to hospital electronic prescribing systems: a qualitative study in English hospitals. BMJ Qual Saf. 2017;26:542–51. https://doi.org/10.1136/bmjqs-2015-005149.

Eikey EV, Murphy AR, Reddy MC, Xu H. Designing for privacy management in hospitals: Understanding the gap between user activities and IT staff's understandings. Int J Med Inform. 2015;84:1065–75. https://doi.org/10.1016/j.ijmedinf.2015.09.006.

Food and Drug Administration. Augmented Reality and Virtual Reality Medical Devices: Questions to Consider | FDA. 2023. https://www.fda.gov/medical-devices/digital-health-center-exc ellence/augmented-reality-and-virtual-reality-medical-devices-questions-consider

Fulmer T, Reuben DB, Auerbach J, Fick DM, Galambos C, Johnson KS. Actualizing better health and health care for older adults. Health Aff. 2021;40:219–25. https://doi.org/10.1377/hlthaff. 2020.01470.

Gephart S, Carrington JM, Finley B. A systematic review of nurses' experiences with unintended consequences when using the electronic health record. Nurs Adm Q. 2015;39:345–56. https:// doi.org/10.1097/NAQ.0000000000000119.

Gephart SM, Bristol AA, Dye JL, Finley BA, Carrington JM. Validity and reliability of a new measure of nursing experience with unintended consequences of electronic health records. 2016.

Goldstein M, Hoffman B, Coleman W, Tu S, Shankar R, O'Connor M, Martins S, Advani A, Musen A. Patient safety in guideline-based decision support for hypertension management: ATHENA DSS. JAMIA. 2002;9:11–6. https://doi.org/10.1197/jamia.M1218.Introduction.

Graham AK, Lattie EG, Powell BJ, Lyon AR, Smith JD, Schueller SM, Stadnick A, Brown CH, Mohr DC. American psychologist. 2020.

Haque SN, DeStefano S, Banger A, Rutledge R, Romaire M. Factors influencing telehealth implementation and use in frontier critical access hospitals: Qualitative study. JMIR Form Res. 2021;5: e24118. https://doi.org/10.2196/24118.

Harrington L, Kennerly D, Johnson C. Safety issues related to the electronic medical record (EMR): Synthesis of the literature from the last decade, 2000–2009. J Healthc Manag. 2011;56:31–43.

Harrison MI, Ross K, Shirly B-L. Unintended consequences of information technologies in health care—an interactive sociotechnical analysis. J Am Med Informatics Assoc. 2007;14:542–9. https://doi.org/10.1197/jamia.M2384.Introduction.

Hooff B Van den, Hafkamp L. 2017. Dealing with Dissonance: Misfits between an EHR System and Medical Work Practices. ICIS 2017 Proc 0–17. 2017.

Horsky J, Gutnik L, Patel VL. Technology for Emergency Care: Cognitive and Workflow Considerations. AMIA Annu Symp Proc. 2006;2006:344–48. 86492 [pii]

Health Information Technology: What is Workflow? In: US Dep. Heal. Hum. Serv. Agency Healthc. Res. Qual. 2017. https://healthit.ahrq.gov/health-it-tools-and-resources/evaluation-res ources/workflow-assessment-health-it-toolkit/workflow. Accessed 24 Jan 2018

Jeffery Reeves J, Ayers JW, Longhurst CA. Telehealth in the COVID-19 era: A balancing act to avoid harm. J Med Internet Res. 2021;23: e24785. https://doi.org/10.2196/24785.

Jonasdottir SK, Thordardottir I, Jonsdottir T. Health professionals' perspective towards challenges and opportunities of telehealth service provision: A scoping review. Int J Med Inform. 2022;167: 104862. https://doi.org/10.1016/j.ijmedinf.2022.104862.

Kashiwagi DT, Sexton MD, Souchet Graves CE, Johnson JM, Callies BI, Yu RC, Thompson JM. All CLEAR? Preparing for IT Downtime. Am J Med Qual. 2017;32:547–51. https://doi.org/10. 1177/1062860616667546.

Kemp MT, Liesman DR, Williams AM, Brown CS, Iancu AM, Wakam GK, Biesterveld BE, Alam HB. Surgery provider perceptions on telehealth visits during the COVID-19 pandemic: room for improvement. J Surg Res. 2021;260:300–6. https://doi.org/10.1016/j.jss.2020.11.034.

Khoshrounejad F, Hamednia M, Mehrjerd A, Pichaghsaz S, Jamalirad H, Sargolzaei M, Hoseini B, Aalaei S. Telehealth-based services during the COVID-19 pandemic: a systematic review of features and challenges. Front Public Heal. 2021;9:1–14. https://doi.org/10.3389/fpubh.2021. 711762.

Kim MO, Coiera E, Magrabi F. Problems with health information technology and their effects on care delivery and patient outcomes: A systematic review. J Am Med Informatics Assoc. 2017;24:246–60. https://doi.org/10.1093/jamia/ocw154.

Kuziemsky CE, Randell R, Borycki EM. Understanding unintended consequences and health information technology: contribution from the IMIA organizational and social issues working group. IMIA Yearb. 2016;25:53–60. https://doi.org/10.15265/IY-2016-027.

Larsen E, Fong A, Wernz C, Ratwani RM. Implications of electronic health record downtime: An analysis of patient safety event reports. J Am Med Informatics Assoc. 2018;25:187–91. https://doi.org/10.1093/jamia/ocx057.

Lawrence K, Singh N, Jonassen Z, Groom LL, Arias VA, Mandal S, Schoenthaler A, Mann D, Nov O, Dove G. Operational implementation of remote patient monitoring within a large ambulatory health system: multimethod qualitative case study. JMIR Hum Factors. 2023;10: e45166. https://doi.org/10.2196/45166.

Laxmisan A, Hakimzada F, Sayan OR, Green RA, Zhang J, Patel VL. The multitasking clinician: Decision-making and cognitive demand during and after team handoffs in emergency care. Int J Med Inform. 2007;76:801–11. https://doi.org/10.1016/j.ijmedinf.2006.09.019.

León MA, Pannunzio V, Kleinsmann M. The impact of perioperative remote patient monitoring on clinical staff workflows: scoping review. JMIR Hum Factors. 2022;9: e37204. https://doi.org/10.2196/37204.

Marcilly R, Ammenwerth E, Vasseur F, Roehrer E, Beuscart-Zephir MC. Usability flaws of medication-related alerting functions: A systematic qualitative review. J Biomed Inf. 2015;55:260–71. https://doi.org/10.1016/j.jbi.2015.03.006.

Maslove DM, Rizk N, Lowe HJ. Computerized physician order entry in the critical care environment: A review of current literature. J Intensive Care Med. 2011;26:165–71. https://doi.org/10.1177/0885066610387984.

Menachemi N, Collum TH. Benefits and drawbacks of electronic health record systems. Risk Manag Healthc Policy. 2011;4:47–55. https://doi.org/10.2147/RMHP.S12985.

Menon S, Murphy DR, Singh H, Meyer AND, Sittig DF. Workarounds and test results follow-up in electronic health record-based primary care. Appl Clin Inform. 2016;7:543–59. https://doi.org/10.4338/ACI-2015-10-RA-0135.

Morimoto T, Kobayashi T, Hirata H, Otani K, Sugimoto M, Tsukamoto M, Yoshihara T, Ueno M, Mawatari M. XR (extended reality: virtual reality, augmented reality, mixed reality) technology in spine medicine: status Quo and Quo Vadis. J Clin Med. 2022;11:470. https://doi.org/10.3390/jcm11020470.

Moy AJ, Hobensack M, Marshall K, Vawdrey DK, Kim EY, Cato KD, Rossetti SC. Understanding the perceived role of electronic health records and workflow fragmentation on clinician documentation burden in emergency departments. J Am Med Informatics Assoc. 2023;30:797–808. https://doi.org/10.1093/jamia/ocad038.

Murphy AR, Reddy MC. Privacy practices in collaborative environments : a study of emergency department staff. Proc 17th ACM Conf Comput Support Coop Work Soc Comput. 2014: 269–282. https://doi.org/10.1145/2531602.2531643

Nanji KC, Rothschild JM, Boehne JJ, Keohane CA, Ash JS, Poon EG. Unrealized potential and residual consequences of electronic prescribing on pharmacy workflow in the outpatient pharmacy. J Am Med Informatics Assoc. 2014;21:481–6. https://doi.org/10.1136/amiajnl-2013-001839.

Niazkhani Z, Pirnejad H, Berg M, Aarts J. The impact of computerized provider order entry systems on inpatient clinical workflow: A literature review. J Am Med Informatics Assoc. 2009;16:539–49. https://doi.org/10.1197/jamia.M2419.

Paper V, Ash JS, Berg M, Coiera E, Ash JS, Berg M, Coiera E. Some unintended consequences of information technology in health care: the nature of patient care information system-related errors. J Am Med Informatics Assoc. 2004;11:104–12. https://doi.org/10.1197/jamia.M1471. Medical.

Pirnejad H, Bal R, Shahsavar N. The nature of unintended effects of Health Information Systems concerning patient safety: A systematic review with thematic synthesis. Stud Health Technol Inform. 2010;160:719–23. https://doi.org/10.3233/978-1-60750-588-4-719.

Powell KR, Alexander GL. Consequences of rapid telehealth expansion in nursing homes: promise and pitfalls. Appl Clin Inform. 2021;12:933–43. https://doi.org/10.1055/s-0041-1735974.

Quinn TP, Senadeera M, Jacobs S, Coghlan S, Le V. Trust and medical AI: the challenges we face and the expertise needed to overcome them. J Am Med Informatics Assoc. 2021;28:890–4. https://doi.org/10.1093/jamia/ocaa268.

Ramaiah M, Subrahmanian E, Sriram RD, Lide BB. Workflow and electronic health records in small medical practices. Perspect Health Inf Manag. 2012;9:1d.

Salahuddin L, Abidin WZ, Ismail Z. A systematic literature review on safe health information technology use. J Teknol. 2016;78:1–7. https://doi.org/10.11113/jt.v78.8225.

Schiff GD, Hickman TTT, Volk LA, Bates DW, Wright A. Computerised prescribing for safer medication ordering: Still a work in progress. BMJ Qual Saf. 2016;25:315–9. https://doi.org/10.1136/bmjqs-2015-004677.

Schriger SH, Klein MR, Last BS, Fernandez-Marcote S, Dallard N, Jones B, Beidas RS. Community mental health clinicians' perspectives on telehealth during the COVID-19 pandemic: mixed methods study. JMIR Pediatr Parent. 2022;5:1–15. https://doi.org/10.2196/29250.

Ser G, Robertson A, Sheikh A. A qualitative exploration of workarounds related to the implementation of national electronic health records in early adopter mental health hospitals. PLoS ONE. 2014;9: e77669. https://doi.org/10.1371/journal.pone.0077669.

Sergeeva A, Aij K, Van Den Hooff B, Huysman M. Mobile devices in the operating room: Intended and unintended consequences for nurses' work. Health Informatics J. 2016;22:1101–10. https://doi.org/10.1177/1460458215598637.

Shaver J. The state of tele health before and after the COVID - 19 Pandemic. 2022;49:517–530.

Sheehan B, Bakken S. Approaches to workflow analysis in healthcare settings. NI 2012 11th Int Congr Nurs Informatics, June 23–27, 2012, Montr Canada Int Congr Nurs Informatics (11th 2012 Montréal, Québec) author 2012:371

Shepard A. Disaster recovery and the electronic health record. Nurs Adm Q. 2017;41:187–9. https://doi.org/10.1097/NAQ.0000000000000213.

Sittig DR, Kaalaas-Sittg KM, J aSH J,. Emotional aspects of computer-based provider order entry : a qualitative study. J Am Med Informatics Assoc. 2005;12:561–8. https://doi.org/10.1197/jamia.M1711.Over.

Steinkamp J, Kantrowitz JJ, Airan-Javia S. Prevalence and sources of duplicate information in the electronic medical record. JAMA Netw Open. 2022;5:E2233348. https://doi.org/10.1001/jamanetworkopen.2022.33348.

Thomas EE, Taylor ML, Banbury A, Snoswell CL, Haydon HM, Gallegos Rejas VM, Smith AC, Caffery LJ. Factors influencing the effectiveness of remote patient monitoring interventions: A realist review. BMJ Open. 2021;11:1–9. https://doi.org/10.1136/bmjopen-2021-051844.

Tingvold L, Moholt JM, Førland O, Jacobsen FF, Tranevåg O. Intended, unintended, unanticipated? Consequences of social distancing measures for nursing home residents during the covid-19 pandemic. Glob Qual Nurs Res. 2023;10:23333936231176204. https://doi.org/10.1177/23333936231176204.

Torous J, Bucci S, Bell IH, Kessing LV, Faurholt-Jepsen M, Whelan P, Carvalho AF, Keshavan M, Linardon J, Firth J. The growing field of digital psychiatry: current evidence and the future of apps, social media, chatbots, and virtual reality. World Psychiatry. 2021;20:318–35. https://doi.org/10.1002/wps.20883.

Triberti S, Durosini I, Pravettoni G. A "third wheel" effect in health decision making involving artificial entities: a psychological perspective. Front: Public Heal; 2020. p. 8.

Tucker AL, Zheng S, Gardner JW, Bohn RE. When do workarounds help or hurt patient outcomes? The moderating role of operational failures. J Oper Manag. 2019.

Vanderhook S, Abraham J. Unintended consequences of EHR systems: a narrative review. Proc Int Symp Hum Factors Ergon Heal Care. 2017;6:218–25. https://doi.org/10.1177/232785791706 1048.

Vishwanath A, Singh SR, Winkelstein P. The impact of electronic medical record systems on outpatient workflows: a longitudinal evaluation of its workflow effects. Int J Med Inform. 2010;79:778–91. https://doi.org/10.1016/j.ijmedinf.2010.09.006.

Voshall B, Piscotty R, Lawrence J, Targosz M. Barcode medication administration work-arounds. JONA J Nurs Adm. 2013;43:530–5. https://doi.org/10.1097/NNA.0b013e3182a3e8ad.

Wu RC, Lo V, Morra D, Wong BM, Sargeant R, Locke K, Cavalcanti R, Quan SD, Rossos P, Tran K, Cheung M. The intended and unintended consequences of communication systems on general internal medicine inpatient care delivery: A prospective observational case study of five teaching hospitals. J Am Med Informatics Assoc. 2013;20:766–77. https://doi.org/10.1136/ami ajnl-2012-001160.

Wu DTY, Xu C, Kim A, Bindhu S, Mah KE, Eckman MH. A scoping review of health information technology in clinician burnout. Appl Clin Inform. 2021;12:597–620. https://doi.org/10.1055/s-0041-1731399.

Ye J. The impact of electronic health record-integrated patient-generated health data on clinician burnout. J Am Med Informatics Assoc. 2021;28:1051–6. https://doi.org/10.1093/jamia/ocab017.

Yen P-Y, Kelley M, Lopetegui M, Rosado AL, Migliore EM, Chipps EM, Buck J. Understanding and visualizing multitasking and task switching activities: a time motion study to capture nursing workflow. AMIA Annu Symp Proceedings AMIA Symp. 2016;2016:1264–73.

Younis HA, Eisa TAE, Nasser M, Sahib TM, Noor AA, Alyasiri OM, Salisu S, Hayder IM, Younis HAK. A systematic review and meta-analysis of artificial intelligence tools in medicine and healthcare: applications, considerations, limitations. Motivation and Challenges Diagnostics. 2024;14:109. https://doi.org/10.3390/diagnostics14010109.

Zadeh PE, Tremblay MC. A review of the literature and proposed classification on e-prescribing: Functions, assimilation stages, benefits, concerns, and risks. Res Soc Adm Pharm. 2016;12:1–19. https://doi.org/10.1016/j.sapharm.2015.03.001.

Zheng K, Haftel HM, Hirschl RB, O'Reilly M, Hanauer DA. Quantifying the impact of health IT implementations on clinical workflow: A new methodological perspective. J Am Med Informatics Assoc. 2010a;17:454–61. https://doi.org/10.1136/jamia.2010.004440.

Zheng K, Haftel HM, Hirschl RB, O'Reilly M, Hanauer D, a,. Quantifying the impact of health IT implementations on clinical workflow: a new methodological perspective. J Am Med Inform Assoc. 2010b;17:454–61. https://doi.org/10.1136/jamia.2010.004440.

Zheng K, Ratwani RM, Adler-Milstein J. Studying workflow and workarounds in electronic health record-supported work to improve health system performance. Ann Intern Med. 2020;172:S116–22. https://doi.org/10.7326/M19-0871.

Part II
The State of the Art of Workflow Research

Chapter 5
A Review of Clinical Workflow Studies and Methods

Philip Payne, Marcelo Lopetegui, and Sean Yu

Abstract It has been well established that the optimization of workflow can have substantial impact on the feasibility, efficiency, quality, safety, and outcomes of healthcare delivery. The process of studying and understanding workflow in support of such optimization has existed for some time, originally developed in the business and industrial research domains, and has been variably applied within the healthcare domain to date. In this chapter, we introduce the basic nomenclature and methods that encapsulate such workflow studies in the healthcare setting and provide a series of examples that demonstrate how such methods can be applied to solving critical problems. We conclude by reviewing open and active areas of inquiries concerning the current and future use of such workflow analysis methodologies.

Keywords Workflow · Workflow analysis · Time motion studies · Process modelling

5.1 Introduction

Workflow is an integral part of healthcare delivery. In this context, <u>workflow</u> can be formally defined as: *"the sequence of steps involved in moving from the beginning to the end of a working process[1]."* Building upon this definition, we can also define a working <u>process</u> as: *"a series of actions or operations conducing to an end.[1]".*

P. Payne (✉)
Institute for Informatics, Data Science, and Biostatistics, Washington University in St. Louis, St. Louis, MO, USA
e-mail: prpayne@wustl.edu

M. Lopetegui
HICAPPS SpA, La Reina, Santiago, Chile
e-mail: marcelo@hicapps.com

S. Yu
Regeneron Pharmaceuticals Inc, Tarrytown, NY, USA
e-mail: sean.yu@regeneron.com

© The Author(s), under exclusive license to Springer Nature Switzerland AG 2025
K. Zheng et al. (eds.), *Reengineering Clinical Workflow in the Digital and AI Era*,
Cognitive Informatics in Biomedicine and Healthcare,
https://doi.org/10.1007/978-3-031-82971-0_5

The ability to observe, instrument, and understand workflow provides critical information for a variety of applications, including but not limited to:

- Enhancing the quality, safety, and outcomes of care delivery
- Identifying opportunities to overcome barriers to technology adoption and adaptation in complex healthcare settings
- Improving the efficiency and timeliness of clinical and translational research

The process of modelling and analyzing workflow is often executed through Time Motion Studies (TMS). TMS, alternatively referred to as "time-motion studies" or "time and motion studies", are defined in the National Library of Medicine Medical Subject Heading system (MeSH) as *"the observation and analysis of movements in a task with emphasis on the amount of time required to perform the task."* TMS methodologies originated as a business efficiency technique through the collective contributions of Frederick Taylor (Time Studies) (Taylor 1914) and Frank and Lillian Gilbreth (Motion Studies) (Baumgart et al. 2009).

The widespread use of TMS in the healthcare setting is a relatively recent development, and has proven to provide a valuable means for collecting quantitative workflow data in a broad spectrum of settings, ranging from evaluating the effectiveness of system implementations (Amusan et al. 2008) and assessment of costs (Schiller et al. 2008), to describing general workflow (Kloss et al. 2010) and utilization of time by clinicians (Kim et al. 2011). In clinical workflow studies, TMS gather quantitative workflow assessments specifically through continuous direct observation, which has been shown to be more accurate than work-sampling (Wirth et al. 1977) and self-reporting (Gordon et al. 2008; Ampt et al. 2007), and is increasingly being accepted as the "gold standard" for measuring and quantifying clinical workflow (Burke et al. 2000; Bratt et al. 1999). The general "design pattern" for the conduct of TMS is illustrated in Fig. 5.1.

5.2 Key Concepts and Definitions Surrounding Time Motion Study Methodologies

As a tool for obtaining quantitative assessments of clinical workflow, TMS have been adapted and used in the healthcare setting since the early twentieth century. Without a unifying standard, however, the definition and scope of TMS have shifted significantly. Although we agree with the definition provided by the Agency for Healthcare Research and Quality, *"an observation method used to determine the timing and duration of tasks or procedures"*, a recent review concluded that the term "TMS" had been used to describe *"a broad spectrum of dissimilar methods whose only common factor is the capture and/or analysis of the duration of one or more events"* (Lopetegui et al. 2014). In the literature, there are many studies reported as TMS but they instead used methods such as self-reports and analysis of automatically generated timestamps. Moreover, among the studies that would be

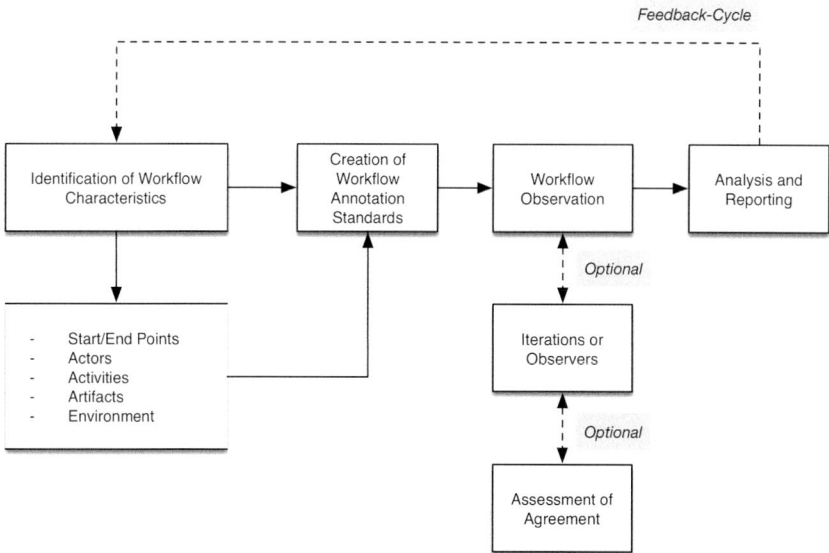

Fig. 5.1 Overview of prototypical workflow study design pattern. In this pattern, the process begins with the identification of key characteristics that serve to define a workflow of interest. Such characteristics are then used to create workflow annotation (or codification) standards that enable the collection of constituent data during various observation types. Subsequently, workflow observations are conducted, and the data generated therein are codified per the preceding annotation standards. Such observations usually include temporal data concerning instances and durations of workflow related activities. In some studies, observations are iterative, or involve multiple observers, necessitating the assessment of inter-observer or inter-observation agreement. Finally, the results of the preceding steps are analyzed and reported on, often employing descriptive statistics, and key findings are "fed back" to inform future workflow studies or optimization efforts

considered TMS, there is significant variability in the implementation and reporting of their findings, making aggregation of results difficult. Therefore, there is a need for researchers to properly categorize and rigorously define their methodologies. In a recent review (Lopetegui et al. 2014), we depicted four major classes of methods used in the literature currently classified as TMS, namely:

(1) Methods that produce time-motion data by external observers (**external observation**)
(2) Methods that produce time-motion data by the participants being studied (**self-observation**)
(3) Methods that produce time-motion data automatically by computerized systems (**automated observation**)
(4) Methods that lead to the creation of models and frameworks that can be used to support and/or enable the interpretation of data and findings generated during the course of TMS (**model formulation**)

Below, we provide a description of each of these methods and exemplary studies that have utilize them.

5.3   External Observation

In this type of studies, dedicated external observers perform the task of collecting time-motion data. Data collection can be done asynchronously by having the observer analyze video recordings of the study participant's behavior in the work environment, also called "time-action analysis" (Minekus et al. 2013; Oldenrijk et al. 2008). More often, it is conducted by having the observer directly shadow and observe the participant in real time.

Studies involving external observers use mainly two data collection methods: continuous observation and work sampling. In continuous observation, the external observer maintains the attention on the study participant and continuously records the time taken to perform one or multiple tasks, implying that the action of recording is triggered by an action performed by the participant. It is a useful approach to collect data for non-centralized tasks, sensible for short tasks, and provides granular and detailed field data. However, this method is resource consuming, and there is opportunity for biases as participants may feel disturbed. Sometimes, participants may also demonstrate improved performance when being observed: a phenomenon known as the Hawthorne effect.[1]

Unlike continuous observation, which measures the elapsed time for a task, work sampling identifies the task being performed at a given instant (Hakes and Whittington 2011), repeating the measure at predefined fixed or random intervals during the observation. It is premised on the repetitive nature of work, and assumes the probabilistic generalization of the sampling findings to describe how workers spend their time overall. Compared to continuous observation, a major benefit of work sampling is that the observer can work with multiple study participants during a single observation period. Further, work sampling has been reported as an efficient approach for studies designed to classify work activities into fewer categories. With more categories describing less frequent tasks, the required number of observations may increase substantially (Burke et al. 2000), thus losing the advantage afforded by this method. Strictly speaking, work sampling estimates the proportion of time spent on an activity based on observations conducted at random time points (Barnett 2008).

The temporality of the sampling methodology has been debated in the literature, concluding that systematic work sampling often results in flawed and biased estimates; and random work sampling is a better approach (Oddone and Simel 1994)

---

[1] This was first reported in Chicago during the 1920s, when after studying methods for increasing productivity it was found that regardless of the change introduced in the working environment, the result was always an increase in productivity. It is now explained as "an increase in worker productivity produced by the psychological stimulus of being singled out and made to feel important" (Franke and Kaul 1978).

especially when assessing tasks that are performed periodically. However, one of the pioneering researchers of TMS argues that the reduction in biases provided by randomization is overweighed by the complexities in scheduling the observations, advocating in favor of fixed periodic intervals (Finkler et al. 1993). We observed this issue in our recent review: all work sampling studies involving external observers used a systematic fixed time interval: e.g., 1 min (Murden and Pintz 2003), 5 min (Deshpande et al. 2012), and so forth. A study used a much higher frequency of sampling at every 15 s, which the authors referred to as "Davis observation code" (Yawn et al. 2003). Under optimal circumstances, work sampling has been proposed as a useful and efficient methodology for analyzing the distribution of work activities in relation to the types of activities they perform (Pelletier and Duffield 2003). This method, however, falls short for questions related to task durations, occurrences, or workflow studies. A highly cited paper concludes that work sampling may not provide an acceptably precise approximation of the results that could be obtained by continuous observation time motion studies (Burke et al. 2000).

5.4   Self-report

In this group of studies, time-related data are generated by study participants themselves. Although self-report can be a low-cost means for measuring work activities, perceptual differences among the participants who self-report their data can lead to discrepancies in how activities are categorized (Keohane et al. 2008). Also, participants may either lie about what they are doing, or change normal routine in order to generate data that they believe to be more favorable (Burke et al. 2000). This shortcoming has been demonstrated outside TMS when comparing self-reported data and observational data in studies of dentists providing preventive services: self-reported frequencies consistently exceeded observed frequencies (Demko et al. 2008).

Self-reports are also considered unreliable because they tend to over-estimate clinicians' contact time with patients and under-estimate their non-productive time, compared to work sampling using an external observer (Bratt et al. 1999). Anecdotally, one study comparing the number of duty-hour violations among residents found no difference between self-reports and computer-recorded timestamps (Todd et al. 2011); however instead of reporting the agreement between the two sources of data, they compared if a threshold of work hours was exceeded, but not the specific durations. This reinforces the need to be aware of the inherent human biases in terms of the design and selection of outcomes when using self-reports as the main source of research data.

Data collection methods used by studies in this group can be first classified as synchronous or asynchronous. Commonly used approaches on the asynchronous side of the spectrum include interviews, focus groups, and surveys. These methods directly solicit information from study participants regarding the time it takes them to perform different tasks and/or different steps of a process. Asynchronous self-report methods are considered limited due to their reliance on participants' subjective account of their workflow and working conditions (Hauschild et al. 2011). It has been widely acknowledged that clinicians are poor estimators of measures commonly found in TMS, such as task durations. For example, when comparing physician recall of event durations in the operating room, self-reported survey responses over-estimated the durations by 30 min on average, from a few minutes up to two hours, when compared to durations extracted from the surgery log (McCall et al. 2006).

Commonly used approaches on the synchronous side of the spectrum are active tracking and self-reported work sampling. In active tracking, study participants are asked to log time motion data based on their work activities, either immediately after completing a task, or at a later time (e.g., by the end of the workday). On the other hand, self-reported work sampling involves repeated recording of work activities at pre-determined or random time points by study participants. As previously discussed, random work sampling is more commonly used (Yee et al. 2012), which is often facilitated by some types of electronic devices that remind participants at random intervals to record data. In a study that compared self-reported work sampling and traditional/external work sampling for measuring nursing tasks (Ampt et al. 2007), the self-reported method was found to be an unreliable means for obtaining an accurate reflection of the work tasks conducted by ward-based nurses. Also, nurses preferred the presence of an external observer, as recording activities while conducting clinical duties can be burdensome (Keohane et al. 2008). Despite the limitation, self-reported work sampling is easier to conduct and is more scalable with relatively low cost. Indeed, one of the largest TMS to date used the self-report work sampling method to study nursing work across 36 hospitals (Hendrich et al. 2008).

5.5 Automated Observation

In this group of studies, timestamps and durations of tasks are captured automatically by sensors or computerized systems. Usually, the physical movement of study participants, or their interaction with clinical IT systems, trigger the recording of time-motion data, providing a rich "motion" dimension and precise "time" measurements. It is important to note that studies of this category do not refer to those that use computerized tools for external observers (e.g., a tablet PC with TMS research data collection software). Instead, in these studies, time-motion data are being recorded automatically without the presence of an external observer, and without any active involvement of study participants.

Automated time-motion data streams may come from a broad range of sources, including indoor or global positioning systems, accelerometers, electrodes, radio frequency identification (RFID), and clinical IT systems. From study participants' perspective, this method provides a passive and non-intrusive means for capturing time-motion data while they perform their usual clinical tasks. Examples include

location-tracking devices (e.g., RFID tags) that record events when the participant approaches sensors, time-stamped logs of interaction events within an electronic health record (EHR) system, and sensor movements on a laparoscopic surgery
training module.

With the availability of such continuous event logs, researchers have better tools
to determine the structure underlying the sequence of events, or a flowchart-like
process model. Markov Models or Hidden Markov Models have been commonly
used to model workflows in the healthcare setting including trauma resuscitations
(Mache et al. 2008) or patient trajectories (Mache et al. 2010); and process mining
techniques have also been employed to discover process models from event logs,
check conformance/deviation of particular event logs, and suggest changes to the
process to enhance workflow (Mache et al. 2009).

Although timestamps recorded by motion sensors have been demonstrated as a
reliable source of data (Marjamaa et al. 2006), time-stamped logs from software
usage need to be interpreted carefully. If the variable of interest is the duration
of interactions with the software system (e.g., charting time), it may constitute an
accurate measure. However, if the variable of interest would need to be deduced from
the computer-recorded timestamp as a proxy (e.g., how long it takes for a patient to
transfer to another unit), it might become problematic. For example, a TMS conducted
in an emergency department compared continuous observation results to timestamps
extracted from the EHR, concluding that on average the EHR-based events were
recorded 2 min before they actually took place (median, interquartile range 31 min
before to 3 min minutes) (Gordon et al. 2008).

5.6 Model Formulation

In this final class of studies, the primary emphasis is not on conducting empirical
investigation using TMS, but rather the creation of conceptual frameworks or equivalent constructs that can support and enable the interpretation of the results of TMS.
These include efforts to create models that define the major characteristics that can be
measured or understood through TMS, such as actors, activities, and environmental
features pertinent to a given workflow (Sittig and Singh 2010). Such efforts can also
include studies that focus on the creation of taxonomies and nomenclatures, as well
as quantitative metrics, that serve to assist in the aggregation and interpretation of
multiple, complimentary TMS (Yen et al. 2016; Lopetegui et al. 2013).

5.7 TMS Data Capture Tools

Since the early 2000s, several research teams have worked on building electronic
data capture tools to facilitate the conduct of TMS. Among them, the most relevant
contributions include:

- **Marc Overhage, Lisa Pizziferri, and Yi Zhang.** Considered the pioneer of TMS in studying clinical workflow, Overhage and his colleagues introduced the Palm Pocket Digital Assistant program in 2001 (Overhage et al. 2016). This tool incorporates multi-level classification of clinical activities with which observers could label visible physical activities (e.g., talking on phone) and then group them into conceptual categories (e.g., direct patient care). Pizziferri et al. further adapted Overhage et al.'s categorization schema by adding new tasks and categories, and created a Microsoft Access-based application that could be deployed on touch-screen tablet computers (Pizziferri et al. 2005). They also introduced the concept of "primary task" to accommodate multitasking. Later, Zhang et al. adapted Pizziferri et al.'s tool by including a nursing activities taxonomy, and requiring certain additional attributes to be captured such as location, whom the activity served, position while performing the task (standing/sitting/walking), admission or discharge, and the clinical purpose of the activity (Zhang et al. 2011). They also extended the tool by adding the capability for recording communication multitasking (when a clinician is performing a clinical task while simultaneously communicating with others). Finally, they manually mapped the task list to the Omaha System which is a comprehensive practice and documentation standardized taxonomy designed to describe client care in combined terms [problem + category + target + care description].
- **Philip Asaro.** Asaro developed a Palm-based application for conducting TMS in an emergency department in 2003. His tool also included a categorization schema for tasks, and allowed simultaneous recording of two activities with independent timing. He also published a novel synchronized data capture method in 2004 to study patient flow (Asaro 2004), wherein multiple data collectors observed different providers using a synchronized timestamp allowing reconstruction of tasks/events of ED care for individual patients. Then, in 2008, he used the tool to evaluate the impact of a computerized prescriber order entry (CPOE) system on nursing documentation workflow (Asaro and Boxerman 2008).
- **Johanna Westbrook.** In 2007, Westbrook and her colleagues developed a Pocket PC application which included ten broad work task categories, additional participants involved in the task, and tools/equipment used to perform the task. It also allows external observers to record concurrent tasks independently, and incorporates a novel interruption module to record broken/resumed tasks and the ability to fix input errors. Westbrook et al. also pioneered on assessing inter-observer reliability using the agreement of overall percentage time in tasks. Their method was named WOMBAT (Work observation Method by Activity Timing), and has since been used in several studies (Ballermann et al. 2011; Westbrook et al. 2008, 2007, 2010; Westbrook and Woods 2009).
- **Stephanie Mache.** In 2008, Mache et al. developed and evaluated a Pocket PC-based "computer-based medical work assessment program" (Mache et al. 2008). They generated a list of tasks that physicians commonly perform across different settings, and their application allows for the recording of primary and secondary tasks for multitasking events, as well as interruptions. In addition, they developed a new inter-observer reliability assessment method based on time and naming of

the tasks. By creating and piloting new taxonomies for specific scenarios, this tool has been used repeatedly in German workflow studies regarding surgeons (Mache et al. 2010), junior OB/GYN's (Kloss et al. 2010), junior gastroenterology physicians (Mache et al. 2009), pediatricians (Mache et al. 2010), oncology residents (Mache et al. 2011), anesthesiologists (Hauschild et al. 2011), and emergency physicians (Mache et al. 2011).

- **Philip Payne.** In 2012, Payne et al. introduced the Time Capture Tool (TimeCaT) (Lopetegui et al. 2012): a comprehensive, flexible, and user-centered web application designed to support data capture for TMS. This tool aimed for widespread adoption by a collaborative network of TMS researchers who would be willing to contribute to further development and standardization of formulations regarding multitasking, inter-observer reliability assessment, and taxonomy selection. The end goal of the project was to create standardized TMS methods and thus the ability to produce comparable results that can be readily aggregated to facilitate knowledge discovery. Continued ongoing efforts of this project include the development and validation of an inter-observer reliability scoring algorithm, the creation of an online clinical task ontology, and a quantitative workflow comparison method.

Some of these tools are described in more depth in Chap. 12: Computer Tools for Recording Clinical Workflow Data.

5.8 Seminal Time Motion Studies in Healthcare

Building upon the concepts and definitions presented earlier in this chapter, in the following section, we summarize a set of seminal papers reporting significant TMS-based studies conducted in healthcare. As shown in Table 5.1, each of these papers is described in terms of the driving problem being investigated, the methods used, as well as intended outcomes or optimization objectives.

5.9 Limitations and Future Directions

Nearly a century after the introduction of TMS to the healthcare arena, there is a genuine interest in aggregating results from TMS studies to generate knowledge regarding healthcare workflow, efficiency, patient safety, and quality. There is also a growing interest in using aggregated TMS results to support decision making on the acquisition and implementation of health information technologies (IT). Regrettably, existing attempts to aggregate results conclude that study comparison is very difficult due to the considerable variation in design, conduct, and reporting of such studies (Zheng et al. 2011). Efforts to summarize findings across TMS are further challenged due to the heterogeneity in activity categorizations and a lack of methodological standardization (Tipping et al. 2011).

Table 5.1 A summary of seminal time motion studies in healthcare, including titles, driving problems, methods used, and outcomes or objectives for those studies

Title	Driving problem	Methods used	Intended outcomes or optimization objectives
A new sociotechnical model for studying health information technology in complex adaptive healthcare systems	To identify the factors the influence or otherwise impact the design and deployment of healthcare information technology platforms in the clinical environment	**Model formulation**	Improving quality and safety of patient care activities
Reference: Sittig DF, Singh H. A new sociotechnical model for studying health information technology in complex adaptive healthcare systems. Quality and Safety in Health Care. 2010;19(Suppl 3):i68–74			
Workarounds to barcode medication administration systems: their occurrences, causes, and threats to patient safety	Understanding how physical work-arounds impact patient safety in the context of medication reconciliation	**External observation**	Improving quality and safety of patient care activities
Reference: Koppel R, Wetterneck T, Telles JL, Karsh BT. Workarounds to barcode medication administration systems: their occurrences, causes, and threats to patient safety. Journal of the American Medical Informatics Association. 2008;15(4):408–23			
A 36-hospital time and motion study: how do medical-surgical nurses spend their time?	Identifying the common tasks and activities that surgical nurses engage in during the course of normal workflow, and any impediments to their effective/efficient execution	**Self-observation**	Managing patient throughput and resource utilization in healthcare delivery environments
Reference: Hendrich A, Chow MP, Skierczynski BA, Lu Z. A 36-hospital time and motion study: how do medical-surgical nurses spend their time? The Permanente Journal. 2008;12(3):25			
How hospitalists spend their time: insights on efficiency and safety	Identifying the common tasks and activities that hospitalists engage in during the course of normal workflow, and any impediments to their effective/efficient execution	**External observation, Automated-observation**	Managing patient throughput and resource utilization in healthcare delivery environments

(continued)

Table 5.1 (continued)

Title	Driving problem	Methods used	Intended outcomes or optimization objectives
Reference: O'leary KJ, Liebovitz DM, Baker DW. How hospitalists spend their time: insights on efficiency and safety. Journal of Hospital Medicine. 2006;1(2):88–93			
Electronic health records in specialty care: a time-motion study	Understanding how clinicians interact with EHRs in specialty care settings and the impact of human-factors associated with said workflow on clinical decision making	**External observation**	Understanding and optimizing clinical decision making
Reference: Lo HG, Newmark LP, Yoon C, Volk LA, Carlson VL, Kittler AF, Lippincott M, Wang T, Bates DW. Electronic health records in specialty care: a time-motion study. Journal of the American Medical Informatics Association. 2007;14(5):609–15			
Primary care physician time utilization before and after implementation of an electronic health record: a time-motion study	Identifying barriers to EHR adoption in primary care setting, using paper-based records as a comparator	**External observation**	Understanding and optimizing clinical decision making
Reference: Pizziferri L, Kittler AF, Volk LA, Honour MM, Gupta S, Wang S, Wang T, Lippincott M, Li Q, Bates DW. Primary care physician time utilization before and after implementation of an electronic health record: a time-motion study. Journal of Biomedical Informatics. 2005;38(3):176–88			

First steps towards standardizing TMS include the work of Zheng et al. who, after analyzing a subset of 24 "time and motion studies" specifically assessing health IT implementations, proposed a checklist aiming at standardizing the reporting of such studies' methods and results (Zheng et al. 2011). Also, methodological standardization has been proposed by Patel et al., by introducing a methodological framework for evaluating clinical cognitive activities in complex real-world environments that provides a guiding framework for characterizing the patterns of activities (Kannampallil et al. 2016). Although these efforts are important initial steps toward standardizing TMS, they do not address the persistent lack of common understanding concerning the definition of what is or is not a "time motion study". Ultimately, a crucial step toward standardization and validation of time motion studies in the healthcare domain involves establishing a common understanding of TMS, accompanied by a proper identification of the distinct techniques it encompasses and aspects of the field that remain open and active areas of investigation. This chapter represents an initial attempt.

Based on the current state-of-the-art practice of the design and execution of TMS, we believe that there are a number of future directions for the field that will serve to enhance or extend the scope and impact of the TMS methodologies. These directions include but are not limited to:

- Leveraging **sensor data** to expand the scope/nature of TMS, so that automated observation methods can incorporate higher volumes of "streaming" data collected from a variety of instrumented artifacts in a given environment. Such use of sensor data could include the tracking of activities performed by individual clinicians, utilization of technology-based tools, and the manipulation of physical environments. Leveraging such data will require the development of new TMS methodologies capable of dealing with data sources that exhibit variable volumes, velocities, and variability (i.e., "big data.")
- Creating **continuous learning environments** based on feedback from workflow studies, wherein we need to shorten the timeframe via which findings from TMS are provided back to the individuals being observed in order to support real-time or near-real-time decision making and workflow redesign. This could be made possible through using sensors to enable automated data collection, as well as improving the computational and data analytics capabilities that support/enable automated interpretation, summarization, and visualization of such TMS data (e.g., disintermediating analysis and reporting stage of TMS adhering to the prototypical design pattern shown in Fig. 5.1).
- Finally, if we are successful in leveraging sensor technologies and creating continuous learning environments, we will be able to deliver **workflow-aware information at the point of care** (e.g., contextual, just-in-time information). Such a paradigm shift would fulfill the primary promise of clinical informatics, which is to deliver right information to the right person in the right format. Given the importance of clinical workflow on human cognition and decision making, increasingly fine-grained understanding of such factors, afforded by TMS and novel data and analytics techniques, provides a basis for achieving this goal.

5.10   Conclusions

The original use of the term Time Motion Studies, which combines the work by Taylor's focusing on "time", and Gilbreths' on "motion" (Gilbreth 1914), refers to a method for improving efficiency and establishing employee productivity standards. In TMS, a task is broken into steps, and the sequence of movements or actions performed by study participants to accomplish those steps is observed to detect motion and to measure precise time taken for each movement or action. The extant literature of TMS includes a broad spectrum of distinct methodologies, including surveys, patient chart reviews, work sampling, and continuous observation. A commonality across these studies is the use of data generated via TMS to improve clinical workflow, with the ultimate objective of improving outcomes such as resource utilization, efficiency, safety, and patient health. As we look forward and envision the future of this stream of TMS-based research, our assessment of the current state of practice suggests the following improvement opportunities:

- Enhancing and extending the methods for evaluating processes and outcomes associated with workflow studies;
- Translating the results of workflow studies into data-driven interventions that could be delivered at the point of care and beyond; and
- Improving the adoption and optimal use of technology in complex healthcare environments based on a better understanding of workflow-related inhibiting or enabling factors.

However, to achieve these goals, it requires us to address several important gaps in knowledge and practice, such as:

- Ensuring the adoption and use of TMS methods become more widespread, and demonstrate the benefits in a variety of empirical settings and practitioner communities;
- Creating a sustainable body of scholarly and applied work surrounding both methodological innovations and applied science relevant to TMS; and
- Perhaps most importantly, ensuring that we use consistent language and nomenclature to describe all of these endeavors, such that a robust, applicable body of knowledge and best practices is being created and maintained.

References

Ampt A, Westbrook J, Creswick N, Mallock N. A comparison of self-reported and observational work sampling techniques for measuring time in nursing tasks. J Health Serv Res Policy [Internet]. 2007 Jan [cited 2012 Feb 14];12(1):18–24. http://www.ncbi.nlm.nih.gov/pubmed/17244393

Amusan AA, Tongen S, Speedie SM, Mellin A. A time-motion study to evaluate the impact of EMR and CPOE implementation on physician efficiency. J Healthc Inf Manag [Internet]. 2008 Jan [cited 2011 Sep 27];22(4):31–7. http://www.ncbi.nlm.nih.gov/pubmed/19267017

Asaro P V. Synchronized time-motion study in the emergency department using a handheld computer application. Stud Health Technol Inform [Internet]. 2004 Jan [cited 2012 Mar 2];107(Pt 1):701–5. http://www.ncbi.nlm.nih.gov/pubmed/15360903

Asaro P V, Boxerman SB. Effects of computerized provider order entry and nursing documentation on workflow. Acad Emerg Med [Internet]. 2008 Oct [cited 2011 Sep 16];15(10):908–15. http://www.ncbi.nlm.nih.gov/pubmed/18785946

Ballermann MA, Shaw NT, Mayes DC, Gibney RTN, Westbrook JI. Validation of the Work Observation Method By Activity Timing (WOMBAT) method of conducting time-motion observations in critical care settings: an observational study. BMC Med Inform Decis Mak [Internet]. 2011 Jan [cited 2012 Mar 2];11:32. http://www.pubmedcentral.nih.gov/articlerender.fcgi?artid=3112380&tool=pmcentrez&rendertype=abstract

Barnett G V. A new way to measure nursing: computer timing of nursing time and support of laboring patients. Comput Inform Nurs [Internet]. 2008;26(4):199–206. http://www.ncbi.nlm.nih.gov/pubmed/18600127

Baumgart A, Neuhauser D. Frank and Lillian Gilbreth: scientific management in the operating room. Qual Saf Health Care [Internet]. 2009 Oct [cited 2011 Sep 27];18(5):413–5. http://www.ncbi.nlm.nih.gov/pubmed/19812107

Bratt JH, Foreit J, Chen PL, West C, Janowitz B, de Vargas T. A comparison of four approaches for measuring clinician time use. Health Policy Plan [Internet]. 1999 Dec [cited 2012 Feb 20];14(4):374–81. http://www.ncbi.nlm.nih.gov/pubmed/10787653

Bratt JH, Foreit J, Chen PL, West C, Janowitz B, de Vargas T. A comparison of four approaches for measuring clinician time use. Health Policy Plan [Internet]. 1999 Dec;14(4):374–81. http://www.ncbi.nlm.nih.gov/pubmed/10787653

Burke TA, McKee JR, Wilson HC, Donahue RM, Batenhorst AS, Pathak DS. A comparison of time-and-motion and self-reporting methods of work measurement. J Nurs Adm [Internet]. 2000 Mar [cited 2011 Dec 19];30(3):118–25. http://www.ncbi.nlm.nih.gov/pubmed/10725940

Demko CA, Victoroff KZ, Wotman S. Concordance of chart and billing data with direct observation in dental practice. Community Dent Oral Epidemiol [Internet]. 2008 Oct [cited 2011 Sep 27];36(5):466–74. http://www.ncbi.nlm.nih.gov/pubmed/18924258

Deshpande GA, Soejima K, Ishida Y, Takahashi O, Jacobs JL, Heist BS, et al. A global template for reforming residency without work-hours restrictions: decrease caseloads, increase education. Findings of the Japan Resident Workload Study Group. Med Teach [Internet]. 2012 Jan [cited 2013 May 8];34(3):232–9. http://www.ncbi.nlm.nih.gov/pubmed/22364456

Finkler SA, Knickman JR, Hendrickson G, Lipkin M, Thompson WG. A comparison of work-sampling and time-and-motion techniques for studies in health services research. Health Serv Res [Internet]. 1993 Dec [cited 2012 Jan 31];28(5):577–97. http://www.pubmedcentral.nih.gov/articlerender.fcgi?artid=1069965&tool=pmcentrez&rendertype=abstract

Franke RH, Kaul JD. The Hawthorne experiments: First statistical interpretation. Am Sociol Rev. 1978;43(5):623–43.

Gilbreth FB. Scientific management in the hospital. Mod Hosp. 1914;3:321–4.

Gordon BD, Flottemesch TJ, Asplin BR. Accuracy of staff-initiated emergency department tracking system timestamps in identifying actual event times. Ann Emerg Med [Internet]. 2008 Nov [cited 2011 Sep 27];52(5):504–11. http://www.ncbi.nlm.nih.gov/pubmed/18313799

Hakes B, Whittington J. Assessing the impact of an electronic medical record on nurse documentation time. Comput Inform Nurs [Internet]. [cited 2011 Sep 27];26(4):234–41. http://www.ncbi.nlm.nih.gov/pubmed/18600132

Hauschild I, Vitzthum K, Klapp BF, Groneberg DA, Mache S. Time and motion study of anesthesiologists' workflow in German hospitals. Wien Med Wochenschr [Internet]. 2011 Sep [cited 2011 Dec 15];161(17–18):433–40. http://www.ncbi.nlm.nih.gov/pubmed/22016065

Hendrich A, Chow MP, Skierczynski BA, Lu Z. A 36-hospital time and motion study: how do medical-surgical nurses spend their time? Perm J [Internet]. 2008 Jan [cited 2011 Nov 24];12(3):25–34. http://www.pubmedcentral.nih.gov/articlerender.fcgi?artid=3037121&tool=pmcentrez&rendertype=abstract

Kannampallil TG, Abraham J, Patel VL. Methodological framework for evaluating clinical processes: A cognitive informatics perspective. J Biomed Inform [Internet]. 2016 Dec [cited 2017 Dec 14];64:342–51. http://linkinghub.elsevier.com/retrieve/pii/S1532046416301617

Keohane CA, Bane AD, Featherstone E, Hayes J, Woolf S, Hurley A, et al. Quantifying nursing workflow in medication administration. J Nurs Adm [Internet]. 2008 Jan [cited 2011 Sep 27];38(1):19–26. http://www.ncbi.nlm.nih.gov/pubmed/18157001

Kim CS, Lovejoy W, Paulsen M, Chang R, Flanders SA. Hospitalist time usage and cyclicality: opportunities to improve efficiency. J Hosp Med [Internet]. [cited 2011 Sep 20];5(6):329–34. http://www.ncbi.nlm.nih.gov/pubmed/20803670

Kloss L, Musial-Bright L, Klapp BF, Groneberg DA, Mache S. Observation and analysis of junior OB/GYNs' workflow in German hospitals. Arch Gynecol Obstet [Internet]. 2010 May [cited 2012 Feb 22];281(5):871–8. http://www.ncbi.nlm.nih.gov/pubmed/19639328

Lopetegui M, Yen P, Lai AM, Embi PJ, Payne PRO. Time capture tool (TimeCaT): Development of a comprehensive application to support data capture for time motion studies . AMIA Annu Symp Proc. 2012.

Lopetegui MA, Bai S, Yen P-Y, Lai A, Embi P, Payne PRO. Inter-observer reliability assessments in time motion studies: the foundation for meaningful clinical workflow analysis. AMIA Annu Symp Proc [Internet]. 2013 Jan [cited 2014 May 27];2013:889–96. http://www.pubmedcentral. nih.gov/articlerender.fcgi?artid=3900222&tool=pmcentrez&rendertype=abstract

Lopetegui M, Yen P-Y, Lai A, Jeffries J, Embi P, Payne P. Time motion studies in healthcare: What are we talking about? J Biomed Inform [Internet]. 2014 Mar [cited 2014 Mar 10]. http://www. sciencedirect.com/science/article/pii/S1532046414000562

Mache S, Scutaru C, Vitzthum K, Gerber A, Quarcoo D, Welte T, et al. Development and evaluation of a computer-based medical work assessment programme. J Occup Med Toxicol [Internet]. 2008 Jan [cited 2012 Feb 2];3:35. http://www.pubmedcentral.nih.gov/articlerender.fcgi?artid= 2628342&tool=pmcentrez&rendertype=abstract

Mache S, Bernburg M, Scutaru C, Quarcoo D, Welte T, Klapp BF, et al. An observational real-time study to analyze junior physicians' working hours in the field of gastroenterology. Z Gastroenterol [Internet]. 2009 Sep [cited 2011 Sep 27];47(9):814–8. http://www.ncbi.nlm.nih.gov/pub med/19750428

Mache S, Vitzthum K, Kusma B, Nienhaus A, Klapp BF, Groneberg DA. Pediatricians' working conditions in German hospitals: a real-time task analysis. Eur J Pediatr [Internet]. 2010 May [cited 2012 Mar 2];169(5):551–5. http://www.ncbi.nlm.nih.gov/pubmed/19774393

Mache S, Kelm R, Bauer H, Nienhaus A, Klapp BF, Groneberg DA. General and visceral surgery practice in German hospitals: a real-time work analysis on surgeons' work flow. Langenbecks Arch Surg [Internet]. 2010 Jan [cited 2011 Sep 20];395(1):81–7. http://www.ncbi.nlm.nih.gov/ pubmed/19618203

Mache S, Vitzthum K, Klapp BF, Groneberg DA. Doctors' working conditions in emergency care units in Germany: a real-time assessment. Emerg Med J [Internet]. 2011 Nov 22 [cited 2011 Dec 15]; http://www.ncbi.nlm.nih.gov/pubmed/22109534

Mache S, Schöffel N, Kusma B, Vitzthum K, Klapp BF, Groneberg DA. Cancer care and residents' working hours in oncology and hematology departments: an observational real-time study in German hospitals. Jpn J Clin Oncol [Internet]. 2011 Jan [cited 2011 Sep 20];41(1):81–6. http:// www.ncbi.nlm.nih.gov/pubmed/20693548

Marjamaa R a, Torkki PM, Torkki MI, Kirvelä O a. Time accuracy of a radio frequency identification patient tracking system for recording operating room timestamps. Anesth Analg [Internet]. 2006 Apr [cited 2012 Aug 2];102(4):1183–6. http://www.ncbi.nlm.nih.gov/pubmed/16551921

McCall N, Cromwell J, Braun P. Validation of physician survey estimates of surgical time using operating room logs. Med Care Res Rev [Internet]. 2006 Dec [cited 2013 May 18];63(6):764–77. http://www.ncbi.nlm.nih.gov/pubmed/17099125

Minekus JPJ, Rozing PM, Valstar ER, Dankelman J. Evaluation of humeral head replacements using time-action analysis. J Shoulder Elbow Surg [Internet]. Jan [cited 2013 May 20];12(2):152–7. http://www.ncbi.nlm.nih.gov/pubmed/12700568

Murden R a, Pintz EE. Housestaff-faculty ratios in ambulatory clinics and patient care and education. Acad Med [Internet]. 2003 Feb;78(2):224. http://www.ncbi.nlm.nih.gov/pubmed/12584105

Oddone E, Simel DL. A comparison of work-sampling and time-and-motion techniques for studies in health services research. Health Serv Res [Internet]. 1994 Dec [cited 2013 May 7];29(5):623–6. http://www.pubmedcentral.nih.gov/articlerender.fcgi?artid=1070031&tool=pmcentrez&ren dertype=abstract

van Oldenrijk J, Schafroth MU, Bhandari M, Runne WC, Poolman RW. Time-action analysis (TAA) of the surgical technique implanting the collum femoris preserving (CFP) hip arthroplasty. TAASTIC trial identifying pitfalls during the learning curve of surgeons participating in a subsequent randomized controlled trial (an ob. BMC Musculoskelet Disord [Internet]. 2008 Jan [cited 2011 Sep 27];9:93. http://www.pubmedcentral.nih.gov/articlerender.fcgi?artid=248 3707&tool=pmcentrez&rendertype=abstract

Overhage JM, Perkins S, Tierney WM, McDonald CJ. Controlled trial of direct physician order entry: effects on physicians' time utilization in ambulatory primary care internal medicine practices. J Am Med Inform Assoc [Internet]. 2001;8(4):361–71. http://www.pubmedcentral.nih.gov/articl erender.fcgi?artid=130081&tool=pmcentrez&rendertype=abstract

Pelletier D, Duffield C. Work sampling: valuable methodology to define nursing practice patterns. Nurs Health Sci [Internet]. 2003 Mar;5(1):31–8. http://www.ncbi.nlm.nih.gov/pubmed/126 03719

Pizziferri L, Kittler AF, Volk L a, Honour MM, Gupta S, Wang S, et al. Primary care physician time utilization before and after implementation of an electronic health record: a time-motion study. J Biomed Inform [Internet]. 2005 Jun;38(3):176–88. http://www.ncbi.nlm.nih.gov/pubmed/158 96691

Schiller B, Doss S, DE Cock E, Del Aguila MA, Nissenson AR. Costs of managing anemia with erythropoiesis-stimulating agents during hemodialysis: a time and motion study. Hemodial Int [Internet]. 2008 Oct [cited 2011 Sep 27];12(4):441–9. http://www.ncbi.nlm.nih.gov/pubmed/ 19090867

Sittig DF, Singh H. A new sociotechnical model for studying health information technology in complex adaptive healthcare systems. Qual Saf Heal Care [Internet]. 2010 Oct 1 [cited 2016 Nov 23];19(Suppl 3):i68–74. http://qualitysafety.bmj.com/lookup/doi/https://doi.org/10.1136/ qshc.2010.042085

Taylor FW. The principles of scientific management. Ney York: Harper & Brothers Publishers; 1914.

Tipping MD, Forth VE, Magill DB, Englert K, Williams M V. Systematic review of time studies evaluating physicians in the hospital setting. J Hosp Med [Internet]. [cited 2011 Sep 20];5(6):353–9. http://www.ncbi.nlm.nih.gov/pubmed/20803675

Todd SR, Fahy BN, Paukert JL, Mersinger D, Johnson ML, Bass BL. How accurate are self-reported resident duty hours? J Surg Educ [Internet]. [cited 2011 Sep 20];67(2):103–7. http://www.ncbi. nlm.nih.gov/pubmed/20656607

Westbrook JI, Woods A. Development and testing of an observational method for detecting medication administration errors using information technology. Stud Health Technol Inform [Internet]. 2009 Jan [cited 2012 Mar 2];146:429–33. http://www.ncbi.nlm.nih.gov/pubmed/19592880

Westbrook JI, Braithwaite J, Georgiou A, Ampt A, Creswick N, Coiera E, et al. Multi-method evaluation of information and communication technologies in health in the context of wicked problems and sociotechnical theory. J Am Med Inform Assoc [Internet]. 2007 [cited 2011 Sep 8];14(6):746–55. http://www.pubmedcentral.nih.gov/articlerender.fcgi?artid= 2213479&tool=pmcentrez&rendertype=abstract

Westbrook JI, Ampt A, Kearney L, Rob MI. All in a day's work: an observational study to quantify how and with whom doctors on hospital wards spend their time. Med J Aust [Internet]. 2008 May 5 [cited 2011 Jul 19];188(9):506–9. http://www.ncbi.nlm.nih.gov/pubmed/18459920

Westbrook JI, Woods A, Rob MI, Dunsmuir WTM, Day RO. Association of interruptions with an increased risk and severity of medication administration errors. Arch Intern Med [Internet]. 2010 Apr 26 [cited 2012 Mar 2];170(8):683–90. http://www.ncbi.nlm.nih.gov/pubmed/20421552

Wirth P, Kahn L, Perkoff GT. Comparability of two methods of time and motion study used in a clinical setting: work sampling and continuous observation. Med Care [Internet]. 1977 Nov [cited 2011 Dec 19];15(11):953–60. http://www.ncbi.nlm.nih.gov/pubmed/926877

Yawn B, Goodwin MA, Zyzanski SJ, Stange KC. Time use during acute and chronic illness visits to a family physician. Fam Pract [Internet]. 2003 Aug [cited 2013 May 20];20(4):474–7. http:// www.ncbi.nlm.nih.gov/pubmed/12876124

Yee T, Needleman J, Pearson M, Parkerton P, Parkerton M, Wolstein J. The influence of integrated electronic medical records and computerized nursing notes on nurses' time spent in documentation. Comput Inform Nurs [Internet]. 2012 Jun [cited 2013 May 8];30(6):287–92. http://www. ncbi.nlm.nih.gov/pubmed/22411414

Yen P-Y, Kelley M, Lopetegui M, Rosado AL, Migliore EM, Chipps EM, et al. Understanding and Visualizing Multitasking and Task Switching Activities: A Time Motion Study to Capture

Nursing Workflow. AMIA . Annu Symp proceedings AMIA Symp [Internet]. 2016 [cited 2018 Jan 16];2016:1264–73. http://www.ncbi.nlm.nih.gov/pubmed/28269924

Zhang Y, Monsen K a, Adam TJ, Pieczkiewicz DS, Daman M, Melton GB. Systematic refinement of a health information technology time and motion workflow instrument for inpatient nursing care using a standardized interface terminology. AMIA Annu Symp Proc [Internet]. 2011 Jan;2011:1621–9. http://www.pubmedcentral.nih.gov/articlerender.fcgi?artid=3243138&tool=pmcentrez&rendertype=abstract

Zheng K, Guo MH, Hanauer D a. Using the time and motion method to study clinical work processes and workflow: methodological inconsistencies and a call for standardized research. J Am Med Inform Assoc [Internet]. 2011 Sep 1 [cited 2011 Sep 27];18(5):704–10. http://www.pubmedcentral.nih.gov/articlerender.fcgi?artid=3168304&tool=pmcentrez&rendertype=abstract

Chapter 6
Recent Developments in Workflow Research in Healthcare

Mustafa Ozkaynak, Zhe Shan, and Danny T. Y. Wu

6.1 Introduction

Workflow can be defined as "the flow of work through space and time" (Karsh 2009)—i. e., temporally organized activities that occur across settings. Workflow is a changing landscape. Workflow can change as the work changes or with changes in the flow of the work. Workflow can also be influenced as our understanding of space and time changes. The purpose of this chapter is to highlight these changes by discussing recent developments in methodology and theory related to workflow research in a clinical setting.

We highlight six recent developments in cognitive informatics that directly and indirectly affect workflow and should be considered in clinical workflow research. These are (1) artificial intelligence applications; (2) automation and workflow monitoring; (3) further integration of clinical and daily living settings; (4) Diversity, equity, and inclusion efforts; (5) climate change and (6) developments in Dissemination and Implementation (D&I) science.

Artificial intelligence and machine learning based technologies (including generative AI such as Chat GPT or Google Gemini) have been increasingly adopted in clinical settings for diagnostic procedures (Yin et al., 2021), documentation (Chi et al., 2021), therapy selection (Lee et al., 2021), and disease outbreak prediction

M. Ozkaynak (✉)
College of Nursing, University of Colorado | Anschutz Medical Campus, Aurora, CO, USA
e-mail: mustafa.ozkaynak@cuanschutz.edu

Z. Shan
Farmer School of Business, Miami University, Oxford, OH, USA

D. T. Y. Wu
Department of Biostatistics, Health Informatics, and Data Sciences, University of Cincinnati College of Medicine, Cincinnati, OH, USA

© The Author(s), under exclusive license to Springer Nature Switzerland AG 2025
K. Zheng et al. (eds.), *Reengineering Clinical Workflow in the Digital and AI Era*,
Cognitive Informatics in Biomedicine and Healthcare,
https://doi.org/10.1007/978-3-031-82971-0_6

97

(Yang et al., 2020). These technologies have the potential to lead to more personalized and efficient patient care, as well as improvements in clinical research and trial design. State-of-the-art AI applications, however, will not reach their full potential unless they are integrated into clinical workflow. There are multiple barriers that were not necessarily a primary focus in previous technologies. They include data privacy concerns, algorithm transparency, data standardization, interoperability, and patient safety concerns (Gretton 2018; Magrabi et al. 2019; Robert Challen et al. 2019; Sujan et al. 2019; Xu et al. 2014). Workflow studies that consider the fragility of AI models in real-world, heterogeneous, and noisy clinical environments, are critical to the integration of AI systems into clinical decision making.

The increased adoption of information technology and the availability of massive amounts of data, provide new opportunities for more effective and efficient workflows through automation (Zayas-Cabán et al. 2023; Zayas-Cabán 2021). In fact, some of these technologies are not new but they are more powerful and sophisticated and enable users for more complex functions. Particularly, the availability of audit logs may play an important role for automation. Automation allows for monitoring and controlling the delivery of products and services (International Society of Automation 2024). Workflow monitoring tools we previously described based on three case studies (Wu et al. 2022a, b), can be essential for automation because they can gather and analyze relevant workflow information and provide real-time feedback and guidance. If clinician workflow patterns are not carefully captured and translated into automation and optimization requirements, workflow automation will have low reliability and user adoption and can introduce unintended negative consequences and even patient harms (Bloomrosen et al. 2011; Cabitza et al. 2017; Harrison et al. 2007; Ogundaini et al. 2022). Workflow monitoring tools (WMOT) can reduce resource burdens and standardize the data collection and analysis process. While a WMOT is not used in clinical care, its results can help improve care routines and enhance local Electronic Health Record (EHR) systems.

Significant advancements in digital health technologies made the boundaries between clinical and daily living settings thinner by (1) Ability to bring clinical data into daily living settings and (2) capturing daily living activities and bringing necessary data into clinical settings. This includes the integration of telemedicine, wearable devices, and remote monitoring tools, which have become increasingly prevalent, and accelerated by the COVID-19 pandemic.

Health care institutions recently have paid more attention to diversity, equity and inclusion (DEI) efforts both for their staff and the patients to which they provide care (Clark et al. 2023; del Pino-Jones et al. 2021; Todić et al. 2022; White et al. 2022). These efforts increase diversity of staff and highlight patient preferences and values. Workflow should accommodate this diversity. Workflow analysis in the future can focus on the identification of diversity gaps among various groups of clinicians and the opportunities to improve DEI. Moreover, new workflows are needed to collect patient preferences and values and integrate them into clinical decisions.

Climate change would affect care delivery and workflow in an unpredictable way. Currently there are limited empirical studies and frameworks available to gauge this effect. One example, the Clinical cLimate InforMAtics acTions for the Environment

(I-CLIMATE) framework (Sittig et al. 2022), illustrates how clinical informatics can help reduce healthcare's environmental pollution and climate-related impacts using 5 actionable components: (1) create a circular economy for health IT, (2) reduce energy consumption through smarter use of health IT, (3) support more environmentally friendly decision making by clinicians and health administrators, (4) mobilize healthcare workforce environmental stewardship through informatics, and (5) Inform policies and regulations for change. Implementation of this framework requires a sociotechnical framework which contains technology as well as people involved, their communication patterns, culture, environment, and external rules and regulations. Workflow is an effective way to capture all these dimensions.

D&I science involves"strategies help systems implement, disseminate, and sustain the improvements and enhancements" (Jackson et al. 2020). It is heavily interested in context, adaptation, and sustainability. Workflow studies allow us to better understand context (Ozkaynak et al. 2020; Scholl et al. 2018), track adaptations in a systematic way (Haley et al. 2021) and ensure sustainability (Malone et al. 2021). Therefore, workflow studies are a critical component of D&I science and a key driver to translate research findings into clinical practice.

In this chapter, we summarized some of the recent methodological and theoretical advances in workflow research that accommodate these six recent developments that affect cognitive informatics. The methodological advances that we summarized are Real Time Locating Systems, Visual Analytics, Workflow Monitoring, Process Mining, Network Analysis. We also discussed four recently developed theoretical frameworks. This chapter ends with a thorough discussion with future directions.

6.2   Recent Developments in Theory

Conceptual theories, model and frameworks are important for workflow research and workflow studies because they (1) provide a useful definition of workflow and identify critical building blocks to focus on; (2) advance science by allowing for creating new knowledge upon foundational knowledge; (3) provide well-validated pathways to link observed clinical or non-clinical health work with current knowledge, thus enhancing efficiency and generalizability (Blijleven et al. 2019).

In this chapter, we highlight four recently (2019–2024) developed frameworks that inform workflow research and workflow studies in research, clinical practice, and design (Table 6.1). We did not include other frameworks that focused on methodology.

SEWA (Blijleven et al. 2019) was based on direct observations and follow-up interviews with physicians, nurses and clerks using their EHR at a large academic hospital. The components of SEWA were grouped under Work System (Persons, Tasks, EHR System, EHR Workarounds, physical environment, and organization) and Outcomes (Scope and Impact). SEWA provides a grounded foundation for performing sociotechnical analyses of EHR workarounds. SEWA can support redesigning the work system. SEWA can support identifying, analyzing,

Table 6.1 Recently developed frameworks that inform workflow research and workflow studies

Name of the framework	Purpose of the framework	Main building blocks of the framework
SEWA (Sociotechnical EHR workaround analysis) (Blijleven et al. 2019)	Address challenges of studying workarounds emerging from electronic health record (EHR) system usage	Persons, tasks, EHR systems, EHR Workarounds, physical environment, organization, scope, & impact
Conceptual model of health IT workflow integration (Salwei et al. 2021)	Improve integration of the technologies into clinical workflow	Time, flow, scope of patient journey, and Level
Conceptual model of shared health informatics for tracking chronic illness management (CoMSHI) (Vizer et al. 2019)	Inform development of effective technologies that aid tracking of health indicators to support chronic illness management	Person with chronic illness, informal carers, health care providers, community members, communication and information, action, collection, integration, & reflection
Conceptual model of the integration of EHR and patient-generated health data (PGHD) with impact on clinician burnout (Ye 2021)	Explain how interactions with EHR-integrated PGHD may result in clinician burnout	Sensors, EHR, PROs, EHR integrated PGHD system, technostress, workflow related issues, time pressure, & clinician burn out

and resolving workarounds. Workflow was a reference point in defining work arounds. Workarounds occur when EHR users face workflow constraints. Discrepancies frequently occur between EHR system-dictated workflows and actual workflows of EHR users, causing impeded workflows that lead to the development and usage of EHR workarounds. The model suggests that person-characteristics, task-characteristics, technology-characteristics, physical environment and organizational factors, contribute to EHR workarounds.

Conceptual model of health IT workflow integration described four dimensions of workflow integration: time, flow, scope of patient journey, and level through interviewing ED physicians (Salwei et al., 2021). Workflow integration involves the entire work system and interactions between the person, tools and technologies (including health IT), tasks, physical environment, and organization. The conceptual model of workflow integration can be used to inform health IT design; this is the purpose of the proposed checklist that can help to ensure consideration of workflow integration during the development of health IT.

CoMSHI (Vizer et al., 2019) was developed through semi structured interviews with 40 adults concerning their chronic illness management practices and transcription of 30 publicly available videos of 24 adults discussing tracking processes for managing their chronic illness. CoMSHI provides a comprehensive viewpoint of tracking in support of chronic illness management and can inform technology design to improve tracking tools to support people in more confident and capable chronic illness management.

Conceptual model of the integration of EHR and patient-generated health data (PGHD) with the impact on clinician burnout is based on FITT (Fit between Individuals, Task and Technology) framework (Ammenwerth et al., 2006). The model highlights that technostress, time pressure, and workflow-related issues need to be addressed to accelerate the integration of PGHD into clinical care.

When comparing and contrasting these four models, three of these models were developed based on field studies and one based on a previous framework. Each model focuses on a specific topic or problem to solve, namely, workarounds, technology integration, chronic illness management, patient-generated health data and burnout. These four models are multilevel, i.e., have organizational and individual components. Studying workflow at multi-levels has various benefits such as revealing complex relationships between factors that affect care delivery and providing guidance to better identify the scope of a workflow study. We envision that these frameworks will guide studies that utilize the methodologies mentioned in the previous section, to study workflow studies. However, these methodologies as well as future methodologies should take the multilevel nature of workflow into account.

Diversity of these conceptual frameworks in terms of their scope (e.g., EHR use, health IT workflow integration, tracking in chronic illness management integration of diverse datasets and its impact on user burden) highlights the diverse use of work analysis studies to understand various work-related phenomena.

6.3 Recent Advances in Workflow Analysis

6.3.1 Overview

This section examines the evolution and application of workflow analysis, detailing four innovative methods that have shaped the field in recent years: Process Mining, Real-time Locating System (RTLS), Network Analysis, and Visual Analytics and Workflow Monitoring. Initially derived from engineering principles, workflow analysis has found robust applications in business process discovery and beyond. Since its formal introduction in 1999, Process Mining has been at the forefront, offering insights into operational efficiencies and decision-making processes. Notably, the techniques discussed from 2019 to 2023 represent advancements that are distinct from earlier theoretical foundations. These methods have emerged as critical tools for dissecting complex workflows, enabling better strategic planning and operational adaptability in various sectors, including during public health crises.

6.3.2 Process Mining

The integration of process mining into clinical workflows has emerged as a significant advancement in healthcare analytics, offering a data-driven approach to understanding, optimizing, and innovating within the healthcare sector. This literature review synthesizes research across five key themes, highlighting the potential of process mining to enhance operational efficiency, support clinical decision-making, address implementation challenges, adapt to the COVID-19 pandemic, and innovate new techniques and applications.

Operational Efficiency and Quality Improvement. The quest for operational efficiency and quality improvement in healthcare is a primary focus of process mining applications. Studies by Durojaiye et al. (2019) and Rojas et al. (2019) reveal how process mining can identify inefficiencies and optimize patient care pathways, leading to improved patient outcomes. Boersma et al. (2019) advocate for the integration of process mining into continuous optimization cycles, highlighting its role in achieving operational excellence. The versatility of process mining is further demonstrated by Martinez-Millana et al. (2019) and Kempa-Liehr et al. (2020), who emphasize its utility in supporting clinical roles and predictive modeling. Collectively, these studies underscore the transformative impact of process mining on operational efficiency and the quality of care.

Clinical Decision Support and Pathway Analysis. Process mining serves as a robust tool for clinical decision support and pathway analysis, as evidenced by the works of Dahlin and Raharjo (2019) and Chiudinelli et al. (2020), which analyze treatment pathways and care patterns in cancer care. Andrews et al. (2020) and Marazza et al. (2020) explored the complexity of pre-hospital care transport pathways and a comparison of process models across patient populations, respectively. These studies illustrate the power of process mining in enhancing clinical decision-making, standardizing care, and personalizing treatment approaches.

Process Mining in the Context of COVID-19. The COVID-19 pandemic has presented unique challenges to healthcare systems, prompting researchers to adapt process mining techniques to rapidly changing conditions. Studies like those by Cuendet et al. (2022) and Leandro et al. (2022) have utilized process mining to analyze therapeutic pathways and stroke patient care, respectively, during the pandemic. These contributions highlight the resilience and adaptability of process mining in times of crisis, offering a means to maintain effective patient care and resource management.

Challenges and Solutions in Process Mining Implementation. The implementation of process mining faces several challenges, including data quality, privacy, and the complexity of healthcare data. Innovative solutions, such as those proposed by Kurniati et al. (2019), Pika et al. (2020), Erdogan and Tarhan (2022), address these challenges by improving data representation, ensuring privacy, and standardizing complex processes. The research within this theme provides valuable insights into overcoming the barriers to effective process mining in healthcare.

Innovations in Process Mining Techniques and Applications. The final theme encompasses a wave of innovation in process mining techniques and applications, pushing the boundaries of what is possible in healthcare analytics. The integration of blockchain technology by Tiftik et al. (2022), the combination of process mining with natural language processing by Fontenla-Seco et al. (2022), and the development of novel predictive models by Theis et al. (2022) are just a few examples of the advancements transforming the landscape of process mining in healthcare. These studies showcase the potential for sophisticated, tailored, and patient-centered applications that can significantly enhance healthcare delivery and management.

In summary, process mining has proven to be a versatile and powerful tool in the healthcare sector, with applications ranging from improving operational efficiency to supporting clinical decisions, overcoming implementation challenges, responding to global health crises, and driving technological innovation. The body of research reviewed herein demonstrates the significant potential of process mining to transform clinical workflow, leading to more informed, efficient, and patient-centric healthcare processes. As the field continues to evolve, future research should build on these findings to further refine process mining techniques and explore their applications in various healthcare contexts.

6.3.3 Real Time Locating Systems (RTLS)

Researchers in recent years have been using Real-Time Locating Systems (RTLS) to improve clinical workflow. A literature search was conducted in PubMed, IEEE Xplore, and ACM Digital Library on papers published between 2019 and 2023. Three themes were identified and summarized below.

Experience Sharing and Implementation Considerations of RTLS. Papers in the first theme shared experience and considerations in implementing RTLS. For example, Memorial Sloan Kettering Cancer Center in 2019 shared its 10-year experience where tens of thousands of RTLS tags were deployed, and outlined strategies for large-scale RTLS/RFID solutions, such as accuracy requirements, program management, and workflow optimization (Frisch 2019). On the other hand, Heller et al. explored the impact of RTLS in the preoperative environment and focused on the understanding of physicians' and family members' perceptions of its functionality and efficiency (Heller et al. 2020). The findings from their semi-structured interviews showed that physicians expected significant improvement on the implementation and use of RTLS to unleash its full potential while family members were very positive about the provision of the tracking information. Bazo et al. surveyed the hospitals on RTLS usage and discussed the need for organizing and understanding key aspects of healthcare-oriented RTLS (Bazo et al. 2021). They provided a taxonomy to guide researchers and developers in addressing challenges for successful implementation. Overmann et al. conducted a systematic review and found that most RTLS were implemented in an emergency department and evaluated in an observational study (Overmann et al., 2021). More analytic methods should be developed to extract insights from experimental studies. Meanwhile, RTLS can be used outside of hospitals and in a long-term care setting. For example, Grigorovich et al. conducted a systematic review to explore the potential of using RTLS to enhance the care and safety of individuals with cognitive disabilities in long-term care homes (Grigorovich et al. 2021). In addition to demonstrating the functionality, efficiency, and effectiveness of RTLS, the authors highlighted the need for future research on the ethics and privacy of monitoring.

Evidence to Support the Efficacy of RTLS. Papers in the second theme conducted studies to determine the efficacy of RTLS. Some studies were conducted in a laboratory setting. For example, Amir et al. used discrete event simulation on RTLS data and found that patient wait time can be reduced by 19.2% in their breast cancer imaging center (Amir et al. 2019). Arunachalam et al., demonstrated the potential of RTLS to optimize patient-care team interactions by examining the correlation between the patient-care team contact time and the patient's length of stay in an emergency department (ED) (Arunachalam et al. 2019). Additionally, Koenig et al., advocated for the importance of evaluating RTLS in a practice setting involving workflow and movement (Koenig et al., 2021). They defined sensitivity and prevision metrics and found high overall evaluation scores (84% and 93%, respectively) in the ED space of the Mayo Clinic. Osman et al., demonstrated that introducing RTLS to ED workflow and tracking patient flow in real-time can significantly reduce patient waiting times by 10.47% and therefore improve the overall service quality of EDs in Malaysia's public hospitals (Osman et al., 2021). During COVID-19, studies focused on analyzing RTLS data to examine any changes faced during patient-provider interactions when using telemedicine. For example, Patel et al. found no significant decrease in the number or duration of in-person interactions despite the increase of telemedicine use in an ED, suggesting further research to optimize the integration of telemedicine into the ED workflow (Patel et al., 2021). In contrast, Vilendrer et al. found that when adopting telehealth in an inpatient setting, the frequency of in-person encounters decreased and the duration of each encounter increased (Vilendrer et al., 2022). However, the total nursing time at the bedside remained unchanged, suggesting that telehealth complements, rather than replaces, in-person care.

Challenges in implementing RTLS. Papers in the third theme addressed various challenges in implementing RTLS. For example, Spini et al. focused on the privacy of the staff members being tracked and proposed a secure solution using an innovative cryptographic technique called Secure Multi-Party Computation (Spini et al., 2019). Newman-Casey et al. targeted the affordability of RTLS implementation and used off-the-shelf RFID readers and tags along with a custom RFID management application in an outpatient glaucoma clinic (Newman-Casey et al., 2020). The authors demonstrated the potential of such a low-cost system in continuous quality improvement using patient wait time as an example. Lim et al., on the other hand, explored whether applying machine learning (ML) techniques on Wi-Fi fingerprinting data can generate accurate real-time location information (Lim et al., 2022). Their study in a comprehensive stroke care unit showed that such ML-based RTLS can achieve 98% accuracy in predicting the different hospital zones relevant in the acute endovascular intervention workflow. Finally, Barrick et al. complimented the strength of RTLS data by combining data with timestamps in electronic health records (Barrick et al., 2021). Their study identified measurable clinical sub-workflows and significant bottlenecks in sedation procedures in a pediatric ED.

6.3.4   Network Analysis

The burgeoning field of social network analysis (SNA) in clinical workflow research is vividly illustrated through recent studies, which can be categorized into three main groups: healthcare communication, pandemic data analysis, and healthcare service systems.

The first group focuses on **healthcare communication**. Kabo et al. (2023) delved into the spatial dynamics of operating rooms, revealing how physical layout affects team communication. Their findings underscore the need for thoughtful spatial design in healthcare settings. Similarly, Festila and Müller (2021) examine information handoffs in critical care. By identifying different types of handoffs (human–human, human-ICT, ICT-human), this study highlights the complex interplay between human and technological actors in healthcare information networks. Additionally, Steitz and Levy (2019) explored the use of EHR messaging in a breast cancer cohort, emphasizing the role of electronic communication in coordinating complex care. These studies collectively shed light on the nuances of healthcare communication, showcasing the utility of SNA in optimizing team dynamics and information flow.

The second category involves **pandemic data analysis**, where SNA is applied to understand disease spread and symptoms. Wu et al. (2023) leveraged social media data to map COVID-19 symptoms, illustrating the potential of unconventional data sources in pandemic monitoring. Similarly, Chu et al. (2021) used air travel data to analyze the interconnectedness of the COVID-19 pandemic on a global scale. These studies demonstrate the applicability of SNA in understanding the dynamics of pandemic spread and symptom evolution on both local and global scales.

The final category relates to **healthcare service systems**. Hagedorn et al. (2019) and Carroll and Richardson (2019) both emphasized the significance of understanding communication networks within healthcare. Hagedorn et al. focused on secure text-messaging platforms in a pediatric center to map inpatient communication networks, while Carroll and Richardson utilized SNA to model the dynamics of healthcare delivery, identifying potential service bottlenecks. These studies highlight the transformative potential of SNA in improving healthcare efficiency and patient care by comprehensively understanding the connectedness within healthcare services.

In conclusion, these diverse applications of SNA in clinical workflow research underscore its pivotal role in enhancing our understanding of healthcare dynamics. From optimizing communication and collaboration among healthcare providers to analyzing large-scale pandemic trends and improving healthcare service systems, SNA offers valuable insights that are crucial for the advancement of healthcare delivery and patient care.

6.3.5 Visual Analytics and Workflow Monitoring

Visual analytics address the information overload problem by processing a large amount of data into meaningful information and make this information transparent for an analytic discourse (Keim et al. 2008). Visual analytics can be a viable way to uncover complex workflow patterns and support the investigation of workflow issues and barriers. Pioneer work that applies visual analytics to analyze clinical workflow includes Zheng et al. who proposed new measures (e.g., average continuous time) and corresponding data visualizations (time-belt, network, and heatmap) (Zheng et al. 2010). Vankipuram et al. combined Hidden Markov Model and virtual reality-based simulation, to analyze workflow data automatically collected using sensor technology (Vankipuram et al. 2011). Ozkaynak et al. developed a 7-step guideline to analyze workflow data from electronic health records using Markov models and EventFlow visualizations (Ozkaynak et al. 2015). EventFlow is a visualization tool that simplifies and aggregates temporal event sequences in a dataset so that users can explore the overall trends and patterns (Monroe et al. 2013). DISCO, a similar tool specifically made for process mining, was designed with high usability, fidelity, and performance to support workflow analysis (Günther and Rozinat 2012). Recently, Wu et al. (2022a, b) applied visual analytics framework and techniques to develop a Clinical Workflow Analysis Tool (CWAT) to explore time and motion data (Wu et al. 2022a, b).

Workflow analysis has been taken to another level for continuous analysis and monitoring. Workflow monitoring is necessary to ensure the quality of care since healthcare organizations constantly adapt to new treatment methods, medications, and technologies (Antunes et al., 2019). Early work involves developing automated methods to unveil hidden patterns in complex workflow data (Liu et al., 2014) and integrate RTLS with business process management (BPM) to infer new states or events in a care process (Baarah and Peyton 2012). Recent advances in sensors, especially computer vision sensors, provide new opportunities to capture granular workflow data (Antunes et al., 2019). More importantly, continuous workflow monitoring requires a well-designed infrastructure to combine multiple data sources and apply complementary analysis methods to draw insight for the stakeholders to act upon and achieve care quality improvement goals (Wu et al. 2022a, b).

6.3.6 New Insights in Workflow Analysis

In summarizing the recent developments in workflow analysis, it is evident that Real-Time Locating Systems (RTLS) stand out by focusing on the collection of novel workflow data—specifically, movement data—that are not captured in Electronic Health Record (EHR) systems. This unique data type offers fresh insights into workflow patterns that are crucial for optimizing healthcare operations. In contrast, other recent advancements primarily enhance the analysis of existing workflow data.

Although there has been a noticeable trend towards employing established methods to enhance operational efficiency and support clinical decisions, there is a noticeable gap in the development of innovative workflow analysis tools. Current research prioritizes practical problem-solving and the dissemination of findings over the invention of new analytical tools.

Furthermore, while the application of these technologies has seen some success, implementing a workflow analysis solution remains fraught with challenges. Among the notable methods, Process Mining continues to be a vital source of techniques in clinical workflow analysis, helping to model and improve patient care pathways effectively. Network Analysis offers a unique perspective by using nodes and edges to model workflow data, which is particularly beneficial in healthcare settings where teamwork and communication are paramount. Meanwhile, Visual Analytics facilitates the exploration of complex workflow data through interactive visualizations, making it easier for users to discern patterns and insights.

These methods, though developed over a decade ago and widely applied in other fields, hold significant potential for direct application and adaptation within healthcare. For example, applying social network analysis to EHR messaging or integrating blockchain with natural language processing could yield new insights and address specific challenges in healthcare. Given the complexity and multifaceted nature of clinical workflows, no single method can suit all needs. Therefore, it is essential for workflow analysis to consider a broad spectrum of methods, adapting and combining them as necessary to address the primary research questions and achieve a holistic understanding of healthcare processes.

6.4 Discussion

This chapter summarizes various advancements in care delivery practice and research (e.g., artificial intelligence, DEI issues) that would require refreshing workflow definitions, workflow methodologies and conceptual frameworks. This refreshment reflects the opportunities as well as the challenges. We provided a brief, but current review of methodological developments and a sample of recent conceptual frameworks.

Workflow is a foundational concept in health informatics. Regardless of technology or other factors or advancements, examining workflow is critical to ensure the quality and safety of care delivery. However, new technologies (e.g., artificial intelligence) and other changes (e.g., environment, involved people, rules) in care delivery can affect how and why workflow is examined. For example, the advances in AI can effectively support the provider's cognitive processes, which is central in decision-making tasks. One recommendation in integrating AI is focusing on interactive solutions for supporting the physicians effectively in their daily activities, by exploiting their unique knowledge and evidence-based reasoning (Rundo et al. 2020). Therefore, workflow studies should focus on this interactivity, to ensure to capture how it affects clinicians' behaviors. This could be accomplished efficiently by using conceptual frameworks that guide workflow studies.

The four conceptual frameworks that we have discussed expectedly overlap with the current trends that were discussed in the introduction section. These frameworks commonly highlight the increasingly complex nature of the implementation of the informatics interventions. Focusing on workflow is an effective strategy to tackle this complexity and ensure the sustainability of these interventions. These frameworks were developed using qualitative approaches. One of the next steps would be testing these frameworks using quantitative approaches. Further frameworks that focus on context can inform future workflow studies. Moreover, workflow studies can support the implementation of systematic intervention by assessing implementation strategies and adaptations.

The recent methodologies that we summarized in this chapter are heavily data-driven. An effective strategy is to be able to use already available data in EHRs and other sources for these methodologies instead of collecting new data. This ability requires close collaboration among researchers, clinicians, and health IT personnel. Researchers may consider these recently developed data collection and analysis methods when planning and executing their workflow studies. Adoption of the new methodologies depends on easiness to apply of these methodologies. Developing guidelines, sharing resources, close collaboration with community can facilitate the dissemination of recent methodologies.

Recent trends suggest that future workflow methodologies and conceptual frameworks will be more data intensive. Diverse data resources should be harmonized to be able study workflow to identify patterns and variations in a reliable and valid way. Sensitivity to context is also critical particularly in care delivery. Context can be patient characteristics (e.g., diagnosis, preferences), provider characteristics (e.g., experience), process characteristics (temporal features), organizational characteristics (leadership, rules) or societal factors (policy, values).

Acknowledgements We thank Ms. Suzanne C Lareau and Himaja Chintalapalli for editorial support.

References

Amir T, Lee B, Woods RW, Mullen LA, Harvey SC. A pilot of data-driven modeling to assess potential for improved efficiency in an academic breast-imaging center. J Digit Imaging. 2019;32(2):221–7.

Ammenwerth E, Iller C, Mahler C. IT-adoption and the interaction of task, technology and individuals: a fit framework and a case study. BMC Med Inform Decis Mak. 2006;6(1):3.

Andrews R, Wynn MT, Vallmuur K, Hofstede AHMT, Bosley E. A comparative process mining analysis of road trauma patient pathways. Int J Environ Res Public Health. 2020;17(10):3426.

Antunes RS, Seewald LA, Rodrigues VF, Costa CAD, Jr LG, Righi RR, Maier A, Eskofier B, Ollenschläger M, Naderi F, Fahrig R, Bauer S, Klein S, Campanatti G. A survey of sensors in healthcare workflow monitoring. ACM Comput Surv. 2019;51(2):1–37.

Arunachalam SP, Asan O, Nestler DM, Heaton HA, Hellmich TR, Wutthisirisart P, Marisamy G, Pasupathy KS, Sir MY. Patient-care team contact patterns impact treatment length of stay in the emergency department. In: Annual international conference of the IEEE engineering in medicine and biology society. IEEE engineering in medicine and biology society. Annual international conference; 2019. p. 345–8.

Baarah A, Peyton L. Engineering a state monitoring service for real-time patient flow management. In: Proceedings of the 9th middleware doctoral symposium of the 13th ACM/IFIP/USENIX international middleware conference. Montreal Quebec Canada: ACM; 2012. p. 1–6.

Barrick L, Wu DTY, Frey T, Shu D, Abbu R, Porter SC, Overmann KM. Improving care delivery: location timestamps to enhance process measurement of a clinical workflow. Pediatr Qual & Saf. 2021;6(5), e475.

Bazo R, da Costa CA, Seewald LA, da Silveira LG, Antunes RS, Righi R, da R, Rodrigues VF. A survey about real-time location systems in healthcare environments. J Med Syst. 2021;45(3):35.

Blijleven V, Koelemeijer K, Jaspers M. SEWA: a framework for sociotechnical analysis of electronic health record system workarounds. Int J Med Informatics. 2019;125:71–8.

Bloomrosen M, Starren J, Lorenzi NM, Ash JS, Patel VL, Shortliffe EH. Anticipating and addressing the unintended consequences of health IT and policy: a report from the AMIA 2009 health policy meeting. J Am Med Inform Assoc: JAMIA. 2011;18(1):82–90.

Boersma HJ, Leung TI, Vanwersch R, Heeren E, van Merode GG. Optimizing care processes with operational excellence & process mining. In: Kubben P, Dumontier M, Dekker A, editors. Fundamentals of clinical data science, Cham (CH): Springer; 2019. http://www.ncbi.nlm.nih.gov/books/NBK543517/

Cabitza F, Rasoini R, Gensini GF. Unintended consequences of machine learning in medicine. JAMA. 2017;318(6):517–8.

Carroll N, Richardson I. Mapping a careflow network to assess the connectedness of connected health. Health Inform J. 2019;25(1):106–25. SAGE Publications Ltd.

Challen R, Denny J, Pitt M, Gompels L, Edwards T, Tsaneva-Atanasova K. Artificial intelligence, bias and clinical safety. BMJ Qual & Saf. 2019;28(3):231.

Chi EA, Chi G, Tsui CT, Jiang Y, Jarr K, Kulkarni CV, Zhang M, Long J, Ng AY, Rajpurkar P, Sinha SR. Development and validation of an artificial intelligence system to optimize clinician review of patient records. JAMA Netw Open. 2021;4(7):e2117391–e2117391.

Chiudinelli L, Dagliati A, Tibollo V, Albasini S, Geifman N, Peek N, Holmes JH, Corsi F, Bellazzi R, Sacchi L. Mining post-surgical care processes in breast cancer patients. Artif Intell Med. 2020;105:101855.

Chu AM, Cha JN, Tsang JT, Tiwari A, So MK. Analyzing cross-country pandemic connectedness during COVID-19 using a spatial-temporal database: network analysis. JMIR Public Health Surveill. 2021;7(3):e27317.

Clark SG, Cohen A, Heard-Garris N. Moving beyond words: leveraging financial resources to improve diversity, equity, and inclusion in academic medical centers. J Clin Psychol Med Settings. 2023;30(2):281–7.

Cuendet MA, Gatta R, Wicky A, Gerard CL, Dalla-Vale M, Tavazzi E, Michielin G, Delyon J, Ferahta N, Cesbron J, Lofek S, Huber A, Jankovic J, Demicheli R, Bouchaab H, Digklia A, Obeid M, Peters S, Eicher M, Pradervand S, Michielin O. A differential process mining analysis of COVID-19 management for cancer patients. Front Oncol. 2022;12:1043675.

Dahlin S, Raharjo H. Relationship between patient costs and patient pathways. Int J Health Care Qual Assur. 2019;32(1):246–61.

del Pino-Jones A, Cervantes L, Flores S, Jones CD, Keach J, Ngov L-K, Schwartz DA, Wierman M, Anstett T, Bowden K, Keniston A, Burden M. Advancing diversity, equity, and inclusion in hospital medicine. J Hosp Med. 2021;16(4):198–203.

Durojaiye AB, Levin S, Toerper M, Kharrazi H, Lehmann HP, Gurses AP. Evaluation of multi-disciplinary collaboration in pediatric trauma care using EHR data. J Am Med Inform Assoc. 2019;26(6):506–515. Oxford Academic.

Erdogan TG, Tarhan AK. Multi-perspective process mining for emergency process. Health Inform J. 2022;28(1):14604582221077195.

Festila MS, Müller SD. Information handoffs in critical care and their implications for information quality: a socio-technical network approach. J Biomed Inform. 2021;122:103914.

Fontenla-Seco Y, Lama M, González-Salvado V, Peña-Gil C, Bugarín-Diz A. A framework for the automatic description of healthcare processes in natural language: application in an aortic stenosis integrated care process. J Biomed Inform. 2022;128:104033.

Frisch PH. RFID in today's intelligent hospital enhancing patient care & optimizing hospital operations. In: 2019 IEEE international conference on RFID technology and applications (RFID-TA), Pisa, Italy: IEEE; 2019. p. 458–63.

Gretton C. Trust and transparency in machine learning-based clinical decision support, human–computer interaction series. In: Zhou J, Chen F, editors. Cham: Springer International Publishing; 2018. p. 279–92.

Grigorovich A, Kulandaivelu Y, Newman K, Bianchi A, Khan SS, Iaboni A, McMurray J. Factors affecting the implementation, use, and adoption of real-time location system technology for persons living with cognitive disabilities in long-term care homes: systematic review. J Med Internet Res. 2021;23(1):e22831.

Günther CW, Rozinat A. Disco: discover your processes. In: International conference on business process management. 2012. https://api.semanticscholar.org/CorpusID:2907725.

Hagedorn PA, Kirkendall ES, Spooner SA, Mohan V. Inpatient communication networks: leveraging secure text-messaging platforms to gain insight into inpatient communication systems. Appl Clin Inform. 2019;10(3):471–8.

Haley AD, Powell BJ, Walsh-Bailey C, Krancari M, Gruß I, Shea CM, Bunce A, Marino M, Frerichs L, Lich KH, Gold R. Strengthening methods for tracking adaptations and modifications to implementation strategies. BMC Med Res Methodol. 2021;21(1):133.

Harrison MI, Koppel R, Bar-Lev S. Unintended consequences of information technologies in health care—an interactive sociotechnical analysis. J Am Med Inform Assoc: JAMIA. 2007;14(5):542–9.

Heller M, Koval J, Miller E, Solomon S. The impact of a real-time locating system within the perioperative environment on physicians and patients' families. Healthc Q (Tor, Ont). 2020;23(SP):25–32.

International Society of Automation. What is automation. 2024. (https://www.isa.org/about-isa/what-is-automation).

Jackson GL, Cutrona SL, Kilbourne A, White BS, Everett C, Damschroder LJ. Implementation science: helping healthcare systems improve. JAAPA: Off J Am Acad Physician Assist. 2020;33(1):51–53.

Kabo FW, Stucky CH, De Jong MJ. Associations of surgical team communication with the layout of physical space: a network analysis of the operating room in a military medical center. HERD. 2023;16(3):134–45.

Karsh BT. Clinical practice improvement and redesign: how change in workflow can be supported by clinical decision support. No. 09–0054-EF, Rockville, Maryland: Agency for Healthcare Research and Quality; 1998.

Keim D, Andrienko G, Fekete JD, Görg C, Kohlhammer J, Melançon G. Visual analytics: definition, process, and challenges. In: Kerren A, Stasko JT, Fekete JD, North C, editors. Information visualization: human-centered issues and perspectives. Berlin, Heidelberg: Springer Berlin Heidelberg; 2008. p. 154–75.

Kempa-Liehr AW, Lin CY-C, Britten R, Armstrong D, Wallace J, Mordaunt D, O'Sullivan M. Healthcare pathway discovery and probabilistic machine learning. Int J Med Informatics. 2020;137:104087.

Koenig KR, Pasupathy KS, Hellmich TR, Hawthorne HJ, Karalius VP, Sir M, Das D, Heaton HA, Nestler DM. Measuring sensitivity and precision of real-time location systems (RTLS): definition, protocol and demonstration for clinical relevance. J Med Syst. 2021;45(1):15.

Kurniati AP, Rojas E, Hogg D, Hall G, Johnson OA. The assessment of data quality issues for process mining in healthcare using medical information mart for intensive care III, a freely available e-health record database. Health Informatics J. 2019;25(4):1878–93.

Leandro GDS, Miura DY, Safanelli J, Borges RM, Moro C. Analysis of stroke assistance in covid-19 pandemic by process mining techniques. Stud Health Technol Inform. 2022;294:48–52.

Lee MH, Siewiorek DP, Smailagic A, Bernardino A, Bermúdez i Badia SB. A human-AI collaborative approach for clinical decision making on rehabilitation assessment. In: Proceedings of the 2021 CHI conference on human factors in computing systems, CHI'21. New York, NY, USA: Association for Computing Machinery, May 7; 2021. p. 1–14.

Lim DZ, Yeo M, Dahan A, Tahayori B, Kok HK, Abbasi-Rad M, Maingard J, Kutaiba N, Russell J, Thijs V, Jhamb A, Chandra RV, Brooks M, Barras C, Asadi H. Development of a machine learning-based real-time location system to streamline acute endovascular intervention in acute stroke: a proof-of-concept study. J Neurointerventional Surg. 2022;14(8):799–803.

Liu C, Ge Y, Xiong H, Xiao K, Geng W, Perkins M. Proactive workflow modeling by stochastic processes with application to healthcare operation and management. In: Proceedings of the 20th ACM SIGKDD international conference on knowledge discovery and data mining. New York New York USA: ACM; 2014. p. 1593–602.

Magrabi F, Ammenwerth E, McNair JB, De Keizer NF, Hyppönen H, Nykänen P, Rigby M, Scott PJ, Vehko T, Wong ZS-Y, Georgiou A. Artificial intelligence in clinical decision support: challenges for evaluating AI and practical implications. Yearb Med Inform. 2019;28(1):128–34.

Malone S, Prewitt K, Hackett R, Lin JC, McKay V, Walsh-Bailey C, Luke DA. The clinical sustainability assessment tool: measuring organizational capacity to promote sustainability in healthcare. Implement Sci Commu. 2021;2(1):77.

Marazza F, Bukhsh FA, Geerdink J, Vijlbrief O, Pathak S, van Keulen M, Seifert C. Automatic process comparison for subpopulations: application in cancer care. Int J Environ Res Public Health. 2020;17(16):5707.

Martinez-Millana A, Lizondo A, Gatta R, Vera S, Salcedo VT, Fernandez-Llatas C. Process mining dashboard in operating rooms: analysis of staff expectations with analytic hierarchy process. Int J Environ Res Public Health. 2019;16(2):199. Multidisciplinary Digital Publishing Institute.

Monroe M, Lan R, Lee H, Plaisant C, Shneiderman B. Temporal event sequence simplification. IEEE Trans Visual Comput Graphics. 2013;19(12):2227–36.

Newman-Casey PA, Musser J, Niziol LM, Shedden K, Burke D, Cohn A. Designing and validating a low-cost real time locating system to continuously assess patient wait times. J Biomed Inform. 2020;106:103428.

Ogundaini O, de la Harpe R, McLean N. Unintended consequences of technology-enabled work activities experienced by healthcare professionals in tertiary hospitals of Sub-Saharan Africa. Afr J Sci, Technol, Innov Dev. 2022;14(4):876–85. Routledge.

Osman MS, Azizan A, Hassan KN, Ghani HA, Hassan NH, Yakub F, Daud SM, Latiff LA. BLE-based real-time location system integration with hospital information system to reduce patient waiting time. In: 2021 International conference on electrical, communication, and computer engineering (ICECCE). Kuala Lumpur, Malaysia: IEEE; 2021. p. 1–6.

Overmann KM, Wu DTY, Xu CT, Bindhu SS, Barrick L. Real-time locating systems to improve healthcare delivery: a systematic review. J Am Med Inform Assoc: JAMIA. 2021.

Ozkaynak M, Dziadkowiec O, Mistry R, Callahan T, He Z, Deakyne S, Tham E. Characterizing workflow for pediatric asthma patients in emergency departments using electronic health records. J Biomed Inform. 2015.

Ozkaynak M, Reeder B, Park SY, Huh-Yoo J. Chapter 13-design for improved workflow. In: Sethumadhavan A, Sasangohar F, editors, Design for health. Academic Press; 2020. p. 251–76.

Patel B, Vilendrer S, Kling SMR, Brown I, Ribeira R, Eisenberg M, Sharp C. Using a real-time locating system to evaluate the impact of telemedicine in an emergency department during COVID-19: observational study. J Med Internet Res. 2021;23(7):e29240.

Pika A, Wynn MT, Budiono S, Ter Hofstede AHM, van der Aalst WMP, Reijers HA. Privacy-preserving process mining in healthcare. Int J Environ Res Public Health. 2020;17(5):1612.

Rojas E, Cifuentes A, Burattin A, Munoz-Gama J, Sepúlveda M, Capurro D. Performance analysis of emergency room episodes through process mining. Int J Environ Res Public Health. 2019;16(7).

Rundo L, Pirrone R, Vitabile S, Sala E, Gambino O. Recent advances of HCI in decision-making tasks for optimized clinical workflows and precision medicine. J Biomed Inform. 2020;108:103479.

Salwei ME, Carayon P, Hoonakker PLT, Hundt AS, Wiegmann D, Pulia M, Patterson BW. Workflow integration analysis of a human factors-based clinical decision support in the emergency department. Appl Ergon. 2021;97:103498.

Scholl I, LaRussa A, Hahlweg P, Kobrin S, Elwyn G. Organizational-and system-level characteristics that influence implementation of shared decision-making and strategies to address them—a scoping review. Implement Sci. 2018;13(1):40.

Sittig DF, Sherman JD, Eckelman MJ, Draper A, Singh H. I-CLIMATE: a 'clinical climate informatics' action framework to reduce environmental pollution from healthcare. J Am Med Inform Assoc. 2022;29(12):2153–60.

Spini G, van Heesch M, Veugen T, Chatterjea S. Private hospital workflow optimization via secure k-means clustering. J Med Syst. 2019;44(1):8.

Steitz BD, Levy MA. Evaluating the scope of clinical electronic messaging to coordinate care in a breast cancer cohort. Stud Health Technol Inform. 2019;264:808–12.

Sujan M, Furniss D, Grundy K, Grundy H, Nelson D, Elliott M, White S, Habli I, Reynolds N. human factors challenges for the safe use of artificial intelligence in patient care. BMJ Health & Care Inform. 2019;26(1):e100081.

Theis J, Galanter WL, Boyd AD, Darabi H. Improving the in-hospital mortality prediction of diabetes ICU patients using a process mining/deep learning architecture. IEEE J Biomed Health Inform. 2022;26(1):388–99.

Tiftik MN, Erdogan TG, Tarhan AK. A framework for multi-perspective process mining into a BPMN process model. Math Biosci Eng: MBE. 2022;19(11):11800–20.

Todic´ J, Cook SC, Spitzer-Shohat S, Williams JS, Battle BA, Jackson J, Chin MH. Critical theory, culture change, and achieving health equity in health care settings. Acad Med. 2022;97(7):977–88.

Vankipuram M, Kahol K, Cohen T, Patel VL. Toward automated workflow analysis and visualization in clinical environments. J Biomed Inform. 2011;44(3):432–40.

Vilendrer S, Lough ME, Garvert DW, Lambert MH, Lu JH, Patel B, Shah NH, Williams MY, Kling SMR. Nursing workflow change in a COVID-19 inpatient unit following the deployment of inpatient telehealth: observational study using a real-time locating system. J Med Internet Res. 2022;24(6):e36882.

Vizer LM, Eschler J, Koo BM, Ralston J, Pratt W, Munson S. 'It's not just technology, it's people': constructing a conceptual model of shared health informatics for tracking in chronic illness management. J Med Internet Res. 2019;21(4):e10830.

White CY, Patel A, Cossari D. Organizational commitment to diversity, equity, and inclusion: a strategic path forward. Am J Health Syst Pharm. 2022;79(5):351–8.

Wu DTY, Barrick L, Ozkaynak M, Blondon K, Zheng K. Principles for designing and developing a workflow monitoring tool to enable and enhance clinical workflow automation. Appl Clin Inform. 2022a;13(1):132–8.

Wu J, Wang L, Hua Y, Li M, Zhou L, Bates DW, Yang J. Trend and co-occurrence network of COVID-19 symptoms from large-scale social media data: infoveillance study. J Med Internet Res. 2023;25:e45419.

Wu, Danny TY, Shu D, Le K, Abbu R, Zheng K. Applying visual analytics to develop a clinical workflow analysis tool (CWAT) to explore time and motion data in healthcare. In: 2022 workshop on visual analytics in healthcare (VAHC). Washington, DC, USA: IEEE; 2022. p. 1–5.

Xu J, Le K, Deitermann A, Montague E. How different types of users develop trust in technology: a qualitative analysis of the antecedents of active and passive user trust in a shared technology. Appl Ergon. 2014;45(6):1495–503.

Yang Z, Zeng Z, Wang K, Wong S-S, Liang W, Zanin M, Liu P, Cao X, Gao Z, Mai Z, Liang J, Liu X, Li S, Li Y, Ye F, Guan W, Yang Y, Li F, Luo S, Xie Y, Liu B, Wang Z, Zhang S, Wang Y, Zhong N, He J. Modified SEIR and AI prediction of the epidemics trend of COVID-19 in China under public health interventions. J Thorac Dis. 2020;12(3):165–74.

Ye J. The impact of electronic health record-integrated patient-generated health data on clinician burnout. J Am Med Inform Assoc. 2021;28(5):1051–6.

Yin J, Ngiam KY, Teo HH. Role of artificial intelligence applications in real-life clinical practice: systematic review. J Med Internet Res. 2021;23(4):e25759.

Zayas-Cabán T, Okubo TH, Posnack S. Priorities to accelerate workflow automation in health care. J Am Med Inform Assoc. 2023;30(1):195–201.

Zayas-Cabán T, Saira HN, Kemper N. Identifying opportunities for workflow automation in health care: lessons learned from other industries. Appl Clin Inform 2021;12(03):686–97. Georg Thieme Verlag KG.

Zheng K, Haftel HM, Hirschl RB, O'Reilly M, Hanauer DA. Quantifying the impact of health IT implementations on clinical workflow: a new methodological perspective. J Am Med Inform Assoc: JAMIA. 2010;17(4):454–61.

Chapter 7
A Workflow Perspective in Aviation

Guy André Boy

7.1 Introduction

Air traffic control (ATC) is shifting toward air traffic management (ATM), where systems and people are immersed in massive software. Workflow is changing because people and systems interact differently, using different cognitive and socio-cognitive processes and functions. Digitalization of the airspace logically leads to other kinds of function allocation.

Since the 1980s, we have consistently pursued the automation of aeronautical systems. Consequently, flying has become more cognitive, moving pilots' cognitive functions from doing to thinking. Today, automation in aviation should be better-called digitalization of air-ground socio-technical systems. Digitalization of the airspace is looking for the right mix of technology, organization, and people's activities that should be concurrently designed and tested to discover emergent patterns that should be incrementally considered.

The massive use of information technology in aviation led to drastic innovations. The main reasons why automation and innovation have been and still are drivers of aviation evolution are a constant increase[1] in the number of aircraft that causes congested networks, higher air traffic complexity, unpredictable delays, and other things that result in severe congestion at critical airports, rising fuel costs, and pollution.

Aircraft cockpits were significantly transformed during the 1980s, involving the development of many embedded systems. The digitalization of aircraft systems

---

[1] This increase was exponential until the COVID period. In March 2023, total air traffic was 88.0% (total domestic air traffic at 98.9%) of March 2019 levels, according to the International Air Transportation Association (https://www.iata.org/en/pressroom/2023-releases/2023-05-04-01).

G. A. Boy (✉)
CentraleSupélec (Paris Saclay University), ESTIA Institute of Technology, Bidart, France
e-mail: guy-andre.boy@centralesupelec.fr

© The Author(s), under exclusive license to Springer Nature Switzerland AG 2025
K. Zheng et al. (eds.), *Reengineering Clinical Workflow in the Digital and AI Era*,
Cognitive Informatics in Biomedicine and Healthcare,
https://doi.org/10.1007/978-3-031-82971-0_7

increased the need for cognitive engineering developments, especially in the digital-ization of commercial aircraft cockpits. More specifically, flying tasks evolved from manual mechanical control to the management of embedded systems.

Likewise, air traffic has moved from control to management. Two significant programs have considered this shift for over two decades: SESAR in Europe (Single European Sky ATM Research) and NextGen (Next Generation Air Transportation System) in the USA. The main goal was to understand better new airspace manage-ment models that consider traffic growth, safety constraints, and capacity manage-ment toward appropriate human systems integration of new multi-agent systems and teams of teams.

Automation in aviation is not new. Autopilots were introduced in commercial avia-tion in the 1930s (e.g., the Boeing 247 commercial aircraft flew with an autopilot in 1933). However, we learned much from aircraft automation during the last three decades of the twentieth century, especially shifting from analog to digital automa-tion. Anytime we automate, we rigidify tasks and, therefore, activities. Automated systems are very context-dependent (i.e., they work fine when operated in well-known contexts but may be dysfunctional outside of them).

The digitalization of embedded systems made us evolve toward cyber-physical systems (CPSs) and the Internet of Things (IoT). We then deal with much larger systems of systems (SoS) requiring new investigation types. More specifically, such new systems, including people and machines, become more autonomous in broader contexts, which must be further understood and subsequently defined. This evolu-tion from automation to autonomy requires that we emphasize flexibility issues. More specifically, if automation is associated with rigidity (i.e., procedure-based), autonomy should be associated with flexibility (i.e., problem-solving-based), where people should be considered at the center (Boy, 2023).

In this chapter, following up our human-centered design (HCD) approach combined with systems engineering, we will provide a human systems integration (HSI) approach rather than the classical corrective human factors and ergonomics (HFE) solutions. This will give us a basis for comparing aviation and healthcare evolutions. A discussion will be started. We will conclude and provide perspectives.

7.2   Using the AUTOS Pyramid to Support Workflow Analysis

Workflow evolved concerning technology (more specifically, automation), organi-zation (in commercial aircraft, we moved from 5 technical crewmembers during the fifties to 4, then 3, and 2 at the beginning of the 1980s), and jobs (different kinds of functions changed drastically because systems were able to execute tasks that were performed by people before).

A typical flight is divided into phases, sub-phases, and so on. For example, after passenger boarding, there is the taxi phase, then the runway rolling phase (before takeoff), takeoff, after takeoff, initial climb, climb, cruise, and so on. These phases are contextual patterns that determine the appropriate set of tasks. To define workflow patterns, we use the AUTOS pyramid for each contextual pattern, which can be normal, abnormal, or emergency.

The AUTOS pyramid was first introduced in HCD as the AUTO tetrahedron (Boy, 1998) to help relate four entities: Artifact (i.e., system), User, Task, and Organizational environment. We subsequently added contextual patterns, called "Situations," representing the various possible events where the artifact could be used (Boy, 2011). The AUTOS pyramid supports HSI, ensuring that all important entities (i.e., Artifacts, Users, Tasks, Organizations, and Situations) are considered, as well as their properties and interconnections (provided on the edges of the pyramid).

7.2.1   Artifacts, Users, and Tasks

An artifact is anything that people build. In this chapter, artifacts will denote systems. A system is a set of interconnected components (i.e., physical parts) and procedures (i.e., software parts) forming a complex whole that is intended to be useful for doing something. For example, artifacts may be aircraft, avionics systems, devices, and components of these systems. Artifacts are often integrated sets of existing technology. Sometimes, they are made of brand-new technology. Here is a short list of interactive artifacts: force feedback, loudspeakers, screens, signals, buttons, keyboard, joystick, mouse, trackball, microphone, 3D mouse, data suit (or interactive seat), metaphor for interaction, visual rendering, 3D sound rendering, 3D geometrical model and so on. These artifacts are usually integrated with mechanical artifacts such as pipes, containers, engines, pressurizers, turbines, flaps, slats, wheels, brakes, etc.

Users may be novices, experienced personnel, or experts from and evolving in various cultures (e.g., pilots, air traffic controllers, dispatchers). They may be tired, stressed, making errors, old or young, and in good shape and mood. HFE was required during the last five decades in the context of technology-centered engineering, generating the necessity of compensating human inadaptation by developing user interfaces and operational procedures and, therefore, adapting people to machines.

Tasks vary from handling quality control, flight management, managing a passenger cabin, repairing, designing, supplying, or managing a team or an organization. Each task involves one or several cognitive functions that users must learn and use. The AUT triangle (Fig. 7.1) enables the explanation of three edges: task and activity analysis (U-T), information requirements and technological limitations (T-A), and ergonomics and training (procedures) (A-U).

Today, almost any system includes software that mediates user intentions and provides appropriate feedback. Automation introduces constraints and, as already said, more rigidity. End-users do not have the final action (automation does). They need to plan more than in the past. Work becomes more cognitive and (artificially) social, i.e., new social activities must be performed for the other relevant actors to do

Fig. 7.1 The AUT triangle

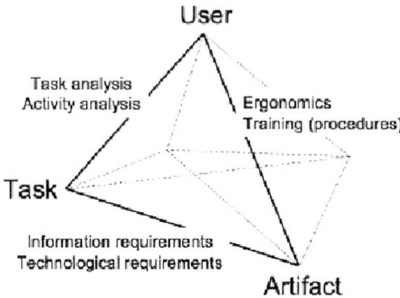

their jobs appropriately. This becomes more obvious when cognition is distributed among many human and machine agents.

Cockpits were incrementally shaped to human anthropometrical requirements to ease the manipulation of the various instruments. This, of course, is always strongly related to technology limitations. Anthropometry developed its language and methods. It is now actively used in design to define workspaces according to human factors such as accommodation, compatibility, operability, and maintainability by the user population. Workspaces are generally designed for 90% to 95% coverage of the user population. Anthropometric databases are constantly maintained to provide appropriate information to designers and engineers. Nevertheless, designers and engineers must be guided to use these databases to make appropriate choices.

Fatigue is a major concern in aviation and strongly depends on work organization. Therefore, it is important to know about circadian rhythms and how people adapt to shift work and long work hours, for example. Consequences are intimately associated with health and safety risks. Fatigue studies provide more knowledge and know-how on proceeding with work time schedules, appropriate training, systematic checks, and health indicators. Of course, this needs to be integrated into regulatory procedures. Useful information can be found in the Handbook of Human–Machine Interaction (Gander et al., 2011).

In aviation, cognitive factors start with workload assessment. This statement may seem restrictive and old-fashioned, but the reader should think twice about workload before starting any work in human factors. On one side, workload is a very difficult concept to define. It is both an output of human performance and a necessary input to optimize performance, i.e., we produce workload to perform better, up to a point where we need to change our work strategy. On the other side, we need to figure out a model that would quantify the degree of load a human being produces while working. Of course, this model should be based on real measurements performed on the human being. Many workload models have been proposed and used in aviation (Bainbridge, 1978; Hart, 1982; Boy & Tessier, 1985). Workload also deals with the complexity of the task being performed. People can do several things simultaneously, in parallel; this involves using several different peripheral resources simultaneously (Wickens, 1992). Sperandio (1980) studied the way air traffic controllers handle several aircraft at the same time and showed that the time spent on radio increased with the number of aircraft being controlled: 18% of their time spent in radio communication for one controlled aircraft, whereas 87% for nine aircraft controlled in parallel. Sperandio showed that task complexity increases human operator efficiency until the workload is unacceptable, forcing controllers to change strategy.

Human–machine interaction moves into human systems cooperation when systems become more autonomous—note that systems may include people. In this case, it is more appropriate to talk about agent-agent cooperation. Hoc and Lemoine studied dynamic task allocation (DTA) of conflict resolution between aircraft in air traffic control on a large-scale simulator. The more assistance, the more anticipative the mode of operation in controllers and the easier the human–human cooperation (HHC). These positive effects of computer support are interpreted in terms of decreased workload and increased shared information space (Hoc & Lemoine, 1998).

Situation awareness (SA) is another useful concept to introduce here, especially as a potential indicator for safety in highly automated human–machine systems. During the last decades, many efforts have been made to assess SA, such as the Situation Awareness Global Assessment Technique (SAGAT) (Endsley, 1988, 1996). Several efforts have been developed to assess SA in the aeronautics domain (Mogford, 1997); the main problem is characterizing the influence of action on situation awareness. Indeed, human operator's actions are always situated, especially in life-critical environments, and SA does not mean the same when actions are intentional as when they are reactive. This is an important issue in human–machine interaction since actions are always intentional (deliberative) and reactive because they are mainly performed in a closed loop (Boy, 2015).

7.2.2   Considering Organizations in Design

The Orchestra model was proposed in aviation to understand better authority sharing (Boy & Grote, 2009; Boy, 2013). Technological design requires multidisciplinary design teams (i.e., a design team must include people with related backgrounds, competence, and experience on each of these relevant artifacts incrementally integrated). In addition, design team members need to understand each other (i.e., they need to be able to read the same music theory, even if they do have the same scores). They must be appropriately coordinated at the task level (i.e., scores need to be harmonized by a composer) and the activity level (i.e., design team members, as musicians, need to be coordinated by a conductor at performance time).

An organizational environment for design includes not only all design team players (i.e., human agents) but also technological means (i.e., system agents). At this point, human systems integration is not only for the sake of the product but also for the design team itself. For this reason, design cards constitute useful support (Boy, 2013). Considering organizations in design introduces three additional edges (Fig. 7.2): social issues (U–O), role and job analyses (T-O), and emergence and evolution (A-O).

Fig. 7.2 The AUTO
tetrahedron

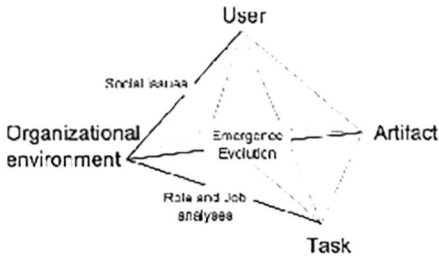

Two research fields have grown independently for the last three decades: aviation crew resource management (CRM) and computer-supported cooperative (CSCW) work in HCI. The former was motivated by the social micro-world of aircraft cockpits, where pilots need to cooperate and coordinate to fly safely and efficiently. CRM started during a workshop on *resource management on the flight deck* sponsored by NASA in 1979 (Cooper et al. 1980). At that time, the motivation was the correlation between air crashes and human errors as failures of interpersonal communications, decision-making, and leadership (Helmreich et al., 1999). CRM training was developed within airlines to change the attitudes and behavior of flight crews. CRM deals with the personalities of the various human agents involved in work situations and is mainly focused on teaching, i.e., each agent learns to understand his or her personality better to improve the overall cooperation and coordination of the working group. The same issues should be considered in design teams, and solutions should be incrementally implemented and evaluated.

Interaction is also influenced by the organizational environment around human(s) and system(s). More explicitly, HSI could focus on someone facing his/her laptop writing a paper; it could also be someone driving a car with passengers; it could be focused on an air traffic management system that includes pilots, controllers, and various aviation systems. People can now interact with computerized systems or with other people via computerized systems. We recently put to the front authority as a major HCD concept. When a system or other parties do the job, or part of the job, for someone, there is delegation. What is delegated? Is it the task? Is it the authority in the execution of this task? By authority, we mean accountability (responsibility) and control. Such questions should find answers within the design team both analytically and experimentally through human-in-the-loop simulations (HITLS).

Organizational complexity is linked to social cognition, agent-network complexity, and, more generally, multi-agent management issues. There are four principles for multi-agent management: agent activity (i.e., what the other agent is doing now and for how long); agent activity history (i.e., what the other agent has done); agent activity rationale (i.e., why the other agent is doing what it does); and agent activity intention (i.e., what the other agent is going to do next and when). Multi-agent management must be understood through a role (and job) analysis. O-factors mainly deal with the required *coupling* between the various purposeful agents to handle the new artifact.

Fig. 7.3 The AUTOS
pyramid

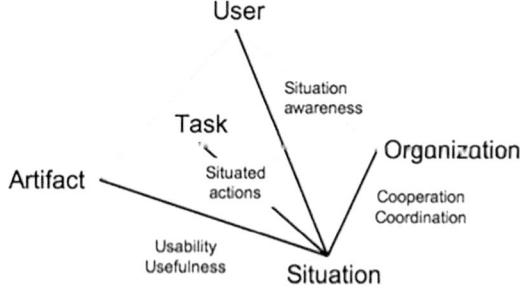

7.2.3   *Testing in a Large Variety of Situations*

The AUTOS framework (Fig. 7.3) is an extension of the AUTO tetrahedron that introduces a new dimension, the "Situation," which was implicitly included in the "Organizational environment." The three new edges are usability/usefulness (A-S), situation awareness (U-S), situated actions (T-S), and cooperation/coordination (O-S).

Interaction depends on the situation where it takes place. Situations could be normal or abnormal. They could even be emergencies. This is why we will emphasize the scenario-based approach to design and engineering. The resulting methods are based on descriptions of people using technology to understand better how this technology is or could be used to redefine their activities. Scenarios can be created early during design and incrementally modified to support product construction and refinement.

Scenarios are good for identifying functions at design time and operations time. They tend to rationalize the way the various agents interact with each other. They enable the definition of organizational configurations and time-wise chronologies.

Situation complexity is often caused by interruptions and, more generally, disturbances. It involves safety and high workload situations. Decomposing contexts commonly analyze it into sub-contexts. The situation is characterized by uncertainty, unpredictability, and various abnormalities within each sub-context. To summarize, situational factors deal with the *predictability* and *appropriate completeness* (scenario representativeness) of the various situations in which the new artifact will be used.

7.2.4   *Using the AUTOS Pyramid in Practice*

Software is very easy to modify. Consequently, design teams develop prototypes that they modify all the time! Interaction is not only a matter of product but also of the agile development process. End-users are not the only ones to interact with a delivered product; designers and engineers also interact with the product to fix it up toward maturity… even after its delivery. This is why agile approaches based on design cards (Boy, 2016) are extremely useful and effective (Schwaber, 1997; Sutherland, 2014). In addition, scenario-based design is an HCD approach that fosters understandability (situation awareness), complexity, reliability, maturity, and induced organizational constraints (rigidity versus flexibility).

Software complexity can be split into internal complexity (or system complexity) and interface complexity. Internal complexity is related to the degree of explanation required for the user to understand what is going on when necessary. Concepts related to system complexity are flexibility (both system flexibility and flexibility of use), system maturity (before getting mature, a system is an accumulation of functions —the "another function syndrome"—and it becomes mature through a series of articulations and integrations); automation (linked to the level of operational assistance, authority delegation, and automation culture); and operational documentation. Technical documentation complexity is directly linked to the explanation of artifact complexity. Technical documentation or performance support is required to provide appropriate assistance at the right time in the right format when the system is hard to use.

What should we understand when we use a product? How does it work? How should it be used? At what level of depth should we go inside the product to use it appropriately? In the early ages of the car industry, most car drivers were also mechanics because when they had a problem, they needed to fix it by themselves; the technology was too new to have specialized people. These drivers were highly skilled engineers, both generalists and specialists in cars. Today, things have drastically changed; drivers are no longer knowledgeable and skilled to fix cars; some specialists do this job because software is far too complex to understand without appropriate help. Recent evolution transformed the job of mechanics into system engineers who know how to use specialized software that enables them to diagnose and fix failures. They can partially understand what is happening inside the engine; a software program does it for them and explains problems to them when the system is well-designed. This would be the ideal case; in practice, most problems come from organizational and situational factors induced by such technology (e.g., appropriate people may need to be available at the right time to fix problems when they arise).

Interface complexity is characterized by content management, information density, and ergonomics rules. Content management is, in particular, linked to information relevance, alarm management, and display content management. Information density is linked to decluttering (Doyon-Poulin et al., 2014), information modality, diversity, and information-limited attractors, i.e., objects on the instrument or display that are poorly informative for the execution of the task but attract user's attention. The "PC screen do-it-all syndrome" is a good indicator of information density (elicited improvement factors were screen size and zooming). Redundancy is always a good rule whether it repeats information for crosschecking, confirmation or comfort or by explaining the "how," "where," and "when" action can be performed. Ergonomics rules formalize user-friendliness, i.e., consistency, customization, human reliability, affordances, feedback, visibility, and appropriateness of involved cognitive functions.

Task complexity involves procedure adequacy, appropriate multi-agent coopera-tion (e.g., air-ground coupling in the aerospace domain), and rapid prototyping (i.e., task complexity can only be properly understood if the resulting activity of agents involved is observable). Task complexity is linked to the number of sub-tasks, task difficulty, induced risk, consistency (lexical, syntactic, semantic, and pragmatic), and the temporal dimension (perception–action frequency and time pressure in partic-ular). Task complexity is due to operations maturity, delegation, and mode manage-ment. Mode management is related to role analysis. To summarize, T-factors mainly deal with *task difficulty* according to a spectrum from best practice to well-identified categories of tasks.

Remember that CFA requires HITLS to observe the activity. Activity analysis could be defined as identifying and describing activities in an organization and eval-uating their impact on its operations. Activity analysis determines (1) what activities are executed, (2) how many people perform the activities, (3) how much time they spend on them, (4) how much and which resources are consumed, (5) what opera-tional data best reflects the performance of activities, and (6) how much value these activities provide to the organization. This analysis is accomplished through direct observation, interviews, questionnaires, and review of the work records addressed to users of prototypes at different stages of design and development.

7.3   Cockpit Evolution: From Control to Management

Twentieth-century engineering was dominated by mechanical engineering. Engi-neers built washing machines, trains, cars, airplanes, and power plants by assem-bling mechanical things. Over the past four decades, computing and information technologies have massively penetrated mechanical machines, gradually creating systems comprising physical hardware and cognitive software. Everything started with the automation around the center of gravity using a yoke or side stick and thrust levers (Fig. 7.4). Early embedded systems were single agents regulating parameters such as speed and heading, one parameter at a time. The feedback time constant was around 500 ms. Pilots have had to adapt to this embedded system, switching from controlling flight parameters to supervising the behavior of the embedded system assigned to a set point.

The guidance system was developed circa the early eighties (Fig. 7.5). This second feedback loop took into account several parameters. Its time constant was around 15 s. Note that this feedback loop was implemented on top of the trajectory control system. High-level automation modes were introduced and managed on the flight control unit panel. At the same time, an integrated digital autopilot and automatic throttle control were installed.

The third embedded system concerned navigation automation, with a time constant of around one minute (Fig. 7.6). Guidance and flight management became integrated. This was the first real revolution in the evolution of aeronautical embedded systems. We were shifting from control of flight parameters to management of

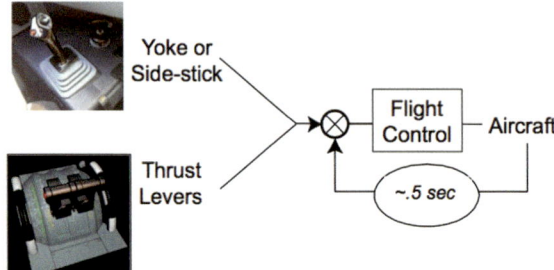

Fig. 7.4 Trajectory control embedded system: flying around the center of gravity[2]

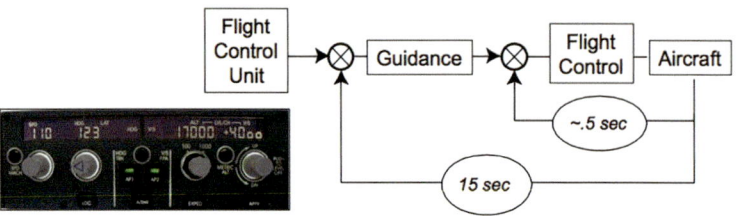

Fig. 7.5 Guidance embedded system: guiding on the basic trajectory

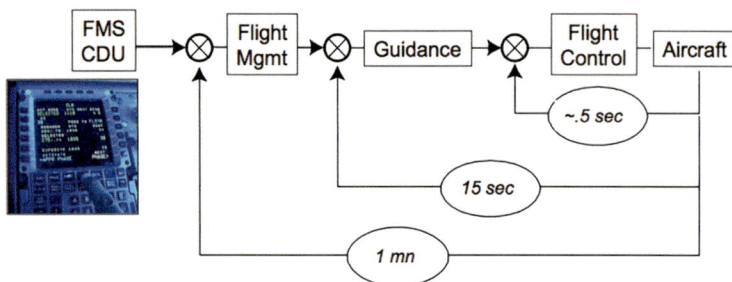

Fig. 7.6 Navigation automation loop: guiding the flight plan

embedded systems. Software became dominant, and the number of artificial agents on aircraft grew exponentially. For that matter, pilots have now to deal with a variety of embedded systems that are not only humans but also software-based agents. Problems may emerge when these software-based agents communicate with each other. This issue will be analyzed later in the chapter.

People increase their performance by extending their capabilities with appropriate embedded systems called "cognitive prostheses" (Hamilton, 2001). However, if these cognitive prostheses use automation to a point that is not clearly understood from an

---

[2] The 4-loop approach to the evolution of aeronautical automation was inspired by Captain Etienne Tarnowski during a keynote he gave at HCI-Aero'06, Seattle, USA.

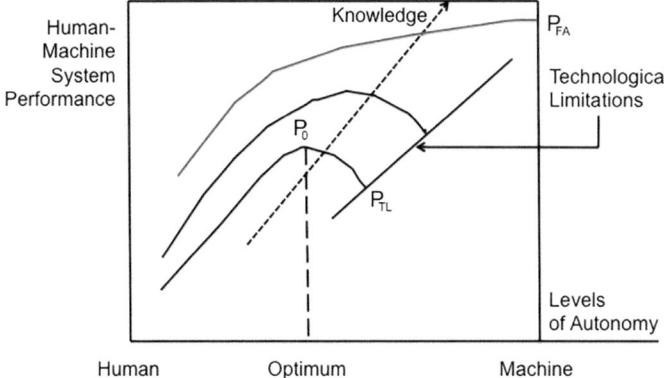

Fig. 7.7 Human–machine system performance versus levels of autonomy (adaptation of boy's NASA technical document, 1988)

operational standpoint, performance may decrease and, in some cases, cause serious problems. Earl Wiener called this "clumsy automation" (Wiener, 1989). When I was working on the Orbital Refueling System of the Space Shuttle in the mid-eighties (Boy, 1987), I found out that there is an optimum P_0 in terms of autonomy level and performance of the overall human–machine system (Fig. 7.7).

Technology-centered engineering typically automates at the point P_{TL} (i.e., on the technological limitations limit). It takes experimental tests and efforts to go back to P_0. HCD considers the existence of P_0 and incrementally tries to find this optimum through creative design and formative evaluation using HITLS. Interestingly, the more we know about the autonomy of the various human and machine agents, the more the optimum P_0 moves to the right and goes up in Fig. 7.7. Of course, if we knew everything about the environment and the agents involved in the various interactions, the optimum P_{FA} would be on the full autonomy of the machine (e.g., in the case of an aircraft, P_{FA} would correspond to a drone).

This shift of optimum P_0 to the right is strongly related to maturity. In HCD, we distinguish between technology maturity and maturity of practice—the former deals with the reliability, availability, and robustness of the technology being designed and developed. The latter deals with people's adaptation to and resilience to the resulting socio-technical system; often, new practices emerge from technology use. We then need to observe usage as early as possible to anticipate surprises before it is too late. HCD proposes methods and tools that enable HCD teams to detect these emergent properties at design time (e.g., using HITLS). In any case, a maturity period is required to assess whether a product can be delivered.

7.4 Organizational Automation and Management

We have seen that the pilot's job moved from control of flight parameters to management of embedded systems during the 1980s. This job revolution in the cockpit is now shifting to air traffic (i.e., air traffic control is moving toward air traffic management). In other words, a single agent's shift from control to management evolves into a multi-agent shift. Why? What are the underlying organizational issues?

The main cause is the number increase effect. According to Boeing's Current Market Outlook 2014–2033, average airline traffic yearly growth is estimated at a rate of 5%. Knowing that most big airports, such as Hartsfield–Jackson Atlanta International Airport, are already over-saturated, the air traffic capacity issue requires complexity science approaches, specifically multi-agent, where agents are aircraft. Connectivity among these agents has to become explicit. If aircraft separation must be reduced during approach and landing, for example, current human-centered air traffic control techniques must be revisited and, in many cases, drastically changed. This is a matter of technology, organizations, and people. On the technology side of the problem to be solved, each aircraft should know about the location and identity of the other aircraft around it. Aircraft should have appropriate sensors and receptors, such as the Automatic Dependence Surveillance–Broadcast (ADS-B) system. Satellite data must be used to identify a clear, dynamic sky model regarding traffic and weather. We can also use weather radar data from all aircraft and fuse them with satellite data to increase the 3D validity of weather models. The same fusion can be done for air traffic using more conventional radar system data. The resulting data can be used to develop an embedded system providing each aircraft with a protection safety net (i.e., each aircraft knows the traffic around it and can decide tactical maneuvers to increase global safety). The protection safety net of each aircraft is an embedded system related to other aircraft equivalents and a coordination ground system that orchestrates the overall traffic.

This approach defines a new kind of organizational automation, which is multi-agent. This multi-agent approach involves interaction among people and systems, among systems, and people (often through information technology). Since there will be a layer of information technology gluing the various air and ground systems, new factors, such as cyber-security, are emerging. Air traffic management of the future will be almost entirely based on highly interconnected cyber-physical systems (CPSs). New kinds of risks will emerge from the activity of this giant airspace CPS-based infrastructure. Malicious actors can attack these systems from anywhere in the world. Consequently, we need to develop further methods and tools to study the security and resilience of such CPS-based infrastructure and find appropriate solutions. Protection will have to be found from technology (safety and security nets), organizations (collaboration among agents), and people (increasing training and expertise).

Air-ground integration is an example of a human systems integration perspective involving function allocation. Since Fitts's law provided the HABA-MABA[3] recommendations for single-agent function allocation, very little has been done on multi-agent function allocation. Function allocation rationale is determining which functions should be carried out by humans and by machines (Fitts, 1951). Cognitive function analysis (CFA) is an effective approach to this problem in a multi-agent environment (Boy, 1998, 2011). CFA also includes physical functions (remember that a cognitive function is defined by a set of resources that may be cognitive and/or physical functions). In addition, the Orchestra model (Boy, 2013) provides a very useful framework to model and simulate the resulting cognitive functions of the human system being developed. Consequently, the agent needs to be further modeled regarding cognitive and physical functions and how they are inter-connected—this is typically doing a CFA. CFA results can be presented as a cognitive/physical function network (or interactive map), which supports studying interaction complexity, distributed situation awareness, and multi-agent decision-making.

7.5 Starting a Discussion

7.5.1 Tangibility

In the beginning of the twenty-first century, embedded systems are reframing the structure–function duality. Instead of functionalizing structures to create automated machines (the twentieth century approach), we are now physically structuralizing software functions. Therefore, automation problems, which were created during the last decades of the twentieth century, are no longer the main issue because software can be tested from the early days of the design process using advanced virtual engineering, making HCD possible (i.e., taking into account human factors at design time). Cognitive function analysis can be validated because activity can be observed in HITLS using virtual prototypes and real users in addition to task analysis. Consequently, early solid function analyses can nurture technological and organizational requirements.

The main issue has then become structure and, therefore, tangibility. Since almost everything can be modeled and simulated on computers, and we now have 3D printing, the structure can be easily obtained. Traditionally, in aeronautics, this was considered by flight tests. This is needed for the validation of any life-critical system. The right balance between cognitive and physical functions should be tested, and between abstractions and physical structures. Tangibility needs to be tested in terms of physical tangibility and figurative tangibility. The former is based on criteria such as simple reachability, complex accessibility, fatigue, noise management, resource availability, and so on. The latter is based on criteria such as monitoring, situation

---

[3] Fitts's HABA-MABA (humans-are-better-at/machines-are-better-at) approach provided generic strengths and weaknesses of humans and machines.

awareness, decision-making, risk-taking, and so on. Of course, these criteria can be detailed concerning the level of granularity required at the current stage of the design process. If digital HITLS at design time contributes to developing more appropriate HSI requirements, effectiveness, and cost, it does not remove the need for actual flight tests once the real system is developed.

7.5.2   Maturity

Much effort and money have been spent to increase system reliability, contributing to aviation safety. As already said, the safety of the future ATM involves increased attention to interactions among its various agents. The qualification of these "new" agents is an issue that concerns this investigation on authority sharing. We want to go beyond the safety-reliability discussion and propose to focus on maturity.

Since the general trend is to manage short-term benefits instead of long-term sustainability, it is common that we currently need to observe a discrepancy in the provision and qualification of human operators. Since human reliability remains critical, the situation will worsen if human operators are even less available and qualified. We are beginning to understand that human factors issues are no longer the result of engineering decisions but economically induced decisions.

Therefore, if we want to keep or improve the current level of safety with an increase in airspace capacity, some drastic changes will need to be made in understanding and managing technology and organizations. Safety–critical systems should be mature for safe use when delivered. The concept of maturity could be misleading because we already have the quality-based Capacity Maturity Model (Paulk et al., 1993) that supports the maturity of manufacturing processes. We are interested in product and practice maturity. Product maturity requires a strong focus on human-centered high-level requirements, as well as participatory design and development all along the life cycle of the product (Boy, 2005). Product maturity engineering involves carefully eliciting the attributes that shape the related maturity of practice. Maturity of practice is reached when a reasonable number of surprises or emerging factors have been identified and associated causes fixed. Product maturity engineering addresses the long-term and is inappropriate for current economy-driven organizations' short-term goals and practices. It should be!

During the early stages of a development process, such as the ATM of the future, the participation of the various representative actors is mandatory. This participatory approach requires that pilots and controllers (i.e., end-users and musicians) and designers and regulators (i.e., the music instrument makers and composers), share a common frame of reference. In addition, the job definitions process must be revised and planned since we know that initial definitions will have to be changed all along the life cycle of the overall ATM development process. Consequently, authority distribution for the design of the various instruments (this is where HCI specialists enter into play) is a matter of incremental development and testing. In PAUSA, we took a scenario-based approach (Carroll, 1995) to carry out such an authority distribution supported by the development of human factors principles and criteria, socio-technical models, and HITLS.

The growing number of interdependencies among ATM agents led us to propose a measure of socio-cognitive stability (SCS) derived from various contributions, including Latour's account on socio-technical stability (Callon, 1991; Latour, 1987), emerging cognitive functions (Boy, 1998), distributed cognition (Hutchins, 1995), and socio-cognitive research and engineering (Hemingway, 1999; Sharples et al., 2002). We make a distinction between local and global SCS. Local SCS is related to the agent's workload, situation awareness, ability to make appropriate decisions, and correct action execution. Appropriate redundancies and cognitive support such as trends, relevant situational information, and possible actions can support it. Global SCS is concerned with the appropriateness of functions allocated to agents, the pace of information flows, and related coordination. It is very similar to the level of synchronization of rhythms in a symphony. Globally, socio-cognitive support could be found in a safety net considering the evolution of interacting agents and proposing a constraining safety envelope in real-time.

Three kinds of metrics have been deduced during the PAUSA project:

- **Complexity** is the number of relevant aircraft managed per appropriate volumetric zone (AVZ) at each time. An AVZ is calculated concerning the type of flow pattern, e.g., aircraft crossing, spacing, and merging. The definition of such an appropriate volumetric zone requires the assistance of operational ATC controllers. From a socio-cognitive perspective in ATM, complexity should be considered together with capacity. This is what the COCA (COmplexity & CApacity) project investigated (Athènes et al., 2002; Cummings & Tsonis, 2006; Hilburn, 2004; Laudeman et al., 1998; Leveson et al., 2009).
- **Time pressure criticality** is the workload that an agent (or a group of agents) requires to stabilize an ATM system after a disturbance. Such workload measure could be assessed as the ratio between the required times for each action and the total available time (Boy, 1983).
- **Flexibility** is defined as the ease of real-time modification of an air-ground contract. Flexibility assessments should guide ATM human-centered automation and organizational setting. Overall, increasing capacity also increases complexity and uncertainty, which must be managed by finding the right balance between reducing uncertainties through centralized planning and coping with uncertainties through decentralized action. Loose coupling requires actors to use their autonomy by system goals (Grote, 2004).

This chapter was written to provide salient workflow aspects and evolutions of human systems integration in aviation. How can we compare these aspects and evolutions with those in healthcare? Can an increase in the number of aircraft be compared to a rise in the number of patients? For sure, complexity analysis is required in both domains. Of course, we cannot substitute aircraft for patients! However, the need for dispatch is similar. In aviation, interconnectivity among various kinds of aircraft must always be considered along with attributes such as long-haul flights, failures, aircraft size, and performance. The same could said in healthcare; interconnectivity among various kinds of patients must always be considered along with attributes such as the seriousness of their health.

Time pressure criticality is also a factor shared by aviation and healthcare, as all in life-critical systems. We tend to plan trajectories (i.e., 4D trajectories), leading to trajectory-based operations (TBO). However, this works fine in normal situations but may fail in abnormal and emergencies where procedure-based planning rigidity becomes an obstacle to problem-solving flexibility requirements. This involves human skills and knowledge not only on basic flying capabilities but also embedded systems and their capabilities. This is why organizational automation, especially workflow automation, should be developed considering appropriate function allocation. Cognitive function analysis is strongly advised.

7.6   Conclusion and Perspectives

Workflow design and management require systems' functions and structures to be articulated correctly. The first difficulty comes from system complexity (i.e., systems of systems, teams of teams, several critical attributes to be considered, emergent phenomena, and properties to be incrementally elicited and re-injected into the overall system). Identifying non-linear processes and bottlenecks (bifurcations in the complexity science sense). For that matter, the AUTOS pyramid and cognitive function analysis greatly supported the analysis, design, and evaluation of highly automated systems in aviation. We started to automate aircraft, and we are now automating air traffic. The actual shift is from rigid (low-level) automation to flexible (high-level) autonomy, where authority sharing has to be considered seriously (i.e., who is in charge and accountable to whom).

The socio-technical evolution of aviation systems has produced excellent results in the exponential decrease in accident fatalities since the 1980s toward zero.[4] This evolution includes automation (now digitalization), regulations, and a unique safety culture. However, digitalization has become the most crucial aviation human systems integration issue. Software is easy to modify but involves us in a virtual world where new phenomena emerge, such as cybersecurity. The good news is that we can carry out HCD development very early during the life cycle of a system (i.e., activity and function analyses can be performed very early using human-in-the-loop simulations) and discover emergent behaviors and properties of the underlying socio-technical system sooner than before. The counterpart is that tangibility testing remains the highest priority (i.e., physical tangibility regarding structures and figurative tangibility regarding functions). The tangibility issue is inherent to digital engineering. Whether in aviation or healthcare, it must be addressed during the whole life cycle of

---

[4] "Airlines recorded zero accident deaths in commercial passenger jets last year, according to a Dutch consulting firm and an aviation safety group that tracks crashes, making 2017 the safest year on record for commercial air travel" (https://www.reuters.com/article/us-aviation-safety/2017-saf est-year-on-record-for-commercial-passenger-air-travel-groups-idUSKBN1EQ17L).

a socio-technical system. More generally, human systems integration is an emerging socio-technical system field at the intersection of three primary disciplines: systems engineering, human factors and ergonomics, and information technology (Boy & Kennedy, 2023; Boy 2023).

References

Athènes S, Averty P, Puechmorel S, Delahaye D, Collet C. ATC complexity and controller workload: trying to bridge the gap. In: Hansman J, Chatty S, Boy G, editors. Proceedings of HCI-Aero'02. Boston (USA). 2002.

Bainbridge L. Forgotten alternatives in skill and workload. Ergonomics. 1978;21:169–85.

Boy GA. Operator assistant systems. Int J Man Mach Studies. 1987;27:541–54.

Boy GA, Grote G. Authority in increasingly complex human and machine collaborative systems: application to the future air traffic management construction. In: The proceedings of the 2009 international ergonomics association world congress, Beijing, China. 2009.

Boy GA. The MESSAGE system: a first step toward computer-supported analysis of human-machine interactions (in French). Le Trav Hum J. 1983;46(2).

Boy GA. Cognitive function analysis. Praeger/Ablex; ISBN 9781567503777. 1998.

Boy GA. Maturity, automation and user experience (Maturité, Automation et Experience des Utilisateurs). In: Proceeding of the French conference on human-computer interaction. New York: ACM-Press;2005.

Boy GA, editor. Handbook of human-machine interaction: a human-centered design approach. UK: Ashgate; 2011. ISBN: 978–0–7546–7580–8.

Boy GA. Orchestrating human-centered design. U.K: Springer; 2013. 978−1−4471−4338−3.

Boy GA. On the complexity of situation awareness. In: Proceedings 19th triennial congress of the IEA. Melbourne, Australia; 2015. p. 9–14.

Boy GA. Tangible interactive systems: grasping the real world with computers. U. K.: Springer; 2016. 978-3-319-30270-6.

Boy GA. An epistemological approach to human systems integration. Technol Soc J (Open Access). 2023;102298 https://doi.org/10.1016/j.techsoc.2023.102298.

Boy GA, Kennedy G, editors. Human systems integration primer volume one. San Diego, CA, USA: INCOSE; 2023. ISBN 978–1–937076–12–2.

Boy GA, Tessier C. Cockpit analysis and assessment by the MESSAGE methodology. In: Proceedings of the 2nd IFAC/IFIP/IFORS/IEA conference on analysis, design and evaluation of man-machine systems, Villa-Ponti, Italy, September 10–12. Oxford: Pergamon Press; 1985. pp. 73–79.

Callon M. Techno-economic networks and irreversibility. In: Law J, editor. A sociology of monsters: essays on power, technology and domination. London: Routledge; 1991. p. 132–61.

Carroll JM. Scenario-based design: envisioning work and technology in system development. New York: Wiley; 1995.

Cooper GE, White MD, Lauber JI. Resource management on the flight deck. In: Proceedings of a NASA/industry workshop held at San Francisco, California June 26–28, 1979. CA: NASA Conference Publication 2120, NASA Ames Research Center; 1980.

Cummings ML, Tsonis CG. Partitioning complexity in air traffic management tasks. Int J Aviat Psychol. 2006;16(3):277–295.

Doyon-Poulin P, Ouellette B, Robert JM. Effects of visual clutter on pilot workload, flight performance and gaze pattern. In: Proceedings of HCI-Aero 2014, Santa Clara, CA. Also in the ACM Digital Library; 2014.

Endsley MR. Automation and situation awareness. In: Parasuraman R, Mouloua M, editors. Automa-
    tion and human performance: theory and applications. Mahwah, NJ: Laurence Erlbaum; 1996.
    p. 163–81.
Endsley MR. Situation awareness global assessment technique (SAGAT). Paper presented at the
    National Aerospace and Electronic Conference (NAECON), Dayton, OH; 1988.
Fitts PM, editor. Human engineering for an effective air navigation and traffic control system.
    Washington, DC: National Research Council; 1951.
Gander P, Graeber C, Belenky G. Operator fatigue: implications for human-machine interaction. In:
    Handbook of human-machine interaction: a human-centered design approach. U.K: Ashgate;
    2011.
Grote G. Uncertainty management at the core of system design. Annu Rev Control. 2004;28:267–74.
Hamilton S. Thinking outside the box at the IHMC. IEEE Computer; 2001; 0018–9162/01, p. 61–71.
Hart SG. Theoretical basis for workload assessment. CA, USA: TM ADP001150, NASA-Ames
    Research Center, Moffett Field; 1982.
Helmreich RL, Merritt AC, Wilhelm JA. The evolution of crew resource management training in
    commercial aviation. Int J Aviat Psychol. 1999;9(1):19–32.
Hemingway CJ. Toward a socio-cognitive theory of information systems: an analysis of key philo-
    sophical and conceptual issues. In: IFIP WG 8.2 and 8.6 joint working conference on information
    systems: current issues and future changes. Helsinki, Finland: IFIP; 1999. p. 275–86.
Hilburn B. Cognitive complexity in air traffic control: a literature review. Project COCA-
    COmplexity and CApacity. EEC Note No. 04/04; 2004.
Hoc JM, Lemoine MP. Cognitive evaluation of human-human and human-machine cooperation
    modes in air traffic control. Int J Aviat Psychol. 1998;8(1):1–32.
Hutchins E. How a cockpit remembers its speeds. Cogn Sci. 1995;19:265–88.
Latour B. Science in action: how to follow scientists and engineers through society. Cambridge,
    MA: Harvard University Press; 1987.
Laudeman IV, Shelden SG, Branstrom R, Brasil CL. Dynamic density. an air traffic management
    metric. California: National Aeronautics and Space Administration, Ames Research Center,
    NASA/TM−1998–112226; 1998.
Leveson N, Dulac N, Marais K, Carroll J. Moving beyond normal accidents and high reliability
    organizations: a systems approach to safety in complex systems. Organ Stud (Sage Publishers).
    2009; 30(2–3).
Mogford RH. Mental models and situation awareness in air traffic control. Int J Aviat Psychol.
    1997;7(4):331–41.
Paulk M, Curtis B, Chrissis M, Weber C. Capability maturity model for software (Version 1.1).
    Technical Report
    CMU/SEI-93-TR-024. 1993.
Schwaber K. Scrum development process. In: Patel D, Casanave C, Miller J, Hollowell G, editors.
    OOPSLA business objects design and implementation workshop proceedings. London, U.K.:
    Springer; 1997.
Sharples M, Jeffery N, du Boulay JBH, Teather D, Teather B, du Boulay GH. Socio-cognitive
    engineering: a methodology for the design of human-centered technology. Eur J Oper Res.
    2002;136(2):310–23.
Sperandio JC. La psychologie en ergonomie (Psychology in ergonomics). Paris: PUF; 1980.
Sutherland J. Scrum: the art of doing twice the work in half the time. Crown Business; 2014.
    ISBN-13: 978–0385346450.
Wickens CD. Engineering psychology and human performance, 2nd ed. New York: Harper Collins
    Publishers Inc; 1992. ISBN: 0673461610.
Wiener EL. Human factors of advanced technology ("glass cockpit") transport aircraft. (NASA
    Contractor Report No. 177528). Moffett Field, CA: NASA-Ames Research Center; 1989.

Chapter 8
Expanding the Characterization of Collaborative Workflow and Health IT

Novia Wong, Craig E. Kuziemsky, Joanna Abraham, Keertana Nambiar, and Madhu C. Reddy

Abstract Despite increased calls for more team-based care delivery, it remains a challenge to implement it in practice. Health information technology (HIT) can support team-based care delivery, but there is currently a gap between the workflow of teams and the technology that we design to support it. To address this gap, we first formalize team-based workflows according to structural and behavioral aspects, including the emerging virtual workspaces. Then, we describe collaborative workflows, and considerations for HIT design to support collaborative workflows. HIT design for collaborative workflow goes beyond just automating the task at hand, as collaborative workflows are a social construction between data, people and processes; and we need to understand how these connections form and evolve before looking to technology to automate it. Collaborative workflows are not static, but rather are dynamic processes with clinical, social and system design implications. Growth of technologies like telehealth offer opportunities to expand team-based care into communities. However, there is no one size fits all model for HIT supported teamwork. HIT design for healthcare teams needs to be flexible so that it can be tailored for the setting and task at hand and also to evolve along with the collaborative processes that it is automating.

N. Wong · K. Nambiar · M. C. Reddy
Department of Informatics, School of Informatics and Computer Science, University of California, Irvine, CA, USA
e-mail: noviaw@uci.edu

K. Nambiar
e-mail: krnambia@uci.edu

M. C. Reddy
e-mail: mreddy@uci.edu

C. E. Kuziemsky (✉)
Office of Research Services, MacEwan University, Edmonton, AB, Canada
e-mail: kuziemskyC@macewan.ca

J. Abraham
Department of Anesthesiology and Institute for Informatics, School of Medicine, Washington University in St. Louis, St. Louis, MO, USA
e-mail: joannaa@wustl.edu

133

Keywords Healthcare teams · Collaboration · Structure · Behavior · Workflow

8.1 Introduction to Healthcare Teamwork

Health system factors such as an increased prevalence of chronic illness, an aging population, increased patient complexity and a strong desire for quality, safety, and coordination of care models have highlighted the need for team-based care delivery (Committee on Patient, Health Information, & Institute of Medicine 2011; Mitchell et al. 2012; Roett & Coleman 2013). The COVID-19 pandemic affirmed the need for increased team-based care delivery (Donnelly et al. 2021). However, it also highlighted existing and new challenges to implementing team-based care delivery models (Bates 2015; Zajac et al. 2021).

Teams can be broadly defined as "a distinguishable set of two or more people who interact dynamically, interdependently, and adaptively toward a common and valued goal/object/mission, who have each been assigned specific roles or functions to perform, and who have a limited life span of membership" (Salas et al. 1992). However, there are in fact many different ways by which teams can be characterized. Information behavior, organizational configuration, duration (e.g., long- vs short-term teams), modality of interaction (e.g., synchronous and asynchronous), individual actors (e.g., human and artificial intelligence, AI), and roles (e.g., primary care vs. supporting teams) are a few ways that teams have been classified (Nancarrow et al. 2013; Xyrichis & Ream 2008; Stowers et al. 2021; Onnasch & Roesler 2021). Despite these differences, a commonality is the need for different degrees of connectivity that varies according to the type of team and the context in which communication and coordination between team members occur.

8.2 Characterizing Healthcare Teams

There are many ways that healthcare teams can be characterized (Martin et al. 2022). The intent of this chapter is not to review all exciting types of classification but rather to characterize healthcare teams with respect to collaborative workflow and health information technology. Characterizing teams starts with its structure and a starting point is whether a team is composed of a singular type of providers (unidisciplinary team) or multiple provider types (multidisciplinary, interdisciplinary or transdisciplinary team). Teams consisting of multiple provider types can be further classified according to the manner in which team members interact with other team members when delivering care. In a *multidisciplinary* team, team members from different disciplines work on a common goal and share information accordingly, but each member stays within the boundaries of their own discipline as they work towards the shared goal (Choi & Pak 2006). Multidisciplinary teams are analogous to swim lanes in that each provider only engages in his/her own care delivery processes with little or no interaction across the lanes (Choi & Pak 2006; Martin et al. 2022). Surgical teams are a common example of multidisciplinary teams in which providers of each type are responsible for performing distinct and highly specialized tasks (Casimiro et al. 2015). In contrast, in an *interdisciplinary* team, team members work across disciplines (i.e., across the swim lanes) as engagement and communication between team members are necessary to accomplishing the team's shared goals. Interdisciplinary teams are common in complex care scenarios such as palliative care (Casimiro et al. 2015). Lastly, in a *transdisciplinary* team, team members are not bound to their disciplines, and may work across roles through shared goals and skill sets (Galvin et al. 2014; Hall et al. 2012). An example of a transdisciplinary team is in remote areas where all provider types may not be available and thus a provider, such as a nurse practitioner, may need to play multiple roles (e.g., dietician, therapist, etc.) when caring for patients.

Teams can also be characterized according to their life cycles and longevity of workflow. Some teams interact only for short durations (e.g., certain teams in the emergency room [ED]) where team is disbanded once the task at hand completes; while other teams (e.g. cancer care or chronic disease management teams) engage in workflows that may extend over months even years (Andreatta 2010; Tang et al. 2015; Rosen et al. 2018). Teams may be assembled with specific needs or ad-hoc workflows; and team personnel can also be characterized as being stable, or dynamic, and may work synchronously or asynchronously (Hollenbeck et al. 2012).

Teams are at times characterized by the degree of collaboration that their members engage in. While it is common to refer to healthcare teams as being 'collaborative,' collaboration is in fact a specific process that carries with it the implications for how a team should operate (Eikey et al. 2015; Reeves et al. 2017). Although collaboration is often used interchangeably with other terms such as communication, coordination and cooperation, collaboration is a distinctive process (Abraham & Reddy 2013) which refers to "planned or spontaneous engagements that take place between individuals or teams of individuals, whether in-person or mediated by technology, where information is exchanged in some way (either explicitly, i.e. verbally or written, or implicitly, i.e. through shared understanding of gestures, emotions, etc.), and often occur across different roles (i.e. physician and nurse) to deliver patient care" (Eikey et al. 2015) (p.263).

The social or behavioral aspects of healthcare teams are also significant (Vos et al. 2020). This is because teams often involve professionals from multiple disciplines and/or medical specialties who contribute with varying roles and responsibilities. For example, physicians are in charge of developing clinical diagnosis and treatment plan; nurses for carrying out the treatment plan; phlebotomists for drawing blood; lab technicians for analyzing patient samples; dieticians for making nutrition recommendations, etc. (Ellingson 2002) Hence, in order to achieve effective teamwork both within and across these various disciplines, all members of the team must demonstrate certain teamwork competencies (e.g. team knowledge, team skill and team attitude) (Baker et al. 2006; Nancarrow et al. 2013). When robotics and AI are integrated into healthcare teams as teammates, further complexities and challenges arise pertaining to social and behavioral aspects, such as trust and adaptability (Stowers et al. 2021).

Table 8.1 shows some of the key behavioral features of a team for ensuring effective teamwork (adapted from Baker et al. 2006).

Finally, teams can be categorized based on geographical and temporal distances. With the rising demands of telehealth and teleconsultation, healthcare teams have shifted to remote and hybrid (i.e., some individuals collaborate in-person while the others participate remotely) collaboration. They may consist of professionals from different countries and cultures (Presbitero 2020), as well as time zones (Morrison-Smith & Ruiz 2020). Healthcare teams, therefore, may experience a shift in leadership and role-expectations (Poitras et al. 2023; Tan et al. 2023). Technologies help mitigate some of these challenges and facilitate communication, leading to a stronger reliance on using technologies for collaborative activities for distributed teams (Morrison-Smith & Ruiz 2020; Belber et al. 2023).

8.3   Health Information Technology and Teams

Teamwork activities are detailed, demanding, time-critical, and collaborative. At the center of this work is the patient whose health is dependent on the effective coordination between physicians, nurses, pharmacists, and a large number of other healthcare roles. In the highly collaborative and information-intensive clinical environments, HIT systems play a crucial role in supporting teamwork activities. They have become an indispensable tool for maintaining communication necessary for the effective and efficient functioning of collaborative healthcare teams.

Table 8.1 highlights the range of structural, social, communicative and other supports needed to support teamwork. Patient care has grown more complex owing to many factors including innovative advances in therapeutics and treatments that allow patients with chronic illness to live longer and more productive lives than in the past. However, the health system innovations needed to support patient complexity, one example being support for team-based care, have not kept pace with clinical innovations (Kuziemsky 2019).

Given the distributed manner in which teams often work, HIT can play a significant role in supporting communication and cooperation between members of a care team. As described above, there is such variation in team structure that understanding the nature of team structure is an essential first step for the design and evaluation of HIT to support team-based care delivery. However, existing research has shown that there is often a gap between the collaborative work practices of teams and the HIT that we design to support them (Leslie et al. 2017; Rudin et al. 2016).

Early HIT systems were developed with a focus on individual users, despite the fact that they are used equally often, or even more often, to support healthcare teams (Berg 1999; Berg et al. 1998). For instance, the core function of electronic health records (EHR) was generally viewed as a repository of patient information used by individual healthcare providers. While EHRs do serve as a patient information repository, they also help to support the collaboration between members of a care team by allowing them to be aware of what has been done for the patient by other team

Table 8.1 Behavioral characteristics of effective teams (adapted from Baker et al. 2006)

Features of effective teams	Supporting function	Potential strategy
Team leadership (Baker et al. 2006; Nancarrow et al. 2013; Klarare et al. 2019; Singer & Kerrissey 2021)	Offers clear direction and management with the ability to coordinate the activities of other team members	Seeking and evaluating information for task coordination among team members
Mutual performance monitoring (Baker et al. 2006; McIntyre & Salas 1995; Salas et al. 1994)	Ability to develop shared understanding of the team environment and apply appropriate task strategies to accurately monitor members' performance	• Identifying mistakes and lapses in other team members' actions • Providing feedback regarding other team members' actions to aid correction
Mutual support (McIntyre & Salas 1995; Porter et al. 2003; Salas et al. 1994)	Ability to support team member needs based on accurate knowledge of their responsibilities	Shifting of tasks to underutilized team members
Adaptability (Cannon-Bowers & Salas 1997; Kozlowski et al., 1999, Stowers et al. 2021, Pype et al. 2018)	Ability to adjust strategies based on information gained from work environment using compensatory behavior and reallocation of shared team resources	Identifying opportunities for growth and innovation for routine practices
Shared mental model (Klimoski & Mohammed 1994; Mathieu et al. 2000; Stout et al. 1996)	Organizes knowledge structure of the relationships between the task and team member interactions	Anticipating and predicting team members' needs
Collaborative competencies (Janssen et al. 2020; McLaney et al. 2022)	Defines core competencies needed to support collaboration including role clarification, interprofessional values & ethics and conflict resolution	HIT can support team development and training to support the transition from individual to group processes
Awareness (Dourish & Bellotti 1992)	Provision of requisite knowledge to integrate individual and team tasks necessary to achieve a shared goal	HIT and other tools to assist with creating awareness of other team members' tasks
Common ground (Clark & Brennan 1991)	Shared knowledge, language and beliefs necessary for team communication and exchange to occur	Team training and use of common terminologies to support the development and maintenance of common ground
Collective orientation (Driskell & Salas 1992; Shamir 1990; Wagner 1995)	Being accountable for one another during team interactions	Appraising teammates' input

(continued)

Table 8.1 (continued)

Features of effective teams	Supporting function	Potential strategy
Mutual trust (Bandow 2001; Weber et al. 2004)	Trusting the ability of the team members to perform their roles and protect the teams' mutual interests	Willingness to admit mistakes and accept feedback
Device integration (Thiebes et al. 2023; Hose et al. 2023)	Integrating tools unobtrusively and seamlessly to support teams across settings and digital literacy	• Acquiring portable and standardized tools for team members in different work environments • Identify superusers and organize team trainig to improve digital literacy
Interdependency (Pype et al. 2018; Tan et al. 2023; Belber et al. 2023; Anderson et al. 2021)	Acknowledging that a team member's individual actions may affect another member's actions	Identifying the non-linear nature of team work to account for various interactions between members

members (Reddy et al. 2003). Clearly, HIT systems such as EHRs or computerized physician order entry (CPOE) could support teamwork far more than what has been originally envisioned by their designers.

Although HIT-facilitated teamwork plays a crucial role in modern care processes, most HIT evaluation studies have focused on how well these systems support *individual* users; for instance, the suitability and effectiveness of their user interface for single-user interaction (Nelson 1992; Shachak et al. 2019). With a few exceptions (Berg 1999; Gorman PN 2000; Reddy et al. 2001, Eikey et al. 2015), evaluating the capability of HIT systems in supporting team collaboration is often neglected. This neglect could have severe consequences. For example, Han et al. demonstrated in their study the danger of implementing a CPOE system without paying adequate attention to collaborative workflows (Han et al. 2005). In their study conducted in a pediatric hospital, the authors found an increased mortality rate that was attributable in part to the implementation of the CPOE system. As they and others (Sittig et al. 2006) pointed out, a key reason for the adverse effect observed was that the system failed to support collaborative work activities, and in some cases prevented collaboration that would normally have taken place at the bedside and elsewhere in the hospital. Poor alignment between HIT design and collaborative teamwork can result in negative unintended consequences (UICs) including patient safety, coordination, and communication UICs.

HIT can support this area via telehealth—teams can share evaluation methods, treatment, and monitoring and screening (Belber et al. 2023). The support HIT provides goes beyond raising awareness of individual conditions as the capabilities of HIT improve. We can also apply the theory of mind model to HIT development, in which HIT uses machine learning and AI to infer what teammates know and the information they hold (Stowers et al. 2021). By supporting service management, predictive medicine, patient data documentation, diagnosis, and decision-making (Secinaro et al. 2021), HIT helps increase risk awareness and allows healthcare teams to deliver better preventive care and collaborative treatments.

8.4   Formalizing Team-Based Workflows

Workflow has been described as the number one pain point between HIT and users (Singh et al. 2013), specifically with regards to the formation and functioning of healthcare teams being a particular challenge (Payne et al. 2016). Although there has been more research on workflows and HIT in recent years (e.g. Unertl et al. 2020), new forms of challenges continue to emerge as healthcare evolves. For example, remote and telehealth teams create challenges related to communication and the functioning of healthcare teams; integrating AI in healthcare prompts the questions of how and where it fits in team-based workflows. Thus, a first step toward mindful HIT design is to formalize team-based workflows so that computerized systems can better support the characteristics of the underlying teamwork. While the above section describes numerous characteristics of healthcare teams, formalizing team-based workflows in clinical settings is still at its early stages. Therefore, we focus on the intricacies of team-based workflows, drawing upon our prior work and recent literature to formalize the above characteristics according to the structural and behavioral aspects of team-based workflows (Press et al. 2012).

In Fig. 8.1, we synthesize the concepts from Table 8.1 to characterize healthcare team workflows into structural and behavioral dimensions. The structure of a team is defined by the degree of interaction, the temporal characteristics of tasks and personnel, and the individual actors involved in team-based workflows. The behavioral aspects define factors such as leadership, trust and collaborative competencies, as well as behaviors that influence how collaborative workflows are actually carried out (Xiao et al. 2013). Characterizing team workflows by structures and behaviors helps us better understand how to link team characteristics to outcomes, and the impact of HIT on team-based workflows. While all structural and behavioral aspects from Fig. 8.1 are important, we focus on collaborative team workflows, which are an integral and often understudied part of team-based care delivery (Kuziemsky 2016).

8.5   Collaborative Workflows

Collaboration is a dynamic system that integrates people, processes, and technology across different settings, policies and other governance structures. Collaboration is different from teamwork as the latter is more about the structure by which patients, healthcare providers and other personnel interact through care delivery while the former refers to the interactive process by which different agents engage to develop a shared understanding (Eikey et al. 2015).

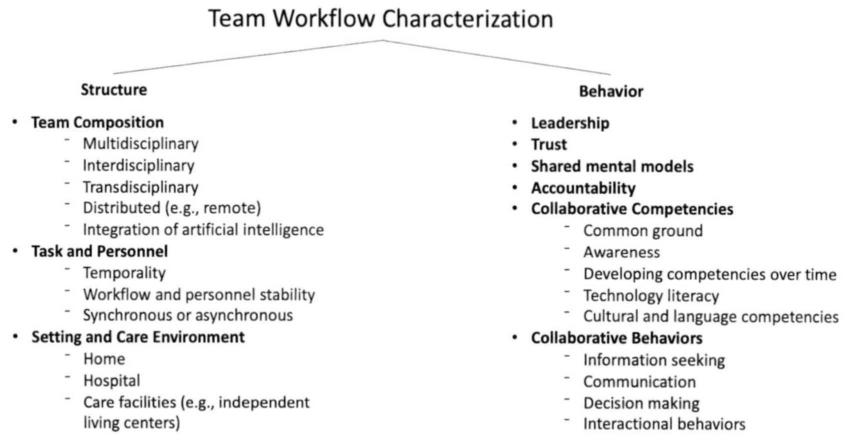

Team Workflow Characterization

Structure	Behavior
• **Team Composition**	• **Leadership**
‾ Multidisciplinary	• **Trust**
‾ Interdisciplinary	• **Shared mental models**
‾ Transdisciplinary	• **Accountability**
‾ Distributed (e.g., remote)	• **Collaborative Competencies**
‾ Integration of artificial intelligence	‾ Common ground
• **Task and Personnel**	‾ Awareness
‾ Temporality	‾ Developing competencies over time
‾ Workflow and personnel stability	‾ Technology literacy
‾ Synchronous or asynchronous	‾ Cultural and language competencies
• **Setting and Care Environment**	• **Collaborative Behaviors**
‾ Home	‾ Information seeking
‾ Hospital	‾ Communication
‾ Care facilities (e.g., independent	‾ Decision making
living centers)	‾ Interactional behaviors

Fig. 8.1 Team-based workflow characterization based on structures and behaviors (Adapted from Kuziemsky, Abraham, and Reddy 2019)

The 3C Collaboration Model (i.e., Communication–Coordination–Cooperation) describes how collaboration involves processes such as communication to exchange information to generate tasks that are then organized via coordination to ensure the successful completion of the overall care task (Hugo et al. 2008; Paul & Reddy 2010; Reddy & Spence 2008).

As described in the previous section, collaboration is challenging for team-based workflows. Clinical processes are often collaborative in nature, and activities and tasks depend on effective management of team-based workflows (Kannampallil et al. 2011; Niazkhani et al. 2009). While individual workflows involve the interaction between an individual care provider and his/her work environment (Malhotra et al. 2007), team-based workflows involve multiple interactions within the healthcare setting including collaboration between multiple providers of a care team. Understanding the movement across the 'individual-collaborative' interchange, and how individual and team needs are reconciled, is a key part of understanding collaborative team-based workflows.

In the following sub-sections, we illustrate how team characteristics are manifested in collaborative team-based workflows. In particular, we highlight key research studies that have been conducted to examine collaborative behaviors related to information seeking, interactions, communication and decision making.

8.5.1 Collaborative Information Seeking (CIS) Behaviors

Collaborative information seeking (CIS), in simple terms, refers to the interactive and mutually beneficial process of seeking information as defined explicitly by and among collaborative team members (Shah 2012). An example of CIS noted in the literature is to communicate evidence with regard to clinical practice using information sought through expert support provided by educators, librarians and other specialists (Hansen et al. 2015).

To understand the context of collaborative information activities of healthcare teams, several researchers have conducted field studies to observe and examine the underlying CIS-related features of team-based workflows. For example, Reddy and Jansen (Reddy & Jansen 2008) conducted ethnographic field studies of patient care teams at a surgical intensive care unit (ICU) of an urban hospital and the ED of a rural hospital. Three major characteristics of CIS behaviors were identified through these studies, including communication, complexity of information need and information retrieval technologies. The authors also compared CIS behaviors to individual information behaviors at different levels (i.e., information behavior, information seeking, information searching), and found that CIS behaviors have more complex characteristics. These complex characteristics encompass interaction between collaborative team members from different specialties and systems, as well as the need to communicate vital information within these interactions. Based on the conceptual understanding of CIS behaviors, the authors designed and developed a prototype collaborative information retrieval system called MUSE (Multi-User Search Engine) to aid communication between team members for more effective information seeking and retrieval.

In another study, Reddy and Spence (Reddy & Spence 2008) conducted ethnographic observations to further understand collaborative information-seeking activities of multidisciplinary patient care teams in the emergency department (ED). Findings from their investigation illustrate that ED team members have both organizational and clinical information needs, which are magnified during information flow breakdowns. They also identified seven categories of information needs as expressed by questions asked by ED care teams. These included patient-specific, organizational, plan of care, miscellaneous, clarification (more details), teaching and medication related questions. They also identified three triggers for CIS activities including lack of expertise, lack of immediate accessible information, and complex information needs.

In a follow-up study, Paul and Reddy (Paul & Reddy 2010) evaluated CIS and sense-making behaviors of healthcare providers, again in an ED setting. This study shows that making sense of information took place during three main occasions: when there was information ambiguity (requiring clarification from different team members); when there was role-based information distribution (unequal distribution of information shared among team members due to their different care roles); and when there was lack of expertise (health professionals lacking expertise on a particular situation, and needing collaborative sense making with other members in a multidisciplinary team). Based on their findings on the sense-making trajectories within CIS, the authors proposed two design principles for creating software systems to facilitate CIS: (1) implementing CIS tools that support the continuity of the process and products of sense making via visualizing the trajectories, using methods such as timelines that show chronological information by the various group members and sense made of the highlighted information; and (2) implementing CIS tools that provide action awareness via notifications, and activity awareness via visualizing timelines of the actions, related to a highlighted activity.

In another study of CIS, Shah and Gonazalez (Shah & González-Ibáñez 2010) adapted Kuhlthau's information search processes (ISP) model and mapped collaborative information-seeking processes to the different stages of the ISP model. The ISP model incorporates a cognitive (thought) and affective (feeling) dimension that reflects user's perspectives on the flow of activities that they engage in when performing an information-seeking task. Based on the six stages of the ISP model (i.e., initiation, selection, exploration, formulation, collection and presentation), the authors analyzed affective feelings (positive or negative) as a result of actions and messages exchanged between team members during CIS. The authors found that positive messages were associated with pleasant feelings (e.g., clarity, satisfaction); and negative messages were associated with unpleasant feelings (e.g., confusions). Their analysis provided additional insights into individual and group dynamics during CIS activities, and also showed a high correlation between initiation (related to uncertainty) and selection (related to optimism); and between exploration (related to confusion/frustration/doubt), formulation (related to clarity) and collection (related to sense of direction/confidence) of information, with participants often switching between these stages while interacting with collaborators. The authors also found a negative correlation between presentation (related to relief/satisfaction/ or disappointment) and exploration, formulation and collection.

Drawing upon the core findings from prior information studies, (Karunakaran et al. 2010) developed a conceptual collaborative information behavior (CIB) model to highlight three distinct phases of CIB in healthcare organizations. Phase 1 involves problem identification based on shared understanding; Phase 2 involves purposely seeking information by two or more individuals in a team in order to satisfy a shared goal; and Phase 3 involves incorporating information gathered into the team's existing knowledge base to achieve a common understanding between individuals in the team. Central activities in these three phases include information sharing and evaluation; collaborative grounding (shared understanding that assimilates and reflects upon available information); and collaborative sense making (individuals with different perspectives making sense of messy information).

CIS behaviors in remote teams revolve around establishing goal similarity, interdependence, coordination, and trust (Chiocchio et al. 2016) through technologies. Remote teams are likely to have a greater variety of cultures compared to co-located teams. To support effective remote CIS, three guiding principles are found to be crucial: practicality, conceptual footing, and technical quality, all relevant to scale construction (Chiocchio et al. 2016). Following such principles allows teams to assess their behaviors to promote self-reflection and maintain efficacy in domains. Furthermore, establishing quality CIS is influenced by the cultural quotient on the team (Presbitero, 2020). Technologies, therefore, need to facilitate cultural-specific expertise exchange.

8.5.2   Collaborative Interactional Behaviors

Lewis (Lewis 2006) used five points of convergence and three points of divergence based on the definitions from the collaboration literature. The five points of convergence are:

- More of an activity rather than a state/object (for example learning collaboratively);
- Team members regard for one another (collaborative interaction only exists when relationships between participants are formed);
- Equalization of team members irrespective of participants' high or low status;
- Process of collaborative interaction with a start, middle and end of the activity which changes at different point in time; and
- Participants are often willing to get involved in the collaborative process and are never coerced.

The three points of divergence are:

- Collaborative activities often occur at different time dimensions such as short or long-time spans with different goals;
- Collaborative interaction serves as a platform to highlight and acknowledge differences in a productive way while taking advantage of similarities among team members.
- Have a shared goal with or without considering individual payoffs.

A few examples of collaborative interactions presented in the literature include:

- A physician collaborates with their patient to decide on the best treatment for the patient's condition; the physician provides their medical expertise and the patient offers knowledge about their body, history and goals (Lewis 2006).
- Healthcare team members encouraging situations that promote collaborative interactions such as: open dialogue, collaborative rounds, implementing pre- and post-operation team briefing, and creating interdisciplinary committees or task forces that discuss challenges (O'Daniel & Rosenstein 2008).
- The collaborative shared healthcare plan provides a framework for collaborative daily life activity recognition, monitoring, location analysis, and developing a shared care plan. It also improves coordination and communication among the healthcare team (Javed et al. 2020).

Numerous studies have been conducted to evaluate the importance of collaborative interactional behavior in team-based workflows, including collaborative interactions among members of a healthcare team, with patients, and with HIT. Apker et al. (2006) conducted an exploratory study to investigate nurses' communication of professionalism during interactions with other members of the care team. Findings from their study showed that the participating nurses used four communication skillsets, including collaboration, credibility, compassion and coordination (4Cs). The authors also identified specific communicative behaviors associated with each of the four skillsets: collaboration is associated with organizing, filtering and providing pertinent information to team members; credibility is associated with clear communication about the information shared; compassion is associated with display of consideration and caring for team member concerns; and coordination involves tasks delegation to other team members while encouraging participants input (Apker et al. 2006). Implications from their study highlighted the pros and cons of varied communication expectations of nursing staff. These varied expectations could serve as a catalyst to embolden nurses on developing new skills to increase their overall productivity. However, varied communication expectations could also lead to tension in the workplace between different clinical roles, which could precipitate stressors that cause nurse burnout, leaving their current positions or completely quitting their nursing profession. Therefore, implementing the 4Cs in nursing education and nursing practice provides an important strategy for improving nurses' communication skills.

In another exploratory study, Hau et al. (2017) investigated the effects of various interaction behaviors of service front liners (i.e., healthcare providers) and customers (i.e., patients), and how they can work together to co-create value. Their investigation depicted a research model with four components of front liner interactions: individuated, relational, ethical and empowered; and customers' interactions with front liners have three components: information seeking, information sharing and responsible behavior. The cumulative effects of these interactions enable value co-creation by both front liners and customers, which has an indirect influence on costumers' perceived value through the 'participation–activating' interaction behavior. Findings from their analyses also identified a significant positive effect of interaction behaviors on patient participation, through which more patient resources are contributed to creating healthcare service. They concluded that the interactions between front liners and customers can be broken down into participation-activating interactions versus value-enhancing interactions, both of which enhance perceived value by customers.

To investigate nurse-physician collaborative interaction behaviors, Lindeke et al. (Lindeke et al. 2005) analyzed workspace collaboration between nurses and physicians, and suggested different collaborative strategies, including self-development, team-development and communication-development, that can be used to improve nurse-physician communication. Self-development strategies are defined as various individual characteristics that influence the level of collaboration between professionals in healthcare settings. These include developing emotional maturity, understanding the perspective of others, and avoiding compassion fatigue/burnout. Team development strategies involve team building, respectful negotiation, conflict management, containment of negative behaviors and workplace design to facilitate collaboration. Finally, communication-development strategies include implementing effective communication tactics (e.g., prioritizing the context with current information and disregarding peripheral data) that are often vital in emergency situations; and using electronic communication means mindfully (e.g., to be courteous and friendly while evaluating and clarifying the messages received).

In a related study on collaborative interaction behaviors, Schadewaldt et al. (2016) examined the experiences and perceptions of nurse practitioners (NPs) and medical practitioners (MPs) working collaboratively in a primary care setting. The authors used mixed research methods such as thematic analyses of qualitative data obtained from observations, work documents describing collaborative practices, and interviews of NPs and MPs; as well as descriptive analyses of quantitative data obtained from questionnaires completed by MPs and NPs. Findings from their study demonstrated intensive collaboration activities between NPs and MPs, which were deemed by the study participants as being beneficial to patients. In addition, their qualitative analysis results highlighted three themes regarding the collaborative experience of NPs and MPs. These themes include: (1) the influence of system structures (i.e. policies and regulations, local infrastructure); for example, the study participants criticized that the current NP reimbursement rates and the available Medicare benefit schedule were inadequate and unfair; (2) influence and consequences of individual role enactment through the coexistence of overlapping, complementary, traditional roles and emerging roles; and (3) participants making adjustments to new routines, and individuals' willingness and personal commitment being crucial to collaborative work. Based on these findings, the authors suggested decision makers of healthcare reform implement strategic support for collaborative clinical work, such as enhancing nurses' sense of autonomy in the workplace to strengthen their positions, and ensuring continuous practice of collaboration.

Besides interpersonal collaborative interactions among members of healthcare teams, researchers have also investigated how collaboration is mediated using HIT systems. Examples include the use of mobile devices during patient rounding and handoff, which has been shown to improve team workflows (Motulsky et al. 2017; Srinivas et al. 2015); and the use of computerized clinical decision-support systems designed to facilitate interactions between physicians and other healthcare professionals (El-Sappagh & El-Masri 2014).

Additionally, interactions mediated by HIT are necessary when team-oriented clinical processes do not afford team members the convenience of face-to-face interactions. Challenges related to communication, trust, and awareness are further exacerbated by barriers such as physical distance in a distributed work environment, or team members working at different points in time (e.g., across different shifts) (Garingo et al. 2016; Marini et al. 2015; Rincon et al. 2012; Morrison-Smith & Ruiz 2020; Poitras et al. 2023). Recent literature further identifies digital literacy and digital accessibility as barriers, especially for teams who are located in the more remote areas (Poitras et al. 2023).

8.5.3 Collaborative Communication Behaviors

Collaborative communication is a concept that embodies a combination of specific relationship-building communication qualities among team members working towards a common goal (Farrelly et al. 2003). This concept is often associated with favorable outcomes such as lower risk-adjusted patient mortality, increased nurse satisfaction with improved professional relationships, and enhanced physician learning, professional relationships and research utilization (Boyle & Kochinda 2004).

For example, one study illustrated the importance of collaborative communication during patient rounds using a Patient's Insight and Views of Teamwork (PIVOT) survey that solicits patient perception of teamwork (Beaird et al. 2017). This study was conducted in an inpatient acute care cardiology ward, and involved implementing an intervention—a structured interdisciplinary bedside rounding initiative called Rounding with Heart (RWH). Based on their observation of specific behaviors recognized in the RWH process, the authors reported multiple benefits associated with the intervention, namely: openness/inclusivity, patient centeredness, attending role/shared leadership, non-confrontational learning, efficacy and team at bedside. The findings of the study also showed that patients had favorable perceptions of the RWH-based teamwork rounding process. The researchers also noted that RWH gave team members an opportunity to build mutual respect and collegiality through daily interactions, and could therefore be used as a means to address negative teamwork behaviors.

Although collaborative communication is an integral part of inpatient rounding, its effectiveness could be diminished due to a number of challenges. Hendricks et al. (Hendricks et al. 2017) conducted a qualitative study to understand such challenges across four acute care units at a large urban hospital. They found that major factors affecting collaborative communication behaviors during interprofessional patient rounds are related to either team members or the healthcare environment, and are best described as opposite manifestations and highlighted in pairs (barriers versus facilitators). For team members, these facilitator–barrier pairs include high versus low turnover of team membership, structured versus unstructured rounding, valuing versus skepticism about interprofessional practice, and confidence versus hesitancy about skills. For the healthcare environment, the facilitator–barrier pairs are: rounding aligned versus mismatched with hospital's mission, time for rounding versus competing demands, geographically co-located versus distributed teams, and readiness for change and innovation versus saturation.

Similar to collaborative communication during inpatient rounds, the effectiveness of patient handoffs also critically depends on seamless team communication to facilitate team-based workflows. To achieve a safe handing-off process of vulnerable patients such as neonates, Vanderbilt et al. (Vanderbilt et al. 2017) suggested use of handoff training and communication practices among neonatal interprofessional teams including members specializing in obstetrics, gynecology and neonatology. They also recommended that the training should involve comprehensive, systematic, and standardized processes within handoff communication and through graduate and continuing medical education.

Another study investigating collaboration during patient handoffs led to the development of a continuity of care model that assesses clinicians' workflow before, during and after handoff in the critical care unit (Abraham et al. 2012). This model highlighted important contextual factors that influence continuity of care provided by interdisciplinary teams. In the study, the authors used clinician-centered data and mixed inductive–deductive approaches to demonstrate the complex and interactive nature of patient handoffs as well as to capture and highlight sources of communication breakdowns. The descriptive framework developed through the study encompasses key features within the handoff communication process such as (1) multiple information flow paths and decision points, (2) non-linear and recursive nature of decision making and collaborative problem-solving activities, and (3) interactive nature of handoffs in a pragmatic critical care environment.

Additionally, it is important to ensure the consistency of the same patient information gathered by different members of the care team. Mamykina et al. (2016) evaluated handoff communication and coordination of patient care teams in a cardiothoracic ICU. Using categorical cluster analysis and a modified pyramid method, the authors assessed the degree of shared mental models between team members. The results revealed emerging patterns in the content and structure of interdisciplinary handoff communication, as well as content overlapping (e.g., patient name and an introductory history of the patient's presenting problem). With regard to the structure of interdisciplinary teams, the authors identified that different provider roles focused on different categories of content during their handoff communication. Based on these findings, they suggested the design of future handoff tools need to be conscious of the differences in clinician roles in order to properly coordinate these roles with existing practice.

In a related handoff study also conducted in the cardiothoracic ICU setting, Collins et al. (2012) analyzed handoff artifacts using semantic coding based on the interdisciplinary handoff information coding (IHIC) framework. The IHIC framework provides lists of handoff content specific to different disciplines and is a particularly useful tool to assist researchers in identifying handoff content important to nurses and physicians within certain clinical environments such as the ICU. Findings from their analysis showed a high degree of overlap in the content of nurses' and physicians' handoff artifacts. There was also a high degree of structure used for organizing and communicating handoff data when coordinating care across multiple disciplines within the critical care unit.

Similarly, Abraham et al. (Abraham et al. 2017) used mixed methods to develop and evaluate the degree of overlap in handoff communication across multiple care providers. Semantic similarity was used as the measure to estimate content overlap between nurse–nurse and resident–resident handoff communication for the same patients. Findings from their analysis showed a substantial amount of overlap for clinical content including active problems, assessments of active problems, patient identifying information, past medical history and medication/treatments; and less overlap for other content categories such as allergies, family-related information, code status and anticipatory guidance.

8.5.4   Collaborative Decision-Making Behaviors

Collaborative decision-making behaviors in healthcare refers to the process of engagement that seeks to devise an optimal plan of actions with a main focus on the highest-priority health-related problems that emerge from the confluence of medical and non-medical issues (O'Grady & Jadad 2010).

An example that depicts the collaborative decision-making process is involving patients in making decisions for cancer treatments after having them review treatment options along with their physicians, which has been shown to improve treatment effectiveness and patient satisfaction (Levit et al. 2013). Another study cited the benefits of collaborative decision making is the implementation of an integrated knowledge translation program involving researchers, managers, policy makers and clinicians in cancer screen and diagnosis (Gagliardi et al. 2014). The study reported an increased level of participation in cancer screening associated with the introduction of the program.

In a more recent study, Bomba et al. (2017) highlighted the value of implementing a shared decision-making model during the course of patient care. They suggested that a shared decision-making process should be patient-centered, and made as a routine practice because of its potential to improve clinicians' ability for managing patients with complex chronic conditions. This shared decision-making process encourages clinicians offer their viewpoint that is aligned with the patient's goals for care. Essentially, all parties involved in the decision-making process, including patients, physicians and other decision makers (e.g., power of attorneys), should actively collaborate in making joint decisions related to care. This activity is particularly vital when a patient lacks the capacity and can no longer make decisions for themselves; or for care planning in advance when the patient would need to make decisions in preparation for an unforeseeable illness or injury.

To make shared decision-making processes less complex and easier to operationalize, Elwyn et al. (2012) introduced a three-step model based on existing conceptual description of collaborative decision making. The three steps are: choice talk, option talk and decision talk. Choice talk is a step to make sure patients understand available options of care; option talk provides detailed information related to the available options; and decision talk helps patients decide what is best for them based on their preferences. Notably, shared decision making requires building good relationships between patients and medical professionals during clinical encounters to encourage information sharing; as well as supporting patients in deliberating and expressing their preferences and views. This shared decision making will eventually help patients make informed decisions in their care process.

Similarly, Holmes-Rovner et al. used qualitative methods to evaluate a shared decision-making program to determine its feasibility in fee-for-service healthcare organizations including physician offices and inpatient facilities (Holmes-Rovner et al. 2000). The program implemented in the study contained a set of interactive videodisks developed by the Foundation for Informed Medical Making (FIMDM), which were designed to improve efficiency in physician and patient treatment selection based on patient preferences. Their investigation showed that the shared decision-making program was perceived favorably by patients, with a right amount of information for patients to review before making an informed decision. Based on the findings from their study, the authors suggested that shared decision making should be incorporated into the informed consent process; and can be used as a quality indicator for provider- or payer-negotiated requirements during routine care procedures (Holmes-Rovner et al. 2000).

Furthermore, to support automation in HIT, Konaté et al. developed an ontology for collaborative decision making with 18 distinct concepts (Konaté et al. 2020), such as decision problem, constraint, alternative, decision result, role, and material. Establishing a validated ontology can create a clear and standardized mapping for HIT designs to support collaborative decision making. More recently, a growing number of healthcare teams have used AI to help with clinical decision making. Compared to mere automation, AI uses machine learning to mimic human cognitive capabilities, such as making predictions by analyzing historical medical records and case studies (Secinaro et al. 2021). Human team members then can agree with or disregard the recommendations provided by AI, dependent on whether the recommendations validate or conflict with their own beliefs and assessments (Jussupow et al. 2021). However, although AI is usually helpful in reducing human errors, their recommendations may still be inaccurate at times; an over-reliance on AI for decision making therefore can also lead to misdiagnosis and patient safety concerns.

Recent advances in telemedicine have transformed collaborative decision-making processes of remote teams. For example, within the context of hospital operating rooms (ORs), Abraham et al. evaluated a telemedicine system implemented in the ORs, Anesthesiology Control Tower (Abraham et al. 2022) that allows the clinical teams to remotely monitor surgeries and provide timely alerts and action plans, which can reduce decision making errors. Decision support with telemedicine teams can help facilitate checks and balances among the clinical team, minimize distractions, and provide additional team members to monitor patient safety during the operation (Abraham et al. 2021). However, new guidelines and policies need to be established for teams to leverage such collaborative decision support technology effectively, including having a backup plan and equipment in case of technological difficulties or delays, as well as increasing patient-provider communication to ensure common ground about the use of telemedicine (Abraham et al. 2021, 2022).

8.6 Theoretical and Methodological Frameworks for Studying Collaborative Workflows

Several theoretical and methodological frameworks have been proposed in the literature for studying collaborative workflows at both micro- and macro-levels. There are also frameworks specifically developed for studying collaboration in the context of HIT.

8.6.1 Micro-Level Approaches

There have been several micro-level frameworks used for studying the empirical aspects of collaboration, including collaborative patterns in which team members specify responsibilities and accountabilities for task completion (Grando et al. 2011; Papapanagiotou & Fleuriot 2014); different collaborative processes performed by teams including communication and decision making (Eikey et al. 2015; Nancarrow et al. 2013; Xyrichis & Ream 2008); and the means by which team leadership is established and tasks are assigned according to competencies and capabilities of team members (Wilk et al. 2016).

Theoretical approaches for studying micro-level aspects of collaboration include Actor Network Theory (McDougall et al. 2016), Activity Theory (Sadeghi et al. 2014), and Complexity Adaptive Systems (Pype et al. 2018).

Micro-level conceptual models also exist, which can be used to guide studies on competencies needed in forming and maintaining collaboration, including common ground; shared knowledge and beliefs that enable collaboration to occur (Collins et al. 2012); and awareness—defined by Dourish and Bellotti as "the understanding of the activities of others which provides a context for your own activity (Dourish & Bellotti 1992)." These conceptual models are not directly relevant to team-based workflows; instead, they look at common knowledge and protocols that need to be developed, and shared among team members, as facilitators of a collaborative workflow.

8.6.2 Macro-Level Approaches

Macro-level frameworks are useful to develop a better understanding of collaborative workflows at the broader team-level by focusing on different approaches by which team members interact over time while completing their designated tasks. One such approach is social network analysis, which studies the degree of interactions and social structures across individuals in a social setting (Flemming et al. 2022). on the degree of social interactions which has been used to study the degree to which provider connectivity is associated with medication errors (Creswick & Westbrook 2015); and also to understand medication information exchange amongst team members (Chan et al. 2017). Other macro-level approaches for studying collaborative workflows include simulation, agent-based modeling; and system dynamic modeling (Isern & Moreno 2015; Rosenman et al. 2017; Truijens et al. 2015; Abildgren et al. 2022).

8.6.3   Moving from Individual to Collaborative Workflow

Central to both micro- and macro-level approaches is the movement from individual to collaborative workflow. This movement can be challenging as it often requires changing the way in which individuals conduct their workflows (Kuziemsky 2015; Reddy & Spence 2008). Thus, an essential part of studies of collaborative workflows is to understand the relationship between individuals and teams (Lingard et al. 2017). A collaborative workflow is not simply the integration of many individual workflows but rather requires the creation of a new set of practices for tasks such as information exchange, communication, and decision making. Individuals often have to make trade-offs when moving between individual and collaborative workflows (Kuziemsky 2015), which emphasizes the need for developing collaborative competencies such as common ground and shared mental models as a precursor to developing collaborative workflows. These competencies can facilitate discussions around the processes, context, actors, and technology needed for collaborative care delivery. Artifacts such as the Collaboration Space Ontology Template and the Collaborative Care Model Canvas can help teams establish common grounds as part of collaborative care delivery (Lakhani et al. 2021). However, collaborative competencies and the rules that govern collaboration are dynamic and constantly evolving and therefore collaborative workflows will need to be monitored and revised as needed (Kuziemsky 2016).

8.7   Expanding the Concept of Teams

Over the past decade, the definition of healthcare delivery has extended from care activities and data collected in clinical environments into patients' homes and everyday settings. Consequently, teams have grown more complex in their composition and characteristics (Larsson et al. 2022). New tools such as AI and wearable technologies can provide a larger volume of patient data (e.g., using sensors to collect vitals outside of a doctor's office) to the healthcare team to facilitate collaboration (Rosen et al. 2018). Although the focus of this chapter is collaboration within a clinical context, we need to start reassessing the conceptualization of "clinical" teams in healthcare. This section provides examples of collaborative activities outside the clinical context, focusing on the integration of patients and AI in collaborative workflows.

Outpatient, post-operative care, and palliative care bring collaboration into patients' home environments. Members of the clinical teams such as home-care nurses may be required to be flexible and make independent decisions, while establishing common grounds outside of their immediate work environment (Klarare et al. 2019; Tan et al. 2023). Yet, HIT that supports home-care collaboration remains under-explored (Larsson et al. 2022) despite its potential shown in remote team collaboration and telehealth.

In addition, researchers are increasingly highlighting the need of a patient-centered or family-centered approach to deliver collaborative care. Involving patients and family members in decision making and knowledge sharing can help provide a sense of control, while giving physicians more context and information about the patient (Wong et al. 2020). Besides data collected through sensors and wearable technologies, patients can also generate their own health data through active self-tracking and self-reporting mechanisms (Mars & Scott 2022). They may use HIT such as mobile health applications or patient portals to collect data to share with their care team. Patients may also provide a point of contact such as a family member to communicate with the physicians synchronously or asynchronously on their behalf (Hart et al. 2020). This is similar to the collaboration and communication within a multidisciplinary team.

As technology advances, patients and their families have more opportunities to interact with robots, AI, and telehealth. Marini et al. observed the impact of robotics tele-rounding in surgical ICU, where patients and families interacting with the intensivists through flat-screen monitors on the robots (Marini et al. 2015). This study showed that although the technology did not meet the nurses' expectations as they deemed that the physical presence of an intensivist was an essential part of surgical ICU care, the use of tele-rounding had no negative effect on patient outcomes, intensivist satisfaction with patient care, and residents' educational experience. Communication, coordination, and adaptation are key aspects to consider when developing effective human–machine teamwork (Stowers et al. 2021). However, current AI has limited cognitive capabilities and machines may sometimes perform worse when partnered with humans (Stowers et al. 2021). Consequently, conducting research that evaluates and designs effective collaboration between human and AI in as part of healthcare teams will be crucial.

8.8 Moving Forward to Support Collaborative Workflows

Increased patient complexity and global health events like the COVID-19 pandemic have highlighted the need for increased team-based care delivery. While AI and other digital health tools can support teamwork, technology alone will not transform the health system into a collaborative system that supports teamwork. We must first understand the nature of teamwork and get the design right before we focus on implementing technology. Although some have suggested that integrating processes and technologies are more of an implementation issue, we believe that it is just as important to properly design HIT to support team-based collaboration (Shachak et al. 2019). A system that is not explicitly designed to support collaboration will have unintended consequences post implementation.

This chapter helps address the above issue by describing collaborative workflows and HIT design considerations to support teamwork. We reviewed collaborative healthcare processes and provided a characterization of collaborative workflows according to structures and processes. We also highlighted that collaborative workflows are a social construction between patients, healthcare providers, clinical processes, and policies and other governance structures and we need to understand how all these factors are integrated prior to introducing technology to support teamwork.

HIT design for collaborative workflows must go beyond simply automating clinical tasks as that misses a great opportunity for digital tools and approaches to enhance the way collaborative care delivery is delivered. There are a variety of technologies that could support the various aspects of collaborative care delivery and it is essential that system design be purposeful for the outcomes we want to achieve. For example, social media tools can improve the connectivity for collaborating providers across disparate locations over the continuum of care. AI tools and approaches can serve as the coordinating entity for teamwork to help with more efficient allocation of tasks, decision making, predictive analysis, and documentation (Ramezani et al. 2023). However, we cannot just introduce HIT or AI systems and hope for the best with respect to supporting collaboration. Establishing connectivity and efficiency are not the same as actively supporting collaboration as it is a dynamic process that requires the establishment and monitoring of collaborative competencies such as common ground and shared awareness. HIT along with training and organizational policies, and programs must all adapt to support collaborative workflows (Buljac-Samardzic et al. 2020).

While team training is currently the most commonly used approach for supporting team-based care delivery, focusing on how to organize teamwork structures and behaviors are equally important (Christofer et al. 2017; Kuziemsky 2023). This chapter contributes to this line of thinking, in that we characterize team workflows according to their structures and associated behaviors. Structures represent different aspects of team configurations such as team composition or the degree of collaboration in a team. Behavioral aspects include the tacit or social workings of a team, and include trust, shared mental models, and collaborative competencies. We cannot.

The adaptive nature of teamwork indicates that collaborative activities are dynamic and reacting to the changing contextual factors (Anderson et al. 2021). As a result, some has suggested a systems approach is necessary to keep up with the complexity of teams (Buse 2022), as well as to understand different healthcare teams and ways to design HIT to support them (Hose et al. 2023). A main takeaway from this chapter is that there is no *one-size-fits-all* strategy for designing HIT that effectively supports collaboration. Instead, the design must be customized to specific team structures and behaviors. Further, this chapter focuses on collaborative workflows, particularly collaborative information-seeking, communication, decision-making and interactional behaviors. All of these behaviors emphasize the need to nurture relationships between team members to develop rules of engagement to achieve and sustain effective team workflows. Rules of engagement are necessary to equalize team members and to reconcile differences in terminology or workflow that may impair collaboration. Drawing upon existing research on common ground and shared awareness can help us develop formalization of rules of engagement to ensure effective and efficient collaborative workflows. Despite healthcare's recent transition to adapting virtual collaboration, the behaviors and rules of engagement discussed in this chapter remain relevant even for remote and hybrid teams.

Healthcare teams will be transformed using technology. The overall challenge is to determine how to get humans and technology to work together? This chapter contributes to that question by providing knowledge on how to understand collaborative workflows and how they develop end evolve over time. In designing for collaboration, it is important to recognize that collaborative processes such as information-seeking or communicative behaviors are not static, but are dynamic and constantly evolving. This is evident in new practices teams have developed to foster effective virtual collaboration. To that end, HIT systems that we design to support collaborative workflows will need to be flexible so that they can adapt to accommodate changes in the collaborative processes.

References

Abildgren, L., Lebahn-Hadidi, M., Mogensen, C.B. et al. (2022). The effectiveness of improving healthcare teams' human factor skills using simulation-based training: a systematic review. Adv Simul 7, 12(2022). https://doi.org/10.1186/s41077-022-00207-2

Abraham J, Kannampallil TG, Patel VL. Bridging gaps in handoffs: a continuity of care based approach. J Biomed Inform. 2012;45(2):240–54.

Abraham J, Kannampallil TG, Srinivasan V, Galanter WL, Tagney G, Cohen T. Measuring content overlap during handoff communication using distributional semantics: An exploratory study. J Biomed Inform. 2017;65:132–44.

Abraham J, Meng A, Holzer KJ, Brawer L, Casarella A, Avidan M, Politi MC. Exploring patient perspectives on telemedicine monitoring within the operating room. Int J Med Inform. 2021;156: 104595. https://doi.org/10.1016/j.ijmedinf.

Abraham J, Meng A, Montes de Oca A, Politi M, Wildes T, Gregory S, Henrichs B, Kannampallil T, Avidan M.S. (2022). An ethnographic study on the impact of a novel telemedicine-based support system in the operating room. J Am Med Inform Assoc. 7;29(11):1919–1930. https://doi.org/10.1093/jamia/ocac138.

Abraham, J., & Reddy, M. C. (2013). *Re-coordinating activities: an investigation of articulation work in patient transfers.* Paper presented at the Proceedings of the 2013 conference on Computer supported cooperative work.

Anderson JE, Lavelle M, Reedy G. Understanding adaptive teamwork in health care: Progress and future directions. J Health Serv Res Policy. 2021;26(3):208–14. https://doi.org/10.1177/135581 9620978436.

Andreatta PB. A typology for health care teams. Health Care Manage Rev. 2010;35(4):345–54. https://doi.org/10.1097/HMR.0b013e3181e9fceb.

Apker J, Propp KM, Ford WSZ, Hofmeister N. Collaboration, credibility, compassion, and coordination: professional nurse communication skill sets in health care team interactions. J Prof Nurs. 2006;22(3):180–9.

Baker, D. P., Day, R., & Salas, E. (2006). Teamwork as an essential component of high-reliability organizations. Health Serv Res, 41(4p2), 1576–1598.

Bandow D. Time to create sound teamwork. J Qual Particip. 2001;24(2):41.

Bates D. Health information technology and care coordination: the next big opportunity for informatics? Yearb Med Inform. 2015;10(1):11–4. https://doi.org/10.15265/IY-2015-020.

Beaird G, Dent JM, Keim-Malpass J, Muller AGJ, Nelson N, Brashers V. Perceptions of teamwork in the interprofessional bedside rounding process. J Healthc Qual. 2017;39(2):95–106.

Belber GS, Vasconcelos RO, Agreli HLF, Haddad AE, Peduzzi M, Leonello VM. Telehealth use in primary healthcare collaborative interprofessional practice: protocol for a scoping review. BMJ Open. 2023;13(3): e069163. https://doi.org/10.1136/bmjopen-2022-069163.

Berg M. Patient care information systems and health care work: a sociotechnical approach. Int J Med Inform. 1999;55(2):87–101.

Berg M, Langenberg C, vd Berg, I., & Kwakkernaat, J. Considerations for sociotechnical design: experiences with an electronic patient record in a clinical context. Int J Med Inform. 1998;52(1–3):243–51.

Bomba P. Supporting the patient voice: building the foundation of shared decision-making. Gener. 2017;41(1):21–30.

Boyle DK, Kochinda C. Enhancing collaborative communication of nurse and physician leadership in two intensive care units. J Nurs Adm. 2004;34(2):60–70.

Bricon-Souf N, Renard JM, Beuscart R. Dynamic workflow model for complex activity in intensive care unit. Int J Med Inform. 1999;53(2–3):143–50.

Buljac-Samardzic M, Doekhie KD, Van Wijngaarden JDH. Interventions to improve team effectiveness within health care: a systematic review of the past decade. Hum Resour Health. 2020;18(1):2. https://doi.org/10.1186/s12960-019-0411-3.

Buse, K. (2022). From health systems to systems for health: much more than semantics. BMJ, o3016. 2022; https://doi.org/10.1136/bmj.o3016

Cannon-Bowers, JA, Salas E. Teamwork competencies: The interaction of team member knowledge, skills, and attitudes. *Workforce readiness: Competencies and assessment*, 1997;151–174.

Casimiro LM, Hall P, Kuziemsky C, O'Connor M, Varpio L. Enhancing patient-engaged teamwork in healthcare: an observational case study. J Interprof Care. 2015;29(1):55–61. https://doi.org/10.3109/13561820.2014.940038.

Chan B, Reeve E, Matthews S, Carroll PR, Long JC, Held F, Hilmer SN. Medicine information exchange networks among healthcare professionals and prescribing in geriatric medicine wards. Br J Clin Pharmacol. 2017;83(6):1185–96. https://doi.org/10.1111/bcp.13222.

Chiocchio F, Lebel P, Dubé J-N. Informational role self-efficacy: a validation in interprofessional collaboration contexts involving healthcare service and project teams. BMC Health Serv Res. 2016;16(1):153. https://doi.org/10.1186/s12913-016-1382-x.

Choi BC, Pak AW. Multidisciplinarity, interdisciplinarity and transdisciplinarity in health research, services, education and policy: 1. Definitions, objectives, and evidence of effectiveness. Clin Invest Med, 29(6), 2006;351–364.

Christofer R, Per O, Anders LP. Organizing for teamwork in healthcare: an alternative to team training? J Health Organ Manag. 2017;31(3):347–62. https://doi.org/doi:10.1108/JHOM-12-2016-0233.

Clark HH, Brennan SE. Grounding in communication. In L. Resnick, L. B, M. John, S. Teasley, & D (Eds.), Perspectives on Socially Shared Cognition (pp. 13--1991): American Psychological Association. 1991.

Collins SA, Mamykina L, Jordan D, Stein DM, Shine A, Reyfman P, Kaufman D. In search of common ground in handoff documentation in an Intensive Care Unit. J Biomed Inform. 2012;45(2):307–15. https://doi.org/10.1016/j.jbi.2011.11.007.

Committee on Patient S, Health Information T, Institute of M. In Health IT and Patient Safety: Building Safer Systems for Better Care. Washington (DC): National Academies Press (US) 2011.

Creswick N, Westbrook JI. Who do hospital physicians and nurses go to for advice about medications? a social network analysis and examination of prescribing error rates. J Patient Saf. 2015;11(3):152–9. https://doi.org/10.1097/pts.0000000000000061.

Donnelly C, Ashcroft R, Bobbette N et al. Interprofessional primary care during COVID-19: a survey of the provider perspective. BMC Fam Pract 22, 31(2021).

Dourish P, Bellotti V *Awareness and coordination in shared workspaces.* Paper presented at the Proceedings of the 1992 ACM conference on Computer-supported cooperative work. 1992.

Driskell JE, Salas E. Collective behavior and team performance. Hum Factors. 1992;34(3):277–88.

Eikey EV, Reddy MC, Kuziemsky CE. Examining the role of collaboration in studies of health information technologies in biomedical informatics: A systematic review of 25 years of research. J Biomed Inform. 2015;57:263–77. https://doi.org/10.1016/j.jbi.2015.08.006.

El-Sappagh SH, El-Masri S. A distributed clinical decision support system architecture. J King Saud Univ-Comput Inf Sci. 2014;26(1):69–78.

Ellingson LL. Communication, collaboration, and teamwork among health care professionals. Commun Res Trends, 21(3). 2002.

Elwyn G, Frosch D, Thomson R, Joseph-Williams N, Lloyd A, Kinnersley P, Rollnick S. Shared decision making: a model for clinical practice. J Gen Intern Med. 2012;27(10):1361–7.

Farrelly F, Quester P, Mavondo F. Collaborative communication in sponsor relations. Corp Commun: Int J. 2003;8(2):128–38.

Flemming R, Schüttig W, Ng F, et al. Using social network analysis methods to identify networks of physicians responsible for the care of specific patient populations. BMC Health Serv Res. 2022;22:462. https://doi.org/10.1186/s12913-022-07807-8.

Gagliardi AR, Webster F, Brouwers MC, Baxter NN, Finelli A, Gallinger S. How does context influence collaborative decision-making for health services planning, delivery and evaluation? BMC Health Serv Res. 2014;14(1):545.

Galvin JE, Valois L, Zweig Y. Collaborative transdisciplinary team approach for dementia care. Neurodegener Dis Manag. 2014;4(6):455–69. https://doi.org/10.2217/nmt.14.47.

Garingo A, Friedlich P, Chavez T, Tesoriero L, Patil S, Jackson P, Seri I. "Tele-rounding" with a remotely controlled mobile robot in the neonatal intensive care unit. J Telemed Telecare. 2016;22(2):132–8.

Gorman PN, A. J., Lavelle M, Lyman J, Delcambre L, Maier D. Bundles in the wild: managing information to solve problems and maintain situation awareness. Libr Trends. 2000;49(2):266–89.

Grando MA, Peleg M, Cuggia M, Glasspool D. Patterns for collaborative work in health care teams. Artif Intell Med. 2011;53(3):139–60. https://doi.org/10.1016/j.artmed.2011.08.005.

Hall KL, Vogel AL, Stipelman B, Stokols D, Morgan G, Gehlert S. A four-phase model of transdisciplinary team-based research: goals, team processes, and strategies. Transl Behav Med. 2012;2(4):415–30. https://doi.org/10.1007/s13142-012-0167-y.

Han YY, Carcillo JA, Venkataraman ST, Clark RS, Watson RS, Nguyen TC, Orr RA. Unexpected increased mortality after implementation of a commercially sold computerized physician order entry system. Pediatrics. 2005;116(6):1506–12. https://doi.org/10.1542/peds.2005-1287.

Hansen P, Shah C, Klas C-P. Collaborative information seeking: Best practices, new domains and new thoughts: Springer. 2015.

Hart JL, Turnbull AE, Oppenheim IM, Courtright KR. Family-Centered Care During the COVID-19 Era. J Pain Symptom Manage. 2020;60(2):e93–7. https://doi.org/10.1016/j.jpainsymman.2020.04.017.

Hau LN, Anh PNT, Thuy PN. The effects of interaction behaviors of service frontliners on customer participation in the value co-creation: a study of health care service. Serv Bus. 2017;11(2):253–77.

Hendricks S, LaMothe VJ, Kara A, Miller J. Facilitators and barriers for interprofessional rounding: a qualitative study. Clin Nurse Spec. 2017;31(4):219–28.

Hollenbeck JR, Beersma B, Schouten ME. Beyond team types and taxonomies: A dimensional scaling conceptualization for team description. Acad Manag Rev. 2012;37(1):82–106.

Holmes-Rovner M, Valade D, Orlowski C, Draus C, Nabozny-Valerio B, Keiser S. Implementing shared decision-making in routine practice: barriers and opportunities. Health Expect. 2000;3(3):182–91.

Hose B-Z, Carayon P, Hoonakker PLT, Brazelton TB, Dean SM, Eithun BL, Kelly MM, Kohler JE, Ross JC, Rusy DA. Work system barriers and facilitators of a team health information technology. Appl Ergon. 2023;113: 104105. https://doi.org/10.1016/j.apergo.2023.104105.

Hugo F, Alberto R, Marco AG, Pimental, Pimental, Mariano, Mariano. The 3C Collaboration Model. In K. Ned (Ed.), *Encyclopedia of E-Collaboration* (pp. 637–644). Hershey, PA, USA: IGI Global. 2008.

Isern D, Moreno A. A systematic literature review of agents applied in healthcare. J Med Syst. 2015;40(2):43. https://doi.org/10.1007/s10916-015-0376-2.

Janssen M, Sagasser MH, Fluit CRMG, et al. Competencies to promote collaboration between primary and secondary care doctors: an integrative review. BMC Fam Pract. 2020;21:179. https://doi.org/10.1186/s12875-020-01234-6.

Javed AR, Sarwar MU, Beg MO, Asim M, Baker T, Tawfik H. A collaborative healthcare framework for shared healthcare plan with ambient intelligence. Abstr Hum-centric Comput Inf Sci. 2020;10(1). https://doi.org/10.1186/s13673-020-00245-7

Jussupow E, Spohrer K, Heinzl A, Gawlitza J. Augmenting medical diagnosis decisions? an investigation into physicians' decision-making process with artificial intelligence. Inf Syst Res. 2021;32(3):713–35. https://doi.org/10.1287/isre.2020.0980.

Kannampallil TG, Schauer GF, Cohen T, Patel VL. Considering complexity in healthcare systems. J Biomed Inform. 2011;44(6):943–7.

Karunakaran A, Spence PR, Reddy MC. Towards a model of collaborative information behavior. 2010.

Klarare A, Hansson J, Fossum B, Fürst CJ, Lundh Hagelin C. Team type, team maturity and team effectiveness in specialist palliative home care: an exploratory questionnaire study. J Interprof Care. 2019;33(5):504–11. https://doi.org/10.1080/13561820.2018.1551861.

Klimoski R, Mohammed S. Team mental model: Construct or metaphor? J Manag. 1994;20(2):403–37.

Konaté J, Zaraté P, Gueye A, Camilleri G, Morais DC, Fang L, Horita M. Group Decision and Negotiation: A Multidisciplinary Perspective 20th International Conference on Group Decision and Negotiation, GDN 2020, Toronto, ON, Canada, June 7–11, 2020, Proceedings
An Ontology for Collaborative Decision Making. Cham: Springer International Publishing; 2020, p. 179–91.

Kozlowski SW, Gully SM, Nason ER, Smith EM. Developing adaptive teams: A theory of compilation and performance across levels and time. Pulakos (Eds.), The changing nature of work performance: Implications for staffing, personnel actions, and development, 1999;240, 292.

Kuziemsky C. A message from the guest editor. healthcare management forum. 2019; 32(3):118–119. https://doi.org/10.1177/0840470419837056

Kuziemsky CE. The role of human and organizational factors in the pursuit of one digital health. Yearb Med Inform. 2023;32(1):201–9. https://doi.org/10.1055/s-0043-1768724.

Kuziemsky C. Decision-making in healthcare as a complex adaptive system. Healthc Manage Forum. 2016;29(1):4–7. https://doi.org/10.1177/0840470415614842.

Kuziemsky CE. Review of social and organizational issues in health information technology. Healthc Inform Res. 2015;21(3):152–60. https://doi.org/10.4258/hir.2015.21.3.152.

Lakhani, R., Peyton, L., & Kuziemsky, C. (2021). Towards an Artifact-Supported Performance Management Framework for Collaborative Care Delivery. *2021 IEEE 9th International Conference on Healthcare Informatics (ICHI)*, 406–414. https://doi.org/10.1109/ICHI52183.2021.00066

Larsson, R., Erlingsdóttir, G., Persson, J., & Rydenfält, C. (2022). Teamwork in home care nursing: A scoping literature review. *Health & Social Care in the Community*, 30(6). https://doi.org/10.1111/hsc.13910

Leslie M, Paradis E, Gropper MA, Kitto S, Reeves S, Pronovost P. An ethnographic study of health information technology use in three intensive care units. Health Serv Res. 2017;52(4):1330–48. https://doi.org/10.1111/1475-6773.12466.

Levit, L., Balogh, E., Nass, S., & Ganz, P. A. (2013). Patient-centered communication and shared decision making.

Lewis LK. Collaborative interaction: Review of communication scholarship and a research agenda. Ann Int Commun Assoc. 2006;30(1):197–247.

Lindeke L, Sieckert A. Nurse-physician workplace collaboration. Online J Issues Nurs, 2005; 10(1).

Lingard L, Sue-Chue-Lam C, Tait GR, Bates J, Shadd J, Schulz V. Pulling together and pulling apart: influences of convergence and divergence on distributed healthcare teams. Adv Health Sci Educ. 2017;22(5):1085–99. https://doi.org/10.1007/s10459-016-9741-2.

Malhotra S, Jordan D, Shortliffe E, Patel VL. Workflow modeling in critical care: piecing together your own puzzle. J Biomed Inform. 2007;40(2):81–92.

Mamykina L, Jiang S, Collins SA, Twohig B, Hirsh J, Hripcsak G, Hum RS, Kaufman DR. Revealing structures in narratives: a mixed-methods approach to studying interdisciplinary handoff in critical care. J Biomed Inform. 2016;62:117–24.

Marini CP, Ritter G, Sharma C, McNelis J, Goldberg M, Barrera R. The effect of robotic telerounding in the surgical intensive care units impact on medical education. J Robot Surg. 2015;9(1):51–6.

Mars, M., & Scott, R. E. (2022). Electronic Patient-Generated Health Data for Healthcare. In UCR Health and UCR School of Medicine, Riverside, CA, USA & S. L. Linwood (Eds.), *Digital Health* (pp. 1–16). Exon Publications. https://doi.org/10.36255/exon-publications-digital-health-patient-generated-health-data

Martin A.K., Green T.L., McCarthy A.L., Sowa P.M., & Laakso E.L. (2022). Healthcare Teams: Terminology, Confusion, and Ramifications. J Multidiscip Healthc. Apr 8;15:765–772. https://doi.org/10.2147/JMDH.S342197.

Mathieu JE, Heffner TS, Goodwin GF, Salas E, Cannon-Bowers JA. The influence of shared mental models on team process and performance. J Appl Psychol. 2000;85(2):273.

McDougall A, Goldszmidt M, Kinsella EA, Smith S, Lingard L. Collaboration and entanglement: An actor-network theory analysis of team-based intraprofessional care for patients with advanced heart failure. Soc Sci Med. 2016;164:108–17. https://doi.org/10.1016/j.socscimed.2016.07.010.

McIntyre, R. M., & Salas, E. (1995). Measuring and managing for team performance: Emerging principles from complex environments. *Team effectiveness and decision making in organizations*, 9–45.

McLaney E, Morassaei S, Hughes L, Davies R, Campbell M, Di Prospero L. A framework for interprofessional team collaboration in a hospital setting: Advancing team competencies and behaviours. Healthc Manage Forum. 2022Mar;35(2):112–7. https://doi.org/10.1177/08404704211063584.E.

Mitchell, P., Wynia, M., Golden, R., McNellis, B., Okun, S., Webb, C. E., . . . Von Kohorn, I. (2012). *Core principles & values of effective team-based health care*: Institute of Medicine Washington, DC.

Morrison-Smith S, Ruiz J. Challenges and barriers in virtual teams: a literature review. SN Applied Sciences. 2020;2(6):1096. https://doi.org/10.1007/s42452-020-2801-5.

Motulsky A, Wong J, Cordeau J-P, Pomalaza J, Barkun J, Tamblyn R. Using mobile devices for inpatient rounding and handoffs: an innovative application developed and rapidly adopted by clinicians in a pediatric hospital. J Am Med Inform Assoc. 2017;24(e1):e69–78.

Nancarrow SA, Booth A, Ariss S, Smith T, Enderby P, Roots A. Ten principles of good interdisciplinary team work. Hum Resour Health. 2013;11(1):19.

Nelson, S. J., Sherertz, D.D., Tuttle, M.S. . (1992). *Issues in the development of an information retrieval system: the Physician's Information Assistant.* Paper presented at the Proc. of the Seventh World Congress on Medical Informatics (Medinfo'92).

Niazkhani Z, Pirnejad H, Berg M, Aarts J. The impact of computerized provider order entry systems on inpatient clinical workflow: a literature review. J Am Med Inform Assoc. 2009;16(4):539–49.

O'Daniel M, Rosenstein AH. Professional communication and team collaboration. 2008.

O'Grady L, Jadad A. Shifting from shared to collaborative decision making: a change in thinking and doing. Journal of Participatory Medicine. 2010;2(13):1–6.

Onnasch L, Roesler E. A Taxonomy to Structure and Analyze Human-Robot Interaction. Int J Soc Robot. 2021;13(4):833–49. https://doi.org/10.1007/s12369-020-00666-5.

Papapanagiotou P, Fleuriot JD. Formal verification of collaboration patterns in healthcare. Behav & Inf Technol. 2014;33(12):1278–93. https://doi.org/10.1080/0144929X.2013.824506.

Paul SA, Reddy MC. Understanding together: sensemaking in collaborative information seeking. Paper presented at the Proceedings of the 2010 ACM conference on Computer supported cooperative work. 2010.

Payne PR, Lussier Y, Foraker RE, Embi PJ. Rethinking the role and impact of health information technology: informatics as an interventional discipline. BMC Med Inform Decis Mak. 2016;16:40. https://doi.org/10.1186/s12911-016-0278-3.

Poitras M-E, Couturier Y, Beaupré P, Girard A, Aubry F, Vaillancourt VT, Carrier J-D, Fortin L, Racine J, Morneau J, Boudreault A, Cormier C, Morin A, McGraw M. Collaborative practice competencies needed for telehealth delivery by health and social care professionals: a scoping review. J Interprof Care. 2023;1–15. https://doi.org/10.1080/13561820.2023.2213712.

Porter CO, Hollenbeck JR, Ilgen DR, Ellis AP, West BJ, Moon H. Backing up behaviors in teams: the role of personality and legitimacy of need. J Appl Psychol. 2003;88(3):391.

Press MJ, Michelow MD, MacPhail LH. Care coordination in accountable care organizations: moving beyond structure and incentives. Am J Manag Care. 2012;18(12):778–80.

Pype P, Mertens F, Helewaut F, Krystallidou D. Healthcare teams as complex adaptive systems: understanding team behaviour through team members' perception of interpersonal interaction. BMC Health Serv Res. 2018;18(1):570. https://doi.org/10.1186/s12913-018-3392-3.

Ramezani M, Takian A, Bakhtiari A, Rabiee HR, Ghazanfari S, Sazgarnejad S. Research agenda for using artificial intelligence in health governance: interpretive scoping review and framework. BioData Mining. 2023;16:31. https://doi.org/10.1186/s13040-023-00346-w.

Reddy M, Pratt W, Dourish P, Shabot MM. Sociotechnical requirements analysis for clinical systems. Methods Inf Med. 2003;42(4):437–44.

Reddy, M. C., Dourish, P., & Pratt, W. (2001). Coordinating Heterogeneous Work: Information and Representation in Medical Care. In W. Prinz, M. Jarke, Y. Rogers, K. Schmidt, & V. Wulf (Eds.), *ECSCW 2001: Proceedings of the Seventh European Conference on Computer Supported Cooperative Work 16–20 September 2001, Bonn, Germany* (pp. 239–258). Dordrecht: Springer Netherlands.

Reddy MC, Jansen BJ. A model for understanding collaborative information behavior in context: A study of two healthcare teams. Inf Process Manage. 2008;44(1):256–73.

Reddy MC, Spence PR. Collaborative information seeking: A field study of a multidisciplinary patient care team. Inf Process Manage. 2008;44(1):242–55.

Reeves S, Pelone F, Harrison R, Goldman J, Zwarenstein M. Interprofessional collaboration to improve professional practice and healthcare outcomes. Cochrane Database Syst Rev. Jun 2017;22; 6(6):CD000072.

Rincon F, Vibbert M, Childs V, Fry R, Caliguri D, Urtecho J, Rosenwasser R, Jallo J. Implementation of a model of robotic tele-presence (RTP) in the neuro-ICU: effect on critical care nursing team satisfaction. Neurocrit Care. 2012;17(1):97–101.

Roett MA, Coleman MT. Practice improvement, part II: collaborative practice and team-based care. FP Essent. 2013;414:11–8.

Rosen MA, DiazGranados D, Dietz AS, Benishek LE, Thompson D, Pronovost PJ, Weaver SJ. Teamwork in Healthcare: Key Discoveries Enabling Safer. High-Quality Care the American Psychologist. 2018;73(4):433–50. https://doi.org/10.1037/amp0000298.

Rosenman, E. D., Dixon, A. J., Webb, J. M., Brolliar, S., Golden, S. J., Jones, K. A., Shah, S., Grand, J. A., Kozlowski, S. W., Chao, G. T., & Fernandez, R. (2017). A Simulation-based Approach to Measuring Team Situational Awareness in Emergency Medicine: A Multicenter, Observational Study. *Academic Emergency Medicine.*

Rudin RS, Schneider EC, Predmore Z, Gidengil CA. Knowledge gaps inhibit health IT development for coordinating complex patients' care. Am J Manag Care. 2016;22(9):e317-322.

Sadeghi, P., Andreev, P., Benyoucef, M., Momtahan, K., & Kuziemsky, C. (2014). Activity theory driven system analysis of complex healthcare processes.

Salas E, Dickinson TL, Converse SA, Tannenbaum SI. Toward an understanding of team performance and training. In: Teams: Their training and performance. Westport, CT, US: Ablex Publishing; 1992. p. 3–29.

Salas, E., Stout, R., & Cannon-Bowers, J. (1994). The role of shared mental models in developing shared situational awareness. *Situational awareness in complex systems*, 297–304.

Schadewaldt V, McInnes E, Hiller JE, Gardner A. Experiences of nurse practitioners and medical practitioners working in collaborative practice models in primary healthcare in Australia–a multiple case study using mixed methods. BMC Fam Pract. 2016;17(1):99.

Secinaro S, Calandra D, Secinaro A, Muthurangu V, Biancone P. The role of artificial intelligence in healthcare: a structured literature review. BMC Med Inform Decis Mak. 2021;21(1):125. https://doi.org/10.1186/s12911-021-01488-9.

Shachak A, Kuziemsky C, Petersen C. Beyond TAM and UTAUT: Future directions for HIT implementation research. J Biomed Inform. 2019;100: 103315. https://doi.org/10.1016/j.jbi.2019.103315.

Shah, C. Collaborative Information Seeking (CIS) in Context. In Collaborative Information Seeking (pp. 25–38): Springer. 2012.

Shah C, González-Ibáñez R. Exploring information seeking processes in collaborative search tasks. Proceedings of the Association for Information Science and Technology. 2010;47(1):1–7.

Shamir B. Calculations, values, and identities: The sources of collectivistic work motivation. Human Relations. 1990;43(4):313–32.

Singer SJ, Kerrissey MJ. Leading Health Care Teams Beyond Covid-19: Marking the Moment and Shifting from Recuperation to Regeneration. *NEJM Catalyst*. 2011. https://catalyst.nejm.org/doi/full/https://doi.org/10.1056/CAT.21.0169

Singh R, Singh A, Singh DR, Singh G. Improvement of workflow and processes to ease and enrich meaningful use of health information technology. Adv Med Educ Pract. 2013;4:231–6. https://doi.org/10.2147/AMEP.S53307.

Sittig DF, Ash JS, Zhang J, Osheroff JA, Shabot MM. Lessons from "Unexpected increased mortality after implementation of a commercially sold computerized physician order entry system." Pediatrics. 2006;118(2):797–801. https://doi.org/10.1542/peds.2005-3132.

Srinivas P, Faiola AJ, Khan B. Supporting information management in ICU rounding a novel mobile system for managing patient-centered notes and action-items. Paper presented at the E-health Networking, Application & Services (HealthCom), 2015 17th International Conference on. 2015.

Stout RJ, Cannon-Bowers JA, Salas E. The role of shared mental models in developing team situational awareness: Implications for training. Training Research Journal. 1996;2(85–116):1997.

Stowers K, Brady LL, MacLellan C, Wohleber R, Salas E. Improving teamwork competencies in human-machine teams: perspectives from team science. Front Psychol. 2021;12: 590290. https://doi.org/10.3389/fpsyg.2021.590290.

Tan AJQ, Chua WL, McKenna L, Tan LLC, Lim YJ, Liaw SY. Interprofessional collaboration in telemedicine for long-term care: An exploratory qualitative study. J Nurs Scholarsh. 2023;55(6):1227–37. https://doi.org/10.1111/jnu.12925.

Tang C, Xiao Y, Chen Y, Gorman PN. Design for Supporting Healthcare Teams. In: Patel VL, Kannampallil TG, Kaufman DR, editors. Cognitive Informatics for Biomedicine: Human Computer Interaction in Healthcare. Cham: Springer International Publishing; 2015. p. 215–39.

Thiebes S, Gao F, Briggs RO, Schmidt-Kraepelin M, Sunyaev A. Design concerns for multiorganizational, multistakeholder collaboration: a study in the healthcare industry. J Manag Inf Syst. 2023;40(1):239–70. https://doi.org/10.1080/07421222.2023.2172771.

Truijens SEM, Banga FR, Fransen AF, Pop VJM, Van Runnard Heimel PJ, Oei SG. The effect of multiprofessional simulation-based obstetric team training on patient-reported quality of care: A pilot study. Simulation in Healthcare. 2015;10(4):210–6.

Unertl KM, Novak LL, Van Houten C, Brooks J, Smith AO, Webb Harris J, Avery T, Simpson C, Lorenzi NM. Organizational diagnostics: a systematic approach to identifying technology and workflow issues in clinical settings. JAMIA Open. 2020;3(2):269–80. https://doi.org/10.1093/jamiaopen/ooaa013.

Vanderbilt AA, Pappada SM, Stein H, Harper D, Papadimos TJ. Increasing patient safety with neonates via handoff communication during delivery: a call for interprofessional health care team training across GME and CME. Adv Med Educ Pract. 2017;8:365.

Vos JFJ, Boonstra A, Kooistra A, et al. The influence of electronic health record use on collaboration among medical specialties. BMC Health Serv Res. 2020;20:676. https://doi.org/10.1186/s12913-020-05542-6.

Wagner JA. Studies of individualism-collectivism: Effects on cooperation in groups. Acad Manag J. 1995;38(1):152–73.

Weber JM, Malhotra D, Murnighan JK. Normal acts of irrational trust: Motivated attributions and the trust development process. Res Organ Behav. 2004;26:75–101.

Wilk S, Kezadri-Hamiaz M, Rosu D, Kuziemsky C, Michalowski W, Amyot D, Carrier M. Using semantic components to represent dynamics of an interdisciplinary healthcare team in a multi-agent decision support system. J Med Syst. 2016;40(2):42. https://doi.org/10.1007/s10916-015-0375-3.

Wong P, Redley B, Digby R, Correya A, Bucknall T. Families' perspectives of participation in patient care in an adult intensive care unit: A qualitative study. Aust Crit Care. 2020;33(4):317–25. https://doi.org/10.1016/j.aucc.2019.06.002.

Xiao Y, Parker SH, Manser T. Teamwork and collaboration. Rev Hum Factors Ergon. 2013;8(1):55–102. https://doi.org/10.1177/1557234x13495181.

Xyrichis A, Ream E. Teamwork: a concept analysis. J Adv Nurs. 2008;61(2):232–41. https://doi.org/10.1111/j.1365-2648.2007.04496.x.

Zajac S, Woods A, Tannenbaum S, Salas E, Holladay CL. Overcoming challenges to teamwork in healthcare: a team effectiveness framework and evidence-based guidance. Front Commun. 2021;6: 606445. https://doi.org/10.3389/fcomm.2021.606445.

Chapter 9
Interruptions and Multitasking in Clinical Work: A Summary of the Evidence

Johanna Westbrook, Magdalena Z. Raban, Joanna Clive, and Scott R. Walter

9.1   Studying Interruptions and Multitasking

Any discussion of interruptions and multitasking needs to consider what is meant by these terms in relation to how they can be defined and measured. Many researchers (Grundgeiger et al., 2016; Rivera-Rodriguez & Karsch, 2010; Walter et al., 2015) have noted the considerable heterogeneity and ambiguity of definitions used in the investigation of these phenomena, despite their common focus on the disruptive aspects of clinical work. Definitions of interruptions in healthcare have largely drawn from those applied to the study of interruptions in controlled experimental psychology settings (Trafton et al., 2003). Much of this psychological experimentation has focused on investigating the cognitive costs to an individual when required to switch between tasks, either as a consequence of multitasking or being interrupted (Douglas et al., 2017). These ideas have been interpreted in a range of ways when introduced into the uncontrolled and more complex healthcare context. Several attempts have been made to review definitions and terms used in the healthcare domain and to either distil them into a universal definition (McFarlane, 1997) or to define a set of common attributes (Brixey et al., 2007; Sasangohar et al., 2012). However, attempts to synthesise several definitions have often resulted in somewhat vague conceptualisations that have not moved this area of study towards definitional consensus. Walter et al. (2018) have instead argued for the need to move away from traditional interruption concepts towards the development of a more context-appropriate conceptualisation centred around the disruptive aspects of clinical work.

J. Westbrook (✉) · M. Z. Raban · J. Clive · S. R. Walter
Centre for Health Systems and Safety Research, Australian Institute of Health Innovation, Faculty of Medicine, Health and Human Sciences, Macquarie University, Sydney, Australia
e-mail: johanna.westbrook@mq.edu.au

Compared to interruptions, multitasking in clinical work has been less well studied, yet it has been identified as another aspect of clinical work that may have workflow and patient safety implications. Two distinct forms of multitasking have been characterised in the literature. Concurrent multitasking (or dual task performance) comprises two or more tasks being simultaneously conducted. This definition of multitasking is the most commonly applied in observational studies of clinical work (Douglas et al., 2017). In contrast, interleaved multitasking involves switching between several tasks that are progressing in parallel. For example, an emergency physician managing two patients at the same time and switching between tasks for these patients. Douglas et al. (2017) discuss both the concepts and definitions associated with the study of multitasking in healthcare, including the crossover between some multitasking and interruption definitions.

Despite the heterogeneity in definitions (Table 9.2), there has been an underlying focus in observational studies of interruption and multitasking on aspects of clinical work that can contribute to individuals' cognitive load. When designing a new study, the central considerations in relation to the definitions to be applied are as follows. First, definitions should address the aims of the investigation and be able to be operationalised; second, both the definitions and the details of how they are operationalised need to be reported clearly. This is rarely done well in studies to date but is essential to allow accurate interpretation of findings and comparison between studies.

9.2   Assessing the Frequency and Characteristics of Interruptions and Multitasking

Direct observational studies have been the main method by which interruptions and multitasking are studied in healthcare. Walter et al. (2015) provide a comprehensive discussion of some of the core challenges to performing quantitative observational studies of clinical work 'in the wild'. To determine the frequency and the relative burden of interruptions and multitasking in clinical work, there is a necessity to identify a denominator. Most commonly interruptions have been reported as a rate using time as the denominator, for example, the number of interruptions per hour. However, when interruptions are examined during specific clinical tasks, studies often report the proportion of these tasks that were interrupted. Studies examining concurrent multitasking have also used time as the denominator, but instead of counting the number of multitasking instances, they often measure the time spent in multitasking and report it as a proportion of the total time.

Table 9.1 provides a summary of the interruption rates and multitasking proportions reported across a range of studies using direct observation of clinical work in different countries. Comparisons of interruption rates across studies can be difficult due to the differences in definitions and observational methodology. The studies summarised in Table 9.1 use broadly similar definitions of interruption, analogous to the first definition presented in Table 9.2, and the same observational technique and data collection tool (Westbrook & Ampt, 2009).

Observational studies of clinicians have shown that interruption rates tend to be higher in critical care settings (Westbrook et al., 2010a; 2018) and inpatient dispensaries (Magee et al., 2023), among specialist consultants (specialists), and for certain types of clinical tasks (Walter et al., 2017, 2011, 2010b; Westbrook et al., 2010a). Most interruptions are generated by other co-workers, rather than patients, and are related to the provision of patient care (Bellandi et al., 2018; Göras et al., 2019; Ratwani et al., 2017; Walter et al., 2017; Weigl et al., 2012). Interruption rates also appear to vary between night and day shifts (Arabadzhiyska et al., 2013), and between weekdays and weekends (Richardson et al., 2016). As may be expected, interruption rates appear to vary by country, with one study from Italy reporting rates over 1.5 times higher for physicians and 3 times higher for nurses on surgical wards, than those reported in studies conducted in other countries (Bellandi et al., 2018).

Similar to interruption rates, the proportions of time spent multitasking vary between healthcare settings, health professionals, and countries (Walter et al., 2014). However, in contrast to interruption rates for the emergency department (ED), which are higher than on wards, ED physicians spend a lower proportion of their time multitasking. This may be indicative of the fact that individuals have greater autonomy over decisions to multitask than over interruptions, the latter of which are almost always in response to an external stimulus. In an environment in which external stimuli are frequent, such as the ED, physicians may choose to multitask to a lesser degree in order to reduce their cognitive load.

Some studies have focused on the frequency of interruptions and multitasking during particular clinical processes. These are often safety critical activities with direct implications for patient care, such as medication administration by nurses. Since interruption rates can vary between the types of clinical activities, understanding the frequency with which they occur during safety critical tasks has been regarded as important under the assumption that high rates are associated with increased safety risk.

Studies that have looked at interruptions during medication administration have used varying measures of interruption rates, making comparisons between studies fraught. Two studies in Australia estimated that between 35 and 53% of medication administrations are interrupted (Westbrook et al., 2017; 2010b). In the UK, nurses were interrupted an average of 2.6 times per medication round (i.e., during the administration of all medications for all the patients under a nurse's care) and in the US, 63% of medication passes (i.e., the administration of all medications to one patient) involved an interruption not relevant to the task at hand.

The reporting of multitasking during medication tasks has also used a variety of measures.

One Australian study reported that multitasking occurred during 25% of medication tasks (Westbrook et al., 2011) with concurrent professional communication occurring in 10.7% of medication tasks. Another Australian study estimated that nurses engaged in an average of 4.6 multitasks per 100 administrations (Westbrook et al., 2017). Other studies have compared multitasking rates in medication tasks to

Table 9.1 Reported interruption rates per hour in studies that used similar interruption definitions and the work observation method by activity timing (WOMBAT) technique and software for data collection

Population studied	Setting	Interruption rate (number of interruptions per hour)	Percentage of time spent in concurrent multitasking	Country	References
Physicians	General wards	2.9	20%	Australia	Westbrook et al. (2008)
Physicians	Surgical wards	13.1	33.5%	Italy	Bellandi et al. (2018)
Junior doctors	General wards on weekends	6.6	20.9%	Australia	Richardson et al. (2016)
Junior doctors	General wards (rounds)	3.1	20%	UK	Bell et al. (2021)
Resident physicians	General wards at night (10pm to 8am)	1.3	6.4%	Australia	Arabadzhiyska et al. (2013)
Physicians	Emergency department	6.6	12.8%	Australia	Westbrook et al. (2010a)
Physicians	Emergency department	7.9	4.6%	Australia	Westbrook et al. (2018)
Physicians	Emergency department	4.3 (during drug related tasks)	17.4% drug related	Norway	Nymoen et al. (2022)
Physicians	Emergency department	4.0 overall	9.8% non-drug related	Norway	Nymoen et al. (2022)
Attending and resident doctors	Intensive care unit	2.5	67%	USA	Hefter et al. (2016)
Registrars	Intensive care unit	4.2	24.4%	Australia	Li et al. (2015)
Physicians	Intensive care unit	3.8	–	Canada	Ballerman et al. (2011)
Surgeons	Operating room	3.0 team overall	53.8%	Sweden	Göras et al. (2019)
Nurses	General wards	2.0	5.8%	Australia	Westbrook et al. (2011)
Nurses	Surgical wards	13.6	15.2%	Italy	Bellandi et al. (2018)
Nurses	General wards	Pre eMS 3.1 Post eMS 1.4	Pre eMS 20.7% Post eMS 5%	Australia	Bingham et al. (2021)
Nurses	Hospital acute & subacute wards	5.0	19%	Australia	Kramer et al. (2023)

(continued)

Table 9.1 (continued)

Population studied	Setting	Interruption rate (number of interruptions per hour)	Percentage of time spent in concurrent multitasking	Country	References
Nurses	Intensive care unit	3.3	–	Canada	Ballerman et al. (2011)
Nurses	Operating room	3.0 team overall	30.1%	Sweden	Göras et al. (2019)
Registered nurse anaesthetists	Operating room	4.6	63.1%	Sweden	Göras et al. (2019)
Registered nurse anaesthetists	Operating room	3.7	62.3%	Sweden	Olin et al. (2022)
Nurses	Nursing homes & private homes	1.2	3.7%	Sweden	Holmqvist et al. (2018)
Pharmacists	General hospital wards	Pre eMS 3.1 Post eMS 4.4	Pre eMS 2.4% Post eMS 8.7%	Australia	Lo et al. (2010)
Pharmacists	Paediatric hospital	3.5	4.4%	Australia	Lehnbom et al. (2016)
Pharmacists	General hospital wards	Pre eMS 4.0 Post eMS 4.0	–	Australia	Westbrook et al. (2019)
Pharmacists	General hospital wards	Pre eMS 3.2 Post eMS 2.5	–	England	Westbrook et al. (2019)
Pharmacists	Inpatient dispensary	6.7	8.6%	Australia	Magee et al. (2023)
Pharmacists	Hospital acute & subacute units	3	19.1%	Australia	Huynh et al. (2022)
Pharmacists	Community pharmacies	3	7.5%	Australia	Karia et al. (2022)
Pharmacy technicians	Inpatient dispensary	5.1	9.50%	Australia	Magee et al. (2023)
Respiratory therapists	Intensive care unit	3.5	–	Canada	Ballerman et al. (2011)
Unit/ward clerks	Intensive care unit	4.4	–	Canada	Ballerman et al. (2011)
Nuclear medicine technologists	General hospital	4.5	16.6%	Australia	Larcos et al. (2016)

eMS = electronic medication system

Table 9.2 Examples of definitions of interruptions and multitasking applied in healthcare studies

Term	Definition	References
Interruption	External stimuli which result in an individual ceasing a task to attend to a new task. For example, ceasing a task to answer a question	Westbrook et al. (2008)
Interruption	Process of coordinating abrupt change in people's activities	McFarlane (1997)
Interruption	A break in performance of a human activity initiated by a source internal or external to the recipients, with the occurrence situated within the context	Brixey et al. (2010)
Concurrent (or dual task) multitasking	The performance of two or more tasks conducted simultaneously. For example, writing notes while also talking	Douglas et al. (2017)
Interleaved multitasking	The management of multiple tasks in which there is switching between tasks that are progressing in parallel	Douglas et al. (2017)
IT interruptions	Perceived, IT-based external events with a range of content that captures cognitive attention and breaks the continuity of an individual's primary task activities	Addas and Pinsonneault (2015)

overall multitasking rates. In the ED, physicians were observed to multitask 4.6% of their overall time, but 20.1% of the time while prescribing (Westbrook et al., 2018). Similarly, ED physicians in Norway were found to multitask during 17.4% of medication tasks but only 9.8% of their time during non-medication tasks (Nymoen et al., 2022).

Interleaved multitasking, which is characterised by iterative task switching, has been identified as a key feature of ED physicians' work with variability between senior and more junior physicians (Augenstein et al., 2021; Walter et al., 2019).

9.3 The Role and Effects of Interruptions in Clinical Work

A considerable body of research on interruptions in healthcare has focussed on their potentially negative role in placing tasks at risk of error, incompletion or in reducing task efficiency. As the previous section illustrates, many descriptive studies have sought to capture the nature, source and occurrence of interruptions, largely in order to inform the design of effective interventions to prevent or ameliorate their potentially negative effects. However, research evidence which directly links the occurrence of interruptions to negative task outcomes in clinical contexts remains limited. A small observational study in operating rooms showed that anaesthetists who immediately engaged with interruptions failed to check blood product details prior to transfusion (Liu et al., 2009). While a study of caesarean section surgeries showed an association between procedure length and interruptions, but not with procedural complications (Willett et al., 2018). In an experimental study of radiologists who were interrupted while reviewing and dictating diagnostic reports, there was no significant impact of interruptions on diagnostic quality. A simulation study of physicians conducting central venous catheter insertion found that interruptions increased the time taken for the task as well as the number of attempts required (Jones et al., 2017). A few studies in the ED have identified a failure of physicians to return to interrupted tasks following interruption, but no specific consequences for care (Fong & Ratwani, 2018; Westbrook et al., 2010a).

A direct observational study in two teaching hospitals, which examined the relationship between medication administration error and interruptions to nurses, found a significant association between interruptions and higher error rates and greater severity of errors (Westbrook et al., 2010b). This relationship was also found in a high-fidelity simulation study of ICU nurses, where nurses who received a higher number of interruptions made more errors in medication administration (Santomauro et al., 2021). Further, a study of emergency physicians demonstrated a significant positive relationship between interruptions and prescribing errors (Westbrook et al., 2018). That said, such studies reporting direct associations between interruptions and errors in clinical settings are still relatively rare (Danesh et al., 2022). The methodological difficulties in identifying and reliably measuring task errors against which to assess the impact of interruptions are a significant and ongoing challenge (Douglas et al., 2017; Walter et al., 2015). Unlike experimental studies, which focus on the association between a stimulus and individual response, studies of interruptions in the wild are very different. Clinical work is highly team-based, and the effects of disruptions on such collaborative work practices are not easily measurable.

In concert with studies attempting to examine the negative effects of interruptions and multitasking on clinical work, there has been increased attention on understanding how both activities may, in fact, be important to clinical workflow. This work has focused more on understanding how interruptions and multitasking can be used effectively in managing the dynamic nature of clinical work. For example, studies by Walter et al. (2017) in the ED demonstrated the ways in which senior clinicians make themselves available to interruption as an integral element in supervising the work of more junior clinicians. Thus, in this context interruptions could be viewed as a key technique to achieve both efficient and effective workflows, which contribute to increased patient safety. For example, interruptions can be a useful strategy by which initiators can obtain and share information, alert others to patient safety risks, obtain assistance, and reduce the likelihood of errors (Knight et al., 2023). Research in other fields on high reliability organisations may be of value in understanding how these work strategies may be beneficial.

One of the ways in which high reliability organisations are able to operate successfully in complex environments is to organise for collective mindfulness. Collective mindfulness has been described as "*a quality of organisational attention that increases the likelihood that people will notice unique details or situations and act upon them*" (Sutcliffe & Vogus, 2014, p. 410). Thus, some of the newer research findings illustrating the ways in which interruptions are used in healthcare point to their potential role in collective mindfulness, particularly in settings such as emergency departments. Further studies are required to explore the more nuanced ways in which interruptions may play an enabling role in safe and efficient care, besides being a potentially negative contributor to cognitive load and task errors.

Excessive rates of interruptions are assumed to negatively impact on clinicians' cognitive loads. Thus, distinguishing between necessary and unnecessary interruptions has been considered in some studies as a way to target interventions more effectively. For example, in a study of interruptions during medication administration, Westbrook et al. (2017) categorised whether observed interruptions were directly related to the medication administration tasks underway. They also excluded any emergency interruptions (e.g., a patient requiring resuscitation, or a patient who fell). Overall, they found that only a small proportion of interruptions were related to the medication tasks in progress. Other studies have asked clinicians the extent to which interruptions were of value (McGillis Hall et al., 2010; Weigl et al., 2017).

In contrast to the negative connotations directed at interruptions, multitasking is often viewed as a prized skill, even to the extent that the ability to multitask has been listed as a necessary skill for US emergency physicians (Perina et al., 2011). Considerably less research has been conducted towards measuring the likely effectiveness of multitasking in clinical settings (Werner et al., 2015). Existing evidence seems to suggest that multitasking may be associated with no improvement in task efficiency during handover (van Rensen et al., 2012) and multitasking among emergency physicians was shown to be associated with task failures during medication prescribing (Westbrook et al., 2018). Further, studies (Augenstein et al., 2021; Weigl et al., 2017) of ED physicians in Germany have found interruptions and multitasking were associated with reported increased stress levels.

9.4   Interventions to Reduce Interruptions to Clinical Work

Drawing upon concepts used in aviation, such as the sterile cockpit, the most common approach to reducing unnecessary interruptions has been the use of barrier or isolation techniques. These have most frequently been trialled in studies designed to reduce interruption rates for nurses, especially during the medication administration process. These interventions have included the use of 'do not interrupt' tabards, sashes or flags, which signal that nurses are involved in a medication task and should not be interrupted; and locating specific medication administration processes in areas demarcated as 'interruption-free' zones. There is some evidence suggesting that such interventions can be effective (Dall'Oglio et al., 2017; Huckels-Baumgart et al., 2017; Raban & Westbrook, 2014). A systematic review in 2014 (Raban & Westbrook, 2014) reported 10 studies of interventions which had undertaken a quantitative assessment of intervention effectiveness in reducing interruptions and/or medication administration errors. Four reported a decrease in interruptions and one an increase. Three studies had multi-component interventions which incorporated a 'do not interrupt' element, and all reported a reduction in error rate. However, none of these studies used a controlled design so that attribution of the change in interruption rate to the respective intervention was not possible (Raban & Westbrook, 2014). A subsequent randomised controlled trial (Westbrook et al., 2017) showed a significant decrease in interruption rate following the introduction of a 'do not interrupt' bundled intervention, but the authors of this study raised questions about the clinical significance of the magnitude of the reduction in interruptions on error rates (from 50 interruptions per 100 administrations to 34/100). Furthermore, issues have been raised about the acceptability and sustainability of this form of intervention in busy clinical environments (Westbrook et al., 2017). A French cluster RCT tested the effects of nurses wearing 'do not interrupt' vests and found no impact on interruption rates or medication administration errors and also reported that nurses generally did not find the intervention useful (Berdot et al., 2021). Thus, despite studies seeking to demonstrate the value of barrier interventions to reduce interruptions there has been limited progress in establishing their effectiveness or long-term sustainability.

Improved understanding of interruptive behaviours in healthcare has prompted the re-conceptualisation of potential interventions in terms of a focus on how they can be used most effectively to support resilient work practices. Gao et al. (2017) suggest alternative approaches. First, the use of resilient engineering, which takes the view that if interruptions are a potential source of negative disruption to work then interventions should be targeted towards assisting clinicians to continue or quickly resume their primary task in the event of disruption. Such interventions might include the provision of cues which allow clinicians to easily resume tasks when interrupted. For example, Prakash et al. (2014) used visual timers to support nurses administering IV medications. Clinical information systems which identify fields remaining unfilled may be another type of cue to alert clinicians to incomplete steps in an interrupted procedure (Georgiou et al., 2017).

Identifying the cause of unnecessary interruptions and specifically addressing them through changes in resources or practices is another approach. For example, several studies of medication administration processes noted interruptions due to a nurse seeking access to the restricted drug keys. The cost to the nurse who is interrupting is low, but for the nurse being interrupted there is no clinical value and the cost may be high in terms of distraction from his/her primary task. Thus, identifying strategies such as considering the way in which drug rounds are organised and the likely demands placed on scarce resources (in this instance the drug keys) provides opportunities for reducing unnecessary interruptions of benefit to all staff.

Consideration of interruptions as an element of behaviours displayed in high reliability organisations is also likely to be a valuable approach. This does not suggest an unfettered use of interruptions, but an examination of the ways in which interruptions contribute to enacting collective mindfulness, and then identifying ways to optimise their use. Further, drawing attention to the role of interruptive behaviours through appropriate training should not be underestimated. In addition, specific training in handling interruptions in different clinical settings is also likely to be beneficial (Cades et al., 2011; Hayes et al., 2017).

9.5   Interruptions and Information Technology

Information technologies both create a source of new interruptions (e.g., in the form of electronic alerts (Baysari et al., 2011) and mobile devices allowing constant communication (Vaisman & Wu, 2017)) as well as potentially reducing the need for some interruptions by providing greater concurrent access to information. Alert fatigue due to the excessive use of computerised alerts, which leads to a large proportion of alerts being ignored, continues to be a significant problem (Poly et al., 2020). However, once again the context in which these disruptions to clinical work occur has been shown to be important. For example, an Australian study (Baysari et al., 2011) showed that less than 20% of interruptive medication alerts generated by a computerised system were read by physicians on ward rounds, yet in the same hospital junior physicians at night considered over 80% of these alerts when prescribing medications (Jaensch et al., 2013). Thus, these interruptions to clinical workflow were deemed to provide variable clinical benefit and other approaches to the design of clinical decision support should be considered (Raban et al., 2023).

Collins et al. (2006; 2007) investigated the impact of distractions and interruptions during clinicians' use of clinical information systems, and suggested that they may introduce new opportunities for errors related to data entry and data retrieval. However, there has been limited research specifically focusing on how interruptions impact clinicians use of clinical information systems. For example, the extent to which interruptions may be a contributor to new IT-related errors (Magrabi et al., 2012; Westbrook et al., 2013), which include incidents such as the incorrect selection of items from drop-down menus, or the opening of the incorrect patient record, is unknown.

As the use of electronic health record (EHR) systems becomes increasingly pervasive, several studies have sought to investigate attention switching by clinicians through the analysis of EHR audit logs (Bartek et al., 2023; Lou et al., 2022). These have demonstrated high rates at which clinicians switch their attention between the records of individual patients, with some evidence of the additional cognitive load that this activity places on clinicians impacting both efficiency and task errors (Bartek et al., 2023; Lou et al., 2022).

9.6   Conclusions

The direction and sophistication of interruption and multitasking research in healthcare has started to change course. There is a continued need to move beyond descriptive studies to those that attempt to account for the complexity of these phenomena and the importance of the contexts in which they occur. Some observational studies have found associations between disruptive aspects of clinical work and errors in care delivery. However, there is some evidence of null effects, along with an emerging body of evidence demonstrating that interruptions, and to a lesser extent multitasking, may be effective strategies for dealing with a dynamic clinical environment and may contribute to greater organisational resilience. The mixed results partly reflect the diversity of healthcare, in that interruptions and multitasking may have different effects depending on the context, the specific scenario, and so on. The varied results may also represent the diversity in how interruptions and multitasking have been defined and conceptualised. By defining a broad range of interactions and behaviours under these terms, we then naturally observe a broad range of effects. Furthermore, evidence to date of the effects of interruptions and multitasking is based on studying the clinical work of individual clinicians. As yet, we have no clear evidence as to how these phenomena affect clinical work at the team or system level, which is an important topic for future research.

The literature suggests that efforts to support clinicians in managing the cognitive load of disruptive environments may be more valuable than blanket interventions to reduce interruptions (Westbrook et al., 2018). Identifying work practice and resource issues to avoid unnecessary interruptions should be considered, along with strategies which support recovery from interruptions such as the use of cues, and increased awareness of, and training about, how to effectively use these strategies to support safe and efficient delivery of care.

References

Addas S, Pinsonneault A. The many faces of information technology interruptions: a taxonomy and preliminary investigation of their performance effects. Inf Syst J. 2015;25(3):231–73. https://doi.org/10.1111/isj.12064.

Arabadzhiyska PN, Baysari MT, Walter S, et al. Shedding light on junior doctors' work practices after hours. Intern Med J. 2013;43(12):1321–6. https://doi.org/10.1111/imj.12223.

Augenstein T, Schneider A, Wehler M, et al. Multitasking behaviors and provider outcomes in emergency department physicians: two consecutive, observational and multi-source studies. Scand J Trauma, Resusc Emerg Med. 2021;29(1):1–9.

Ballerman M, Shaw N, Mayes D, et al. Validation of the work observational method by activity timing (WOMBAT) method of conducting time-motion observations in critical care settings: an observational study. BMC Med Inform Decis Mak. 2011;11. https://doi.org/10.1186/1472-6947-1111-1132.

Bartek B, Lou SS, Kannampallil T. Measuring the cognitive effort associated with task switching in routine EHR-based tasks. J Biomed Inform. 2023;141:104349.

Baysari M, Westbrook J, Richardson K, et al. The influence of computerized decision support on prescribing during ward-rounds: are the decision-makers targeted? J Am Med Inform Assoc. 2011;18:754–759. https://doi.org/10.1136/amiajnl-2011-000135

Bell CL, Allan JL, Ross S, et al. How can we better prepare new doctors for the tasks and challenges of ward rounds?: an observational study of junior doctors' experiences [Article]. Med Teach. 2021;43(11):1294–301. https://doi.org/10.1080/0142159X.2021.1940912.

Bellandi T, Cerri A, Carreras G, et al. Interruptions and multitasking in surgery: a multicentre observational study of the daily work patterns of doctors and nurses. Ergonomics. 2018;61(1):40–7. https://doi.org/10.1080/00140139.2017.1349934.

Berdot S, Vilfaillot A, Bezie Y, et al. Effectiveness of a 'do not interrupt' vest intervention to reduce medication errors during medication administration: a multicenter cluster randomized controlled trial. BMC Nurs. 2021;20(1):153.

Bingham G, Tong E, Poole S, et al. A longitudinal time and motion study quantifying how implementation of an electronic medical record influences hospital nurses' care delivery [Article]. Int J Med Inform 2021;153, Article 104537. https://doi.org/10.1016/j.ijmedinf.2021.104537

Brixey JJ, Tang Z, Robinson D, et al. Interruptions in a level one trauma center: a case study. Int J Med Informatics. 2007;77(4):235–41.

Brixey JJ, Robinson DJ, Turley JP, et al. The roles of MDs and RNs as initiators and recipients of interruptions in workflow. Int J Med Inform. 2010;79(6):e109–115. https://doi.org/10.1016/j.ijmedinf.2008.08.007

Cades DM, Boehm-Davis DA, Trafton JG, et al. Mitigating disruptive effects of interruptions through training: what needs to be practiced? J Exp Psychol Appl. 2011;17(2):97–109. https://doi.org/10.1037/a0023497.

Collins S, Currie L, Bakken S, et al. Interruptions during the use of a CPOE system for MICU rounds. AMIA Annu Symp Proc. 2006;895.

Collins SA, Currie L, Patel VL, et al. Multitasking by clinicians in the context of CPOE and CIS use. In: Kuhn K, Warren J, L TY, editors, MEDINFO 2007;2007. p. 958–62.

Dall'Oglio I, Fiori M, Di Ciommo V, et al. Effectiveness of an improvement programme to prevent interruptions during medication administration in a paediatric hospital: a preintervention-postintervention study. BMJ Open. 2017;7(1):e013285. https://doi.org/10.1136/bmjopen-2016-013285.

Danesh V, Sasangohar F, Kallberg A-S, et al. Systematic review of interruptions in the emergency department work environment. Int Emerg Nurs. 2022;63:101175.

Douglas HE, Raban M, Walter S, et al. Improving our understanding of multi-tasking in healthcare: drawing together the cognitive psychology and healthcare literature. Appl Ergon. 2017;59:45–55.

Fong A, Ratwani RM. Understanding emergency medicine physicians multitasking behaviors around interruptions. Acad Emerg Med. 2018;25(10). https://doi.org/10.1111/acem.13496

Gao J, Rae AJ, Dekker SWA. Intervening in interruptions: what exactly is the risk we are trying to manage? J Patient Saf. 2017. https://doi.org/10.1097/pts.0000000000000429.

Georgiou A, McCaughey EJ, Tariq A, et al. What is the impact of an electronic test result acknowledgement system on emergency department physicians' work processes? a mixed-method pre-post observational study [Article]. Int J Med Informatics. 2017;99:29–36. https://doi.org/10.1016/j.ijmedinf.2016.12.006.

Göras C, Olin K, Unbeck M, et al. Tasks, multitasking and interruptions among the surgical team in an operating room: a prospective observational study [Article]. BMJ Open. 2019;9(5), Article 026410. https://doi.org/10.1136/bmjopen-2018-026410

Grundgeiger T, Dekker S, Sanderson P, et al. Obstacles to research on the effects of interruptions in healthcare. BMJ Qual Saf. 2016;25(6):392–5. https://doi.org/10.1136/bmjqs-2015-004083.

Hayes C, Jackson D, Davidson PM, et al. Calm to chaos: engaging undergraduate nursing students with the complex nature of interruptions during medication administration. J Clin Nurs. 2017;26(23–24):4839–47. https://doi.org/10.1111/jocn.13866.

Hefter Y, Madahar P, Eisen LA, et al. A time-motion study of ICU workflow and the impact of strain*. Crit Care Med. 2016;44(8):1482–9. https://doi.org/10.1097/ccm.0000000000001719.

Holmqvist M, Ekstedt M, Walter SR, et al. Medication management in municipality-based healthcare: a time and motion study of nurses [Article]. Home Healthcare Now. 2018;36(4):238–46. https://doi.org/10.1097/NHH.0000000000000671.

Huckels-Baumart S, Niederberger M, Manser T, et al. A combined intervention to reduce interruptions during medication preparation and double-checking: a pilot-study evaluating the impact of staff training and safety vests. J Nurs Manag. 2017;25(7):539–48. https://doi.org/10.1111/jonm.12491.

Huynh S, Rush L, Dadalias D, et al. Time and motion study quantifying the activities of the cardiology, respiratory, and geriatric clinical pharmacist [Article]. J Pharm Pract Res. 2022;52(5):382–9. https://doi.org/10.1002/jppr.1825.

Jaensch SL, Baysari MT, Day RO, et al. Junior doctors' prescribing work after-hours and the impact of computerized decision support. Int J Med Informatics. 2013;82(10):980–6. https://doi.org/10.1016/j.ijmedinf.2013.06.014.

Jones J, Wilkins M, Caird J, et al. An experimental study on the impact of clinical interruptions on simulated trainee performances of central venous catheterization. Adv Simul (London, England). 2017;2:5. https://doi.org/10.1186/s41077-017-0038-1.

Kannampallil TG, Abraham J, Patel VL. Methodological framework for evaluating clinical processes: a cognitive informatics perspective. J Biomed Inform. 2016;64:342–51. https://doi.org/10.1016/j.jbi.2016.11.002

Karia A, Norman R, Robinson S, et al. Pharmacist's time spent: space for pharmacy-based Interventions and consultation TimE (SPICE)—an observational time and motion study. BMJ Open. 2022;12(3):e055597.

Knight E, Sanderson P, Neal A, et al. Interruptions in healthcare: modeling dynamic processes and effects at a team level. Appl Ergon. 2023;112:104051.

Kramer S, Raymond MJ, Hunter P, et al. Understanding the workflow of nurses in acute and subacute medical wards: a time and motion study. J Clin Nurs. 2023;32(21–22):7773–82. https://doi.org/10.1111/jocn.16835.

Larcos G, Prgomet M, Georgiou A, et al. A work observation study of nuclear medicine technologists: interruptions, resilience and implications for patient safety. BMJ Qual Saf. 2016. https://doi.org/10.1136/bmjqs-2016-005846.

Lehnbom E, Li L, Prgomet M, et al. Little things matter: a time and motion study of pharmacists' activitites in a paediatric hospital. In: Georgiou A, Schaper L, Whetton S editors. Studies in health technology information: digital health innovation for consumers, clinicians, connectivity and community, vol. 227. IOS Press; 2016. p. 80–6. https://doi.org/10.3233/978-1-61499-666-8-80.

Li L, Hains I, Hordern A, et al. What do ICU doctors do?: a multisite time and motion study of the clinical work patterns of registrars. Crit Care Resusc. 2015;17(3):159–66.

Liu D, Grundgeiger T, Sanderson PM, et al. Interruptions and blood transfusion checks: lessons from the simulated operating room. Anesth Analg. 2009;108(1):219–22.

Lo C, Burke R, Westbrook JI. Electronic medication management systems' influence on hospital pharmacists' work patterns. J Pharm Pract Res. 2010;40(2):106–10.

Lou SS, Kim S, Harford D, et al. Effect of clinician attention switching on workload and wrong-patient errors. Br J Anaesth. 2022;129(1):e22–24.

Magee K, Fromont M, Ihle E, et al. Direct observational time and motion study of the daily activities of hospital dispensary pharmacists and technicians [Article]. J Pharm Pract Res. 2023;53(2):64–72. https://doi.org/10.1002/jppr.1852.

Magrabi F, Ong M, Runciman W, et al. Using FDA reports to inform a classification for health information technology safety problems. J Am Med Inform Assoc. 2012;19:45–53.

McFarlane D. Interruption of people in human-computer interaction: a general unifying defintion of human interruption and taxonomy (NRL/FR/5510–97–9870). Naval Research Laboratory, Issue. 1997.

McGillis Hall L, Pedersen C, Hubley P, et al. Interruptions and pediatric patient safety. J Pediatr Nurs. 2010;25(3):165–75.

Nymoen LD, Tran T, Walter SR, et al. Emergency department physicians' distribution of time in the fast paced-workflow-a novel time-motion study of drug-related activities [Article]. Int J Clin Pharm. 2022;44(2):448–58. https://doi.org/10.1007/s11096-021-01364-6.

Olin K, Göras C, Nilsson U, et al. Mapping registered nurse anaesthetists' intraoperative work: tasks, multitasking, interruptions and their causes, and interactions: a prospective observational study [Article]. BMJ Open. 2022;12(1). Article e052283. https://doi.org/10.1136/bmjopen-2021-052283.

Perina DG, Brunett CP, Caro DA, et al. The 2011 model of the clinical practice of emergency medicine. Acad Emerg Med. 2012;19(7):e19−40. https://doi.org/10.1111/j.1553-2712.2012.01385.x.

Poly TN, Islam MM, Yang H-C, et al. Appropriateness of overridden alerts in computerized physician order entry: systematic review. JMIR Med Inform. 2020;8(7):e15653.

Prakesh V, Koczmara C, Savage P, et al. Mitigating errors caused by interruptions during medication verification and administration: interventions in a simulated ambulatory chemotherapy setting. BMJ Qual Saf. 2014;23(11):884–92.

Raban M, Westbrook J. Are interventions to reduce interruptions and errors during medication administration effective?: a systematic review. BMJ Qual Saf. 2014;23:414–21.

Raban MZ, Gates PJ, Gamboa S, et al. Effectiveness of non-interruptive nudge interventions in electronic health records to improve the delivery of care in hospitals: a systematic review. J Am Med Inform Assoc. 2023;30(7):1313–22.

Ratwani RM, Fong A, Puthumana JS, et al. Emergency physician use of cognitive strategies to manage interruptions. Ann Emerg Med. 2017;70(5):683–7. https://doi.org/10.1016/j.annemergmed.2017.04.036.

Richardson LC, Lehnbom EC, Baysari MT, et al. A time and motion study of junior doctors' work patterns on the weekend: a potential contributor to the weekend effect? Intern Med J. 2016;46(7):819–25. https://doi.org/10.1111/imj.13120.

Rivera-Rodriguez A, Karsch B. Interruptions and distractions in healthcare: review and reappraisal. Qual Saf Health Care. 2010;19:304–12.

Santomauro C, Powell M, Davis C, et al. Interruptions to intensive care nurses and clinical errors and procedural failures: a controlled study of causal connection. J Patient Saf. 2021;17(8):e1433–40.

Sasangohar F, Donmez B, Trbovich P, et al. Not all interruptions are created equal: positive interruptions in healthcare. Proc Hum Factors Ergon Soc Annu Meet. 2012;56(1):824–8. https://doi.org/10.1177/1071181312561172.

Sutcliffe K, Vogus T. Organizing for Mindfulness. In: Ie A, Ngnoumen C, Langer E, editors. The wiley blackwell handbook of mindfulness. Wiley Blackwell;2014. p. 407–23.

Trafton JG, Altmann E, Brock D, et al. Preparing to resume an interrupted task: effects of propsective goal encoding and retrospective rehersal. Int J Hum Comput Stud. 2003;58(5):583–603.

Vaisman A, Wu RC. Analysis of smartphone interruptions on academic general internal medicine wards: frequent interruptions may cause a 'crisis mode' work climate. Appl Clin Inform. 2017;8(1):1–11. https://doi.org/10.4338/aci-2016-08-ra-0130.

van Rensen EL, Groen ES, Numan SC, et al. Multitasking during patient handover in the recovery room. Anesth Analg. 2012;115(5):1183–7. https://doi.org/10.1213/ANE.0b013e31826996a2.

Walter SR. Interruptions in emergency medicine: things are not always what they seem. Acad Emerg Med. 2018;25(10):1178–80. https://doi.org/10.1111/acem.13505.

Walter SR, Li L, Dunsmuir WTM, et al. Managing competing demands through task-switching and multitasking: a multi-setting observational study of 200 clinicians over 1000 hours. BMJ Qual Saf. 2014;23(3):231–41. https://doi.org/10.1136/bmjqs-2013-002097.

Walter SR, Dunsmuir WTM, Westbrook JI. Stuyding interruptions and multitasking in situ: the untapped potential of quanititative observational studies. Int J Hum Comput Stud. 2015;79:118–25.

Walter SR, Raban MZ, Westbrook JI. Visualising clinical work in the emergency department: understanding interleaved patient management. Appl Ergon. 2019;79:45–53.

Walter SR, Raban MZ, Dunsmuir WTM, et al. Emergency doctors' strategies to manage competing workload demands in an interruptive environment: an observational workflow time study. Appl Ergon. 2017;58, 454–60. https://doi.org/10.1016/j.apergo.2016.07.020

Weigl M, Müller A, Vincent C, et al. The association of workflow interruptions and hospital doctors' workload: a prospective observational study. BMJ Qual Saf. 2012;21(5):399–407. https://doi.org/10.1136/bmjqs-2011-000188.

Weigl M, Beck J, Wehler M, et al. Workflow interruptions and stress atwork: a mixed-methods study among physicians and nurses of a multidisciplinary emergency department. BMJ Open. 2017;7(12):e019074. https://doi.org/10.1136/bmjopen-2017-019074.

Werner NE, Cades DM, Boehm-Davis DA (2015). Multitasking and interrupted task performance: from theory to application. In: Rosen L, Cheever N, Carrier L, editors, The wiley handbook of pyschology, technology and society. John Wiley & Sons.

Westbrook J, Ampt A. Design, application and testing of the work observation method by activity timing (WOMBAT) to measure clinicians' patterns of work and communication. Int J Med Informatics. 2009;78S:S25–33.

Westbrook JI, Ampt A, Kearney L, et al. All in a day's work: an observational study to quantify how and with whom doctors on hospital wards spend their time. Med J Aust. 2008;188(9):506–9.

Westbrook JI, Coiera E, Dunsmuir WT, et al. The impact of interruptions on clinical task completion. Qual Saf Health Care. 2010a;19(4):284–9. https://doi.org/10.1136/qshc.2009.039255.

Westbrook JI, Woods A, Rob MI, et al. Association of interruptions with an increased risk and severity of medication administration errors. Arch Intern Med. 2010b;170(8):683–90.

Westbrook JI, Li L, Hooper TD, et al. Effectiveness of a 'Do not interrupt' bundled intervention to reduce interruptions during medication administration: a cluster randomised controlled feasibility study. BMJ Qual Saf. 2017;26(9):734–42. https://doi.org/10.1136/bmjqs-2016-006123.

Westbrook JI, Raban MZ, Walter SR, et al. Task errors by emergency physicians are associated with interruptions, multitasking, fatigue and working memory capacity: a prospective, direct observation study. BMJ Qual Saf. 2018. https://doi.org/10.1136/bmjqs-2017-007333.

Westbrook JI, Li L, Shah S, et al. A cross-country time and motion study to measure the impact of electronic medication management systems on the work of hospital pharmacists in Australia and England [Article]. Int J Med Informatics. 2019;129:253–9. https://doi.org/10.1016/j.ijmedinf.2019.06.011.

Westbrook JI, Duffield C, Li L, et al. How much time do nurses have for patients? a longitudinal study of hospital nurses' patterns of task time distribution and interactions with other health professionals. BMC Health Serv Res. 2011;11(319).

Westbrook JI, Baysari MT, Li L, et al. The safety of electronic prescribing: manifestations, mechanisms, and rates of system-related errors associated with two commercial systems in hospitals. J Am Med Inform Assoc. 2013;20(6):1159–67. http://jamia.bmj.com/content/20/6/1159.abstract.

Willett M, Gillman O, Shin E, et al. The impact of distractions and interruptions during Cesarean Sections: a prospective study in a London teaching hospital. Arch Gynecol Obstet. 2018;298(2):313–8. https://doi.org/10.1007/s00404-018-4810-9.

Chapter 10
Reengineering Approaches for Learning Health Systems: Learning from Safety Information Gaps and Workarounds to Develop Effective and Usable Health IT Systems

Jennifer Thate, Sarah Rossetti, Po-Yin Yen, Patricia C. Dykes, Kumiko Schnock, and Kenrick Cato

10.1   Introduction

A learning health system can drive safer and more efficient care by adapting and aligning individual structures (e.g., applications) and processes (e.g., workflows) to optimize outcomes (e.g., patient safety), within a system of systems. Health systems engineering is an approach to facilitate a learning health system. A **learning health system** is defined as "a health system in which internal data and experience are systematically integrated with external evidence, and that knowledge is put into practice" (Systems 2023). Electronic clinical systems, inclusive of electronic health records (EHRs), that are used to capture patient care data for outcomes reporting and to support safer care decisions, particularly in the hospital setting, are heavily reliant on nursing data capture and **workflows**. These data can then be leveraged within a learning health system. Poor system designs that disrupt workflows results in the

J. Thate (✉)
Siena College, Albany, NY, USA
e-mail: jthate@siena.edu

S. Rossetti
Department of Biomedical Informatics, School of Nursing, Columbia University, New York City, NY, USA
e-mail: sac2125@cumc.columbia.edu

P.-Y. Yen
Institute for Informatics, Data Science, and Biostatistics, Washington University School of Medicine in St. Louis, St. Louis, MO, USA

Goldfarb School of Nursing, Barnes-Jewish College, BJC HealthCare, St. Louis, MO, USA
e-mail: yenp@wustl.edu

© The Author(s), under exclusive license to Springer Nature Switzerland AG 2025
K. Zheng et al. (eds.), *Reengineering Clinical Workflow in the Digital and AI Era*,
Cognitive Informatics in Biomedicine and Healthcare,
https://doi.org/10.1007/978-3-031-82971-0_10

development of **workarounds** by clinicians to maintain efficiency in completing care related tasks. When workarounds occur, key data and information may be lost and therefore not available to inform new practice knowledge. As such, health systems engineering approaches that include attention to nursing workflows and the inclusion of nurses as domain experts are essential to creating high performing learning health systems.

The interdisciplinary field of systems engineering focuses on the design and management of complex systems over the system development life cycle (Yen and Bakken 2012a), and includes five iterative phases: **problem analysis, design, development, implementation, and evaluation**. Systems engineering consists of a broad set of process analysis, design, and modeling methods that identify and prioritize potential high-impact problems, and implement system optimization solutions (Fanjiang et al. 2005). As such, systems engineering methods can be applied to a broad range of healthcare processes to model workflow, data, and information flow (Foster et al. 2010; Benneyan and Bond 2013; Peck et al. 2013; Benneyan et al. 2012). These activities optimize system design, prevent development of information silos, and ensure overall integration of health information technology (IT) components into a well-integrated "system-of-systems" (Mathews and Pronovost 2011; Pronovost and Bo-Linn 2012).

This chapter will begin with a discussion of health IT and patient safety, including the development of workarounds when new information technologies disrupt workflows. Further we will discuss how disrupted workflows and workarounds impact patient safety and effective learning health systems. Next, three broad approaches that can be triangulated and applied within a systems engineering framework to reengineer patient care workflows, and to overcome information silos by actively learning from safety information gaps and workarounds within a health system will be presented. These approaches include: (1) "In the lab" participatory design, (2) "In the wild" observations, and (3) "In the metadata" models of health care processes. Usability evaluation, as part of "in the lab" participatory design and "in the wild" observations will also be discussed. To further understand how health IT is used "in the wild", a sociotechnical perspective is considered. We will also give an overview of sociotechnical theory and the associated frameworks important to understand when applying systems engineering approaches. Health systems engineering can leverage these complementary approaches for the development and redesign of applications and their integration within a "system of systems". Finally, use cases will be presented

P. C. Dykes · K. Schnock
Department of Medicine, Division of General Internal Medicine and Primary Care, Brigham and Women's Hospital, Harvard Medical School, Boston, MA, USA
e-mail: pdykes@bwh.harvard.edu

K. Schnock
e-mail: kschnock@bwh.harvard.edu

K. Cato
School of Nursing, University of Pennsylvania, Philadelphia, PA, USA
e-mail: kcato@nursing.upenn.edu

and aligned with phases of the systems development life cycle to illustrate how the various approaches have been applied in nursing to promote learning, reengineering, and safer care, as a part of a learning Health System.

10.2 Background

A. Health Information Technology and Patient Safety

The 1999 Institute of Medicine (IOM) Report "To Err is Human" called for a nationwide effort to eliminate preventable medical errors (Institute of Medicine (IOM) 1999) and yet preventable errors persist (Bates et al. 2023). Among errors reported, it has been noted that 25% of medication-related injuries could have been prevented (Aspden 2007). Healthcare organizations have been tasked with addressing ongoing patient safety challenges and improving the quality of care. A variety of health information technology (IT) systems are increasingly being deployed within healthcare organizations to improve the safety and quality of care and support clinicians' workflows. Healthcare IT such as EHRs with clinical decision support (CDS), computerized provider order entry (CPOE) (Bates et al. 1998), electronic medication administration records (eMAR), and barcode medication administration (BCMA) have been touted as promising strategies for preventing medication errors (Bates 2000; Bates and Gawande 2003), and are particularly relevant to nursing care and workflows. A more recent systematic review of the value of EHRs and the associated applications suggest both positive and negative impacts on clinical outcomes (Modi and Feldman 2022). Abraham and colleagues conducted a review of systematic reviews and found that CPOE was shown to have statistically significant impact on reducing medication errors and adverse drug events (Abraham et al. 2020). Further, a systematic review of studies of BCMA using prospective, before-and-after designs found that there is evidence demonstrating the positive impact of BCMA on preventing medication errors (Hutton et al. 2021).

Although there is evidence for improved medication safety with health IT systems, the IOM noted that health IT products are expected to improve patient safety only if the products are well-designed and strategically implemented (Committee on Patient Safety Technology, 2011). And, as previously noted, inspite of advances, adverse events, of which 22.7% were deemed preventable, still occur (Bates et al. 2023). Further, health IT systems can negatively impact organizational culture, workflow processes, siloed communication, and medical errors due to poor design and lack of integration with the clinical workflow (Gates et al. 2021; Sittig et al. 2020; Niazkhani et al. 2009; Leslie et al. 2017). The need for a good fit between the health IT systems and routine clinical practice is recognized as essential (Bates et al. 2003; Ammenwerth et al. 2003; Kuhn and Giuse 2001), and still largely unaddressed (Detmer and Gettinger 2023). One aspect of this is the integration of the health IT systems into nursing workflows to optimize patient care delivery and to support safe care, decision-making, and continuous learning.

Workflow is the "sequence of physical and mental tasks" performed by, in this case, clinicians (What is workflow 2024) and can be evaluated both by the *efficiency* and *effectiveness* of completing the task. As noted previously, electronic clinical systems that capture data both relevant to direct patient care and data that can be used in a learning health system are heavily reliant on nursing data capture and **workflows**. As such, clinical data capture and documentation should be of high quality, efficient, usable, and clinically pertinent while supporting multiple downstream uses as a byproduct of recording care delivery (Cusack et al. 2013). Further clinical documentation should bridge information silos to enable shared decision-making and collaboration (Thate et al. 2020a, 2020b), enable collection and interpretation of information from multiple sources, and be automated whenever appropriate (Cusack et al. 2013).

Evaluating efficiency of task completion is one way to assess impacts on workflow. Observational studies conducted by Westbrook et al. using the Work Observation Method By Activity Timing (WOMBAT) identified a distribution of the time spent on different nursing tasks and clinician's patterns of professional communication and documentation after introducing health IT systems (Ballermann et al. 2011; Westbrook and Ampt 2009; Westbrook et al. 2013). While qualitative data supported some improvement of time efficiency on nursing documentation, other studies pointed out a lack of user acceptance, and staff attitudes have been cited as a factor that hinders the implementation of health IT systems (Ash and Bates 2005; Ball and Lillis 2000; Robles and Karnas 2007; Clemmer 2004). For example, one study investigated nurses' perceptions of the EHR and found that 64% of nurses reported that the EHR system did not decrease nursing workload. Additionally, only 44% of nurses thought the current system was functionally optimzed, and 61% indicated frustration with multiple EHR documentation workflows (Moody et al. 2004). When a misfit between the new IT system implementation and existing work processes occurs, it creates a frustration for clinicians and could result in workarounds while using the systems (Ignatiadis and Nandhakumar 2009).

B. Workarounds as a Result of Misfit Between Health IT and Workflows

Within the clinical domain, efficient nursing workflows are essential processes that enable effective nursing practice and patient care. Workarounds have been defined as alternative procedures employed by users to accomplish a task in response to a misfit between computer-based and existing clinical processes (Koopman and Hoffman 2003). Workarounds have been identified as creating negative consequences for the system implementation and may lead to violations or deviations from safe operating procedures and standards, which can compromise a key objective of implementing these healthcare IT systems (Blijleven et al. 2022). The root causes of and rationales for workarounds are diverse and include inefficient process design, poor system usability, inadequate user training, and inflexible clinical guidelines (Blijleven et al. 2022; Halbesleben et al. 2008). The efforts to eliminate workarounds are recognized as difficult (Hayes 2000).

Learning health care systems can be directly impacted by documentation workarounds that have unintended negative consequences, including information loss. Information loss impacts the effectiveness of a learning health care system that depends on these internal data coupled with external evidence to inform future actions. For example, in a study conducted by Koppel et al. (Koppel et al. 2005) they described the role of CPOE in facilitating prescription error risk. The study investigators found that workarounds such as post hoc documentation and the use of parallel paper systems for documenting medication administration caused confusion and the risk of information loss within the electronic system (Koppel et al. 2005). Another study conducted by Andersen et al. regarding clinician device choice identified a different type of workaround, that resulted in transcribing medication orders from the computer to paper (Andersen et al. 2009). Workarounds of this type could result in medication errors as well as information loss.

The effectiveness of health IT systems may be reduced when workarounds performed by users in response to the issues negate the system's benefits, however, workarounds may also point to the limitations of EHR systemes (Flanagan et al. 2013). When workarounds have been observed after implementing health IT systems, healthcare organizations need to re-evaluate the implementation and how the system fits in the current clinical practice in terms of improving patient safety, workflow efficiency, and perceptions of the clinical staff. We should assume new health IT systems will change the current workflows, processes, procedures, and policies. Attention to the re-design of workflows to preclude resulting negative workarounds is required as preparation for system implementation, as well as when assessing for successful implementation. It is also important to note that while workarounds are most commonly seen as negative, when viewed as source of clinician innovation to support complex tasks (Flanagan et al. 2013), workarounds can be leveraged to effectively re-design systems and improve health IT applications, as was seen during the COVID-19 pandemic (Grange et al. 2020). Further, workarounds may also be an indicator of nurses' information needs and should be evaluated with this in mind. Therefore, careful attention to workflows during the systems life cycle is paramount in order to promote a learning health system. Applying and triangulating a variety of approaches provides data to inform the process through each phase: problem analysis, design, development, implementation, and evaluation.

10.3 Triangulation of Approaches Within a Systems Engineering Framework

The use of a variety of methodological approaches during the five phases of the systems engineering framework supports successful implementation of health IT solutions that promote a learning healthcare system. We categorize these methodologies into three broad approaches: (1) "In the lab" participatory design, (2) "In the wild" observations, and (3) "In the metadata" models of health care processes. Each of these broad approaches can uncover various aspects of workflow mismatches or disruptions, the formation of workarounds, and the resultant data-driven insights captured in the metadata. When these are used throughout the systems development life cycle, they can be triangulated to both prospectively and retrospectively reengineer patient care workflows, and to overcome information silos by actively learning form safety information gaps and workarounds.

A. In the Lab: Participatory and User-Centered Design for Continuous Learning

The pace of adoption of IT in healthcare is rapidly increasing and the types of IT solutions vary widely. Nurses are a key clinician group who are facing challenges adapting to the use of clinical IT systems. A focus on the interrelationship between nurses, IT and the healthcare environment are fundamental to achieving a learning healthcare system. The need to investigate the impact of health IT from the sociotechnical perspective has been broadly recognized, (Blijleven et al. 2022; Sittig and Singh 2010; Westbrook et al. 2009) which advises that people-focused (socio) elements, organizational and human, and information technology elements (technical) are interdependent and must be evaluated together. Sittig et al. outlined eight dimensions of assessment in their sociotechnical model for studying health IT: (1) hardware and software computing infrastructure, (2) clinical content, (3) human–computer interface, (4) people, (5) workflow and communication, (6) internal organizational policies, procedures and culture, (7) external rules, regulations and pressures, and (8) system measurement and monitoring (Sittig and Singh 2010). Several researchers have adopted sociotechnical evaluation frameworks (Sittig and Singh 2010; Westbrook et al. 2004), using a range of methods (e.g. surveys, interviews, focus groups, task analysis, work sampling, results mapping, and outcome indicator data analysis) to understand the inter-dependency of these elements. Many of these can be applied "in the lab" in support of participatory design, however, to fully explore workflows and workarounds, researchers must also collect data through direct observations of practice.

B. In the Wild: Observational Methods for Continuous Learning

Most concepts included in the sociotechnical frameworks only emerge "in the wild". While some problematic features of health IT applications can be identified and modified during the design phase to avoid disruptions in workflow, many will not be identified until implemented in real-world practice settings. In fact, sociotechnical theory asserts that context is critical and that organizations are nonlinear and comprised of (social) groups within the organization negotiating change in the face of new challenges (Westbrook et al. 2007a). These new challenges include adapting to new technologies. Thus, sociotechnical evaluation frameworks illustrate the importance of addressing the interdependent relationship between the health IT and its social context where health IT is implemented. Health IT usability evaluations, and observations "in the wild" using time and motion studies and nursing workflow assessment are needed to ensure that health IT is compatible with existing nursing workflow, and that any workflow changes do not result in unintended consequences from health IT implementation.

C. **In the Metadata: Using Metadata for Continuous Learning**

Reliable and computable data capture (i.e., data collected consistently and using standard formats) within commercially available EHRs is critical to building a Learning Health System (Collins, 2016) and achieving the Healthcare Quadruple Aim of improving patient experience, health of populations, reducing healthcare costs, and improving the work life of health care providers (Bodenheimer and Sinsky 2014). Reliable and computable data do not naturally emerge, even within the same clinical information system, without proper clinical governance and technical oversight that maximizes the value of data points captured by nurses while minimizing unnecessary burden (Collins, 2016; Collins et al. 2013). Analysis of EHR metadata for usage patterns within a health systems engineering framework can identify nursing practice domains where EHRs impose a high documentation burden and domains where the data captured by nurses is: (1) siloed from other clinical data and (2) characterized by low reliability and computability for reuse.

A central goal of the Learning Health System is to generate knowledge rapidly and inform decisions to improve health (Friedman et al. 2014). To achieve these aims, nursing researchers are utilizing data science approaches to analyze large complex data sets to support nursing practice. Westra and colleagues reviewed the existing literature on big data nursing research and found three main purposes of these data science analyses–knowledge discovery, prediction, and evaluation (Westra et al. 2017). The knowledge discovery studies attempted to find new meaning in patient specific factors (Lee et al. 2011, 2012; Merrill et al. 2015; Monsen et al. 2011; Topaz et al. 2016; Collins et al. 2013), and identify associations or patterns of patient outcomes by utilizing data mining and natural language processing of electronic patient records (Topaz et al. 2016; Hyun et al. 2009). Prediction approaches sought to improve on existing algorithms or develop tools to predict risk factors or patient outcomes (Monsen et al. 2012; Cho et al. 2015; Kontio et al. 2014; Raju et al. 2015; Olson et al. 2014). Large data sets and big data analyses were utilized in evaluation studies to assess and evaluate new tools (Cho et al. 2013) or frameworks for patient outcomes, such as decision support systems (Bowles et al. 2015), care coordination (Topaz et al. 2017; Buis et al. 2013; Popejoy et al. 2015), or internet based portals (Shaw and Ferranti 2011). Within a systems engineering framework, data science approaches applied to EHR evaluation, particularly those with an emphasis on knowledge discovery of novel documentation patterns and nursing sensitive indicators, can complement usability evaluation and observational studies to identify opportunities for reengineering nursing workflows, information silos, documentation burden, and safer patient care.

10.4   Systems Engineering Approaches for Health IT Applications

The interdisciplinary field of systems engineering focuses on the design and management of complex systems over the system development life cycle: **problem analysis, design, development, implementation, and evaluation**. Health systems engineering approaches can be applied to support the development of health IT applications as well as their integration into a larger system of systems. Evaluation methods within a sociotechnical framework, such as workflow observations, task analysis, participatory design, and usability testing are important systems engineering tools.

Usability evaluation methods are conducted where appropriate during each phase of the information technology (IT) development life cycle, from conception through design and evaluation (Johnson et al. 2011, 2005; Schumacher and Lowry 2010; Saleem et al. 2009; Landman et al. 2014; Goodman et al. 2012; Kushniruk and Patel 2004). Integration of health systems engineering activities ensures that the role of the user (i.e., patients, family, healthcare providers) in system design is considered, specifically the user's relationship and interface with the environment, the technology, and the system as a whole. The goal is to understand the user's role and behaviors in identifying and mitigating risks in relationship to the system and the environment, so that workflow and IT system usability constraints can be addressed proactively. Specific theoretical and methodological usability evaluation frameworks will be discussed in detail later in this chapter. The following section provides an overview of systems engineering approaches and tools applied across all phases of the IT system development life cycle, followed by use case examples. Examples of systems engineering and human factor approaches that are useful across the system development life cycle are included in Table 10.1.

A.   Phase 1-Problem Analysis: Using Levels of Health IT Evaluation

Several models and frameworks have been proposed to identify factors influencing health IT usability. A stratified view of health IT usability evaluation (Yen and Bakken 2012b) (Fig. 10.1) presents levels of health IT evaluation which incorporate both the system development life cycle (Stead et al. 1994) and sociotechnical considerations. Level 1 of this model targets health IT specifications to understand user-task interaction to inform heath IT development. Level 2 examines the task performance to assess health IT validation and human–computer interaction. Level 3 addresses environmental factors to identify work processes and system impact in real-world settings. Task/expectation complexity, user variances, and organizational support are factors discovered during problem analyses and are factors that can influence the use of the health IT. Computer supported cooperative work (CSCW) (Pratt et al. 2004) and contextual design (Holtzblatt and Beyer 1997) involving structured observations and interviews of individuals and groups are used in the problem analysis phase to inform the design of health IT. Workflow assessment aims at detecting changes on the constructs of nursing practice.

Table 10.1   Systems engineering and usability tools by project phase

Problem analysis	Design	Development	Implementation	Evaluation
Systems engineering approaches				
• Process mapping and observation • Workflow analysis • Work sampling • Data analysis • Workflow observation • Critical incident Interviewing • Task analysis	• Engineering design methods/life cycle • Reliability science design methods • Measurement alignment • Simulation and queuing models • Work, space, and flow design • Storyboards • Participatory design • Usability testing • Usability roundtables		• Learning and tests of change cycles • Compliance control charts and analysis • Lean and process simplification tools • Focus groups • Workflow observations	• Analytics of outcomes and usage data • Root cause analysis • Redesign 'what if' modeling • Control charts for local improvements • Critical incident interviewing • Surveys
"In the wild" & "In the metadata"	"In the lab"		"In the wild"	"In the metadata"

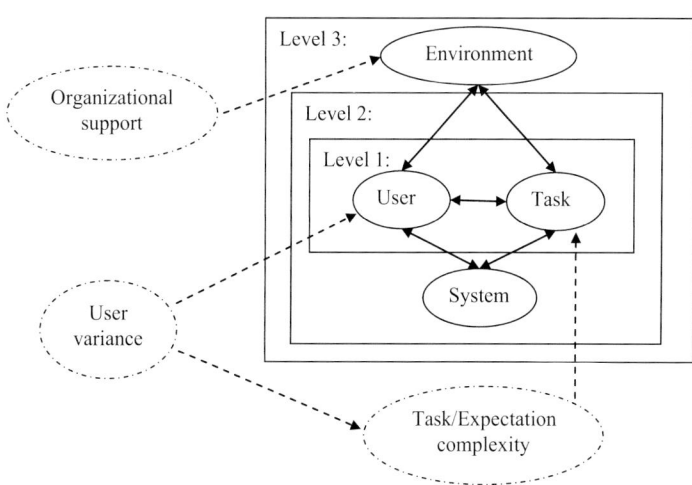

Fig. 10.1   Stratified view of health IT usability evaluation (Yen and Bakken 2012a)

To assess the impact of health IT on nursing practice, workflow assessment can be conceptualized from two perspectives: (1) workflow within the scope of human–computer interaction, and (2) workflow in the social context (environment). They can be represented by the Level 2 and Level 3 evaluation respectively in the stratified view of the health IT usability evaluation model. Investigation with a clearer explication of interactions at the Level 2 and Level 3 evaluations help develop suitable solutions for issues discovered.

1. **Assessing Nursing Workflow Within the Scope of Human–Computer Interaction**

Human–computer interaction studies focus on the relationship between human and computers (or health IT). Cognitive walkthrough (Wharton et al. 1994) and Think Aloud Protocol (Jaspers et al. 2004) are two common usability methods, commonly referred to as human-factors approaches, to assess health IT (Jaspers 2009), and to discover the interactive workflow. Cognitive walkthrough identifies actions and goals needed to accomplish tasks, and is often conducted by Human–computer interaction experts. Think aloud protocol, conducted by end-users, encourages end-users to express out loud what they are looking at, thinking, doing, and feeling, as they perform a task (Lewis 1982).

For example, one study evaluated an electronic perioperative nursing documentation system using cognitive walkthrough, and identified usability problems in the interactive process (Usselman et al. 2015). Another study extended the traditional cognitive walkthrough approach to groupwise walkthrough, and described the collaborative workflow between nurses and case managers in home care (Pinelle and Gutwin 2002). A systematic review of usability evaluation studies reported that cognitive walkthrough and think aloud protocol were used in 49 (26%) studies (Ellsworth et al. 2017). In a think aloud protocol study evaluating a nursing information system, participating nurses expressed their thoughts about the interactive process as well as how the system might impact their workflow, such as team communication, and the efficiency or effectiveness of their work (Rogers et al. 2013). The study identified usability issues in the interface design as well as nurses' concerns about work processes (Rogers et al. 2013).

Assessing the human computer interaction process has become a standard process to identify interactive issues in health IT. Unified Modeling Language (UML) (Booch et al. 1998), a graphical representation approach, can be used to illustrate the interactive workflow between health IT and end-users and inform prototype design (Machno et al. 2015). As usability evaluation is an iterative process, problems identified at Level 2 should be addressed before moving on to the Level 3 evaluation. Once a health IT has been demonstrated to be usable at the human computer interaction stage, the Level 3 evaluation would further incorporate environmental factors to satisfy the sociotechnical model where technology should be investigated within the social context.

2. **Assessing Nursing Workflow in the Social Context and Clinical Environment**

Interviews can be used to elicit user's needs and preferences to provide a deeper understanding of their experience and identify additional social-technical factors. Workflow analyses can then be applied to validate interview findings and to explore opportunities for use of health IT applications in the current practice of care on patient care units. Observational studies, such as time and motion studies, inform how health IT is being used in practice as well as among other competing tasks. Time and motion studies have been used to examine nurse' work patterns, workload, and time allocation of nursing activities (Westbrook et al. 2013, 2011). Through understanding the time allocation of nursing activities, new strategies could be developed to improve care quality. However, most time and motion studies have not specified the time period of the observation (Westbrook et al. 2011, 2007b; Abbey et al. 2012; Sakai et al. 2016; Wright et al. 2015). When the time period is underspecified, it is unclear if the data might be skewed due to observers' time availability, or if the observer's fatigue was taken into account for quality control if a longer observation (8–12 h) was required. In addition, although task definitions are typically provided, the start and the end time point of each activity are often not reported, thus limiting the replication of time-motion studies. Other methodological limitations also include randomly selected observation time (Westbrook et al. 2007b; Tuinman et al. 2016; Gartemann et al. 2012), self-report approach (Hendrich et al. 2008), manual paper-based & stop watch data collection (Abbey et al. 2012), and focusing on a single nursing activity (e.g. documentation (Wong et al. 2017; Read-Brown et al. 2013), medication administration (Elganzouri et al. 2009; Qian et al. 2015, 2016), communication (Popovici et al. 2015), glycemic control (Gartemann et al. 2012)). The time and motion use case described later in the chapter will address some of these methodologic limitations.

B. Phase 2-Design

Design is informed by findings from the problem analysis phase and may include definition of the content, display, and workflow integration strategies most likely to address requirements and overcome barriers identified in Phase 1. Participatory design should ensure that requirements for health IT applications address differing stakeholder (e.g., patients, family, nurse, physicians) goals and the tasks necessary to achieve those goals. Common themes for requirements specification are then prioritized, mapped to new processes and tools, and used to inform the development of prototypes. Low fidelity prototypes of processes and tools are developed and iteratively refined in collaboration with stakeholders using develop-test-revise iterations "in the lab" to identify components to be included in the detailed design for high fidelity prototypes.

C. Phase 3-Development

Once the design of a tool is finalized, iterative testing and evaluation is conducted with stakeholders, including nurses. In this phase, initial testing may be conducted using focus groups and interviews iteratively refining the prototypes until a working prototype is accepted by the stakeholders. Testing and further development "in the lab" with stakeholders continues until the final product is developed. An iterative process of prototype refinement and usability testing whereby the prototypes are tested by representative users (Usability.gov. 2013) continues until sufficiently mature and implementation-ready versions of processes and tools are developed and validated by stakeholders.

D. Phase 4-Implementation

Implementation may begin with a series of pilot implementations to continue learning and to guide refinement within a learning health system. For example, health systems engineering methods and tools used as part of the piloting and implementation phase include process-flow mapping and analysis, work design and simplification, root cause analysis, workload estimation, and general principles from Lean and Six Sigma to evaluate the impact and to refinement of the intervention on workflow and patient care. During this phase, the identification and understanding of the emergence of new tasks, procedures and workflow patterns provide an opportunity to enhance workflow processes to facilitate system use and to correct any "bugs" or unintended consequences of health IT that could lead to workarounds and impede adoption.

E. **Phase 5-Evaluation**

In the phases above we describe specific usability evaluation methods for work-flow reengineering, which should be iteratively applied so that problems identified at each level (Fig. 10.1) are addressed before moving on to the next level. Broadly within a health systems engineering framework, evaluation also includes a range of process and outcome measures. Such measures may include clinical outcomes, such as adverse event rates, or usage analytics to evaluate end-user engagement with the system being evaluated. A continuous learning cycle for iterative evaluation to comprehensively identify system weaknesses and inform optimization can be complemented with data science methodologies to understand the amount, quality, and metadata patterns of system usage and data captured within clinical systems. In studying nursing documentation workflows, data science methodologies evaluating usage data and documentation patterns provide valuable tools for the analysis of EHR interactions.

Critical to this data science process is the contribution of nursing domain knowledge to provide context to these data (Westra and Peterson 2016). As the title of Bakken and Brennan's work "Nursing Needs Big Data and Big Data Needs Nursing" (Brennan and Bakken 2015) asserts, while data science is useful for processing big data, nursing science and practice encapsulates expertise in diagnosis and treatment of human responses. Therefore, clinical nursing domain experts that understand nursing practice and workflows are essential when determining what data are appropriate and particularly helpful for clinical analytics. Data science methods are essential to track patient states across settings, health professionals, and research databases, however these methods require common data definitions to group similar patients across sites and providers, enabling the identification and tracking of patient need and outcome patterns.

Nurse-sensitive patient indicators are defined as "those outcomes that are relevant, based on nurses' scope and domain of practice, and for which there is empirical evidence linking nursing inputs and interventions to the outcome for patients" (Doran and Almost 2003). Nursing-sensitive quality indicators reflect the structure (e.g., nursing education or certification at an institution), process (e.g., nursing assessments, nurse job satisfaction), and outcomes (e.g., patient falls, pressure ulcers) of nursing care (Montalvo 2007). There are a number of nationally recognized quality indicators (Owens and Koch 2015), however the National Database of Nursing Quality Indicators (NDNQI®) (Montalvo 2007) is the most widely used and influential set of nursing outcomes. Capturing data on care and/or outcomes most impacted by nursing practice provides essential outcome measurements to support learning health system analytics which should be a driving focus to standardize nursing data sets for capture in EHRs. Beyond a standard set of nurse-sensitive quality indicators, to better measure the impact of nursing contributions to clinical outcomes there has been a call for the implementation of a unique nurse identifier (UNI) (Sensmeier et al. 2020). Further, standardized (or minimum) data sets, can be used to represent EHR data, such as non-standard flowsheet data, and can be enhanced for capturing relevant documentation workflows that impact and enable effective data analytics (Ahn et al. 2015; Delaney and Westra 1991; Delaney et al. 2015; Ranegger et al. 2015; Williams 1991; Werley et al. 1991). Standardized data sets that identify a specific collection of data elements necessary to represent a given clinical domain or topic are referred to as a "detailed clinical model" or more simply a "reference model" (Moreno-Conde et al. 2015; Kim et al. 2011; Park et al. 2011). Openly available resources of existing reference models are available for use to guide iterative optimization of system design and analytics of clinical data (openEHR Foundation 2016; Healthcare et al. 2015; Health Level 7 International 2025; Hoy et al. 2009; Oniki et al. 2016; Pedersen et al. 2015). In summary, standards are critical to effectively measure nursing care and resultant outcomes to facilitate meaningful evaluation.

10.5 Use Cases of Pragmatic Applications Grounded in Theoretical and Methodological Approaches Within Systems Engineering Framework

In the following section we present use cases from four studies. These use cases will highlight how various approaches were applied in select phases of the systems engineering life cycle, as well as, how these methodologies can be used to better understand workflows and the sociotechnical implications of health IT applications.

A. Brigham and Women's Hospital (BWH)/Northeastern University Systems Engineering (NUSyE) Patient Safety Learning Lab Use Case

The BWH/NUSyE Patient Safety Learning Lab was established in order to apply a systems engineering approach to design safer and more reliable healthcare processes and to improve patient and family engagement in their safety plan during an acute hospitalization. Key stakeholders, in addition to patients and family members, were the nurses and physicians on the acute care clinical units targeted in this lab. Using health systems engineering approaches, an electronic Patient-Centered Safety Plan (PCSP) IT infrastructure was developed to address patient safety threats in real-time and to support continuous learning. The PCSP IT infrastructure included the following: (1) A Patient-Centered Safety Plan Portal to provide patients and family with the core set of information needed to participate in their personal safety plan during a hospitalization, (2) A Patient-Centered Fall Prevention app to engage patients, family, and care team members in the fall prevention process, and (3) MySafeCare, an application to facilitate patient reporting of real-time safety concerns. This BWH/NUSyE Patient Safety Learning Lab use case illustrates methods applied over the five phases: problem analysis, design, development, implementation, and evaluation.

1. Problem Analysis

Interviews and Workflow Observations to Assess Nursing workflow in the Social Context and Environment. In the BWH/NUSyE Patient Safety Learning Lab individual interviews and focus group sessions using semi-structured interview guides (Fig. 10.2) were used to learn about the needs and preferences of patients and healthcare providers and other social-technical factors related to patient engagement in developing their safety plan. The goals of the interviews and observations were twofold: (1) to inform investigators' understanding of the current state of patient engagement in developing their safety plan (e.g., formal plan to keep them safe during an acute hospitalization) and, (2) to identify core requirements for developing a set of tools and processes to facilitate routine engagement of patients in identifying areas of risk and a risk mitigation plan. The interviews informed the current state of existing processes of care from the perspectives of stakeholders. After conducting these sessions, project investigators followed basic content analysis methods (Krippendorff 2012) to interpret descriptive data obtained from the interviews. The focus group sessions were recorded, transcribed, and evaluated to identify perspectives about the degree to which patients are engaged in developing a safety plan in the current state, perceived barriers and facilitators to patient engagement, and core system requirements for tools to facilitate engagement.

A workflow analysis was completed to: (1) identify and document current workflow patterns, (2) consider how they might be impacted by technology, and (3) identify the types of tools and or processes needed to ensure end-user buy-in and workflow integration (see Fig. 10.3). This information was then used to inform the configuration of the intervention and to anticipate needs for training.

Within the BWH/NUSyE Patient Safety Learning Lab interviews and workflow analyses revealed that patients and family were not routinely engaged in their safety plan during an acute hospitalization. We learned that workforce training related to the value of patient engagement was needed. In addition, we learned that the Patient-Centered Safety Plan tools needed to be integrated with the electronic health record and patient safety event reporting systems to facilitate workflow. We also learned that a range of low (e.g., paper-based materials) to high technology (e.g., mobile apps, patient portal, electronic whiteboard) tools were needed to ensure that all patients, even those who were not willing to use technology, were able to engage in their safety plan.

2. Design Phase

An interdisciplinary project team ensured that differing perspectives were captured in the design phase. Findings from Phase 1, Problem Analysis were used to identify requirements for health IT applications that address stakeholder goals and the

Pt./Family Study ID#: _____ Unit#:_____ Interview Date:_____ Interviewer:_____

Topic 1 Background Information	To begin, we would like to learn some background information related to your knowledge about falls. - Could you tell me how often and what time of the day your family usually visits you in the hospital? a. PROBE: How engaged or involved are they with your care? - Have you fallen before and in what setting? a. PROBE: Did you suffer any injuries? b. PROBE: Has anyone close to you fallen before? - Are you afraid of falling at home or at the hospital? a. PROBE: Tell me what you do to actively prevent falls? - How many people do you think fall during a hospital stay each year? *(Comment #1: Researcher states that "1/3 of people above age 65 fall, and regardless of age being hospitalized increases risks for falling and fall injuries.")*
Topic 2 Fall Risks	Now, we would like to ask you about risks for falling. - Did your nurse communicate with you about your risks for falling? a. PROBE: When was this communicated and how often? b. PROBE: To what extent were you involved and in what way? c. PROBE: Was your family involved in any way? - Tell us your risks for falling as suggested by your nurse *(Comment #2: Researcher states "nurses fill out a fall risk assessment form upon your admission based on an established fall scale")* - Would you be willing to complete a fall risk assessment form with your nurse that would identify why you're at risk for falling and subsequently develop a fall prevention plan? *(Comment #3: If patient isn't willing to, then researcher explains "evidence from research shows filling out a risk assessment form with your nurse can reduce risks for falling at hospital" and asks "tell me your concerns about participating in the fall risk assessment")* a. PROBE: Would you be willing to do this every day? b. PROBE: To what extent would you want to be involved and in what way? c. PROBE: Would you want to involve your family in this process? - Tell us what your family knows about your fall risks. a. b. PROBE: Would you want the nurse to communicate the risks to your family?

Fig. 10.2 Sample interview guide

tasks necessary to promote patient engagement in their safety plan. As a part of the design process, team members defined the content, display, and workflow integration strategies most likely to address requirements and overcome barriers identified in Phase 1. Common themes were prioritized, mapped to the new processes associated with the planned intervention and then used to inform the development of the tool prototypes. An initial mockup of each tool was developed and refined by the project team. Prototypes were then further refined though focus groups and interviews with stakeholders (patients, family, and care team members) using develop-test-revise iterations to identify components to be included in the detailed design.

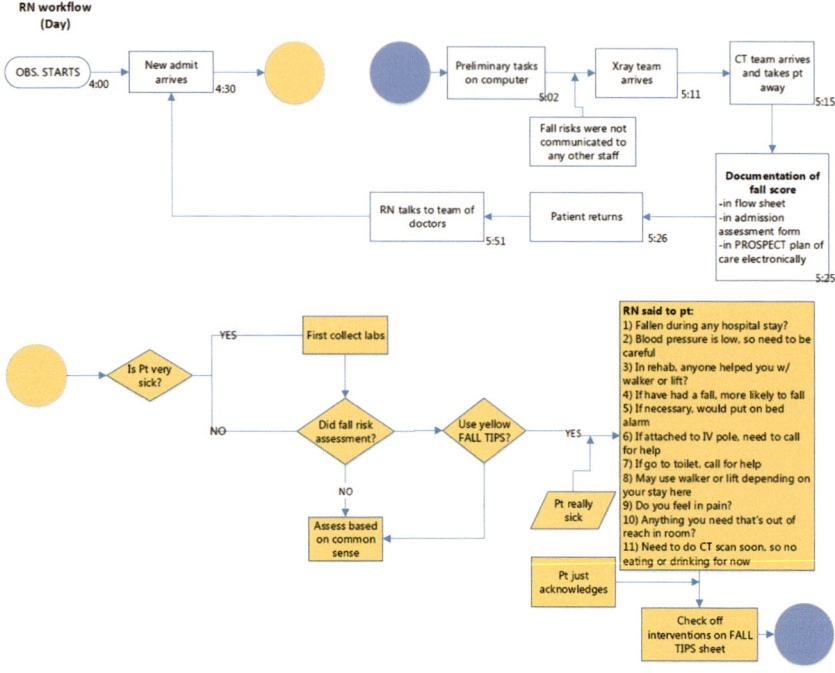

Fig. 10.3 Sample workflow observation related to patient engagement in 3-step fall prevention process

After this process, a detailed design was developed by mapping out the core and interdependent functions of the Patient-Centered Safety Plan tools along with the specific patient requirements. Prototype graphical user interfaces were used to engage with stakeholders and to get direct feedback from the users.

3. **Development Phase**

Once the design of the tools from the BWH/NUSyE Patient Safety Learning Lab were finalized, iterative testing and evaluation of the Patient-Centered Safety Plan tools were conducted with patients, family, and other stakeholders, including nurses. In this phase, a project team did initial testing using focus groups and interviews until a working prototype was accepted by the stakeholders. Testing and further developing with hospitalized patients continued until the final product was developed. An iterative process of prototype refinement and usability testing continued until sufficiently mature versions of the Patient-Centered Safety Plan tools were developed and validated by stakeholders. To perform usability testing, we developed case scenarios that included a set of tasks associated with engaging patients in identifying safety risk factors and identifying an evidence-based prevention plan. We asked end users (nurses and patients) to use the tools to complete the tasks. The usability sessions were monitored by a research team member who observed the participants to see whether they could complete the tasks without instruction. The observer recorded areas of difficulty and asked questions about the process and use of the tools at the end of the session. Data from these sessions were used to refine the Patient-Centered Safety Plan tools. The final version of the Patient-Centered Safety Plan tools, which included both "low-tech" and "high-tech" tools was then formally implemented in Phase 4. See Fig. 10.4.

4. **Implementation Phase**

Implementation of the Patient-Centered Safety Plan tools in the BWH/NUSyE Patient Safety Learning Lab started with a series of pilot implementations. The project team used systems engineering methods and tools including process-flow mapping and analysis, work design and simplification, root cause analysis, workload estimation, and general principles from Lean and Six Sigma to evaluate the impact and to refine the Patient-Centered Safety Plan tools. For example, the project team looked for the emergence of new tasks, procedures, and workflow patterns. The pilot implementation provided an opportunity to enhance the software and to correct any "bugs" that could lead to workarounds and impede adoption. The project team conducted a human factors evaluation regarding use of the Patient-Centered Safety Plan tools by patients, nurses, and physicians. The goals of these observations were to determine: (1) the facilitators of and barriers to effective use; and (2) how communication and collaboration process changed from the pre-intervention to intervention period. This information was used to refine the tools and educate patients and care team members about the tools over the course of implementation process. Failure Modes and Effects Analysis (FMEA) was used to analyze the potential failure modes, the effects of failure, and causes with evaluating their severity, probability, and detectability of the failures. See Table 10.2. The pilot implementation also provided an opportunity to test the integrated system in the wild and identify both sociotechnical factors to inform system versioning or unintended workflow consequences that may have been unrecognized that could limit effectiveness or create excessive work burden on care team members.

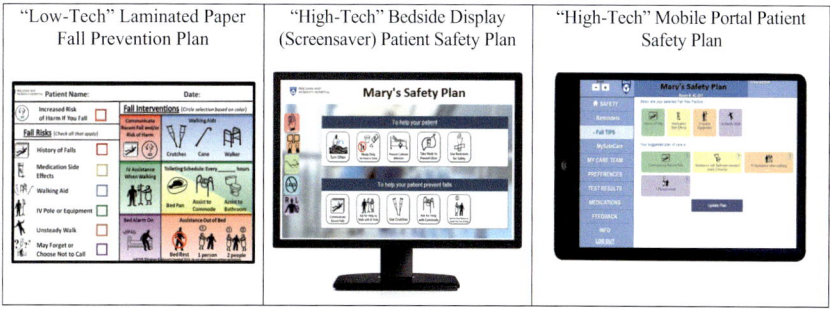

| "Low-Tech" Laminated Paper Fall Prevention Plan | "High-Tech" Bedside Display (Screensaver) Patient Safety Plan | "High-Tech" Mobile Portal Patient Safety Plan |

Fig. 10.4 The patient-centered safety plan sample "low-tech" and "high-tech" tools for engaging patients in their safety plan during and acute hospitalization

Table 10.2 Failure modes and effects analysis (FMEA) for the patient-centered safety plan tools

Item/function	Potential failure mode(s)	Potential effect(s) of failure	Severity	Potential cause(s)/mechanism(s) of failure	Probability	Current design controls	Detectability
Organization	Patient lack of education	Patient doesn't understand use of display	6	Delirium, clinicians not doing enough to educate, patients not always receptive to ed.; pt might not 'receive' that the info has to do with them	7	Engagement rounds	7
Users	Patient not physically able to see the screen saver (visual impairment)	They can't see it/ understand their safety plan; fall	4	Physical impairment; environment; mobility issues	5	None	3
Environment	Screen facing away from the patient	They can't see it/ understand their safety plan; fall	3	Requested it off, moved it away, screen is also used for charting (competing priorities)	9	Staff trained to rotate screen toward patients	2
Technology	User interface	Not understanding safety plan	4	Font size, colors, understanding	3	Usability testing	7

5. Evaluation Phase

Evaluation of the Patient-Centered Safety Plan tools in the BWH/NUSyE Patient Safety Learning Lab included pilot implementations and clinical trials to broadly assess the impact of the newly introduced tools on patient outcomes. For example, before implementing the patient-centered approaches to fall prevention more broadly, our team conducted a pilot study on two units in three different healthcare systems to assess and correct workflow disruptions and to fully develop the implementation protocol. Through the pilot study we learned the specific workflows that nurses recommended for use of the tools. We found that patients' using the tools were more activated and engaged in their patient safety plan (Christiansen et al. 2020) and less likely to experience a fall or related injury (Dykes et al. 2017a). We also piloted the high tech to low tech fall prevention tools to assess their effectiveness in engaging patients and family in the three-step fall prevention process sand found that all were effective in increasing patient knowledge of their personal fall prevention risk factors and fall prevention plan (Duckworth et al. 2019). Moreover, we conducted an evaluation of the patient-centered toolkit to explore the characteristics of patients and families that choose to use the patient safety tools and the barriers to enrollment and use. We also looked at the frequency with which patients and caregivers used the tools to record their goals, review educational content, medications and test results and their use of the patient/provider messaging features. The system usability and satisfaction ratings were favorable (Duckworth et al. 2019). We also conducted a prospective evaluation of the impact of the patient safety tools on patient outcomes including urinary catheter associated urinary tract infection, central line infections, falls and pressure ulcers and found that the risk of developing these adverse events was reduced by 28% after implementation of the Patient-Centered Safety Plan tools in intensive care units (Dykes et al. 2017b). In a nonrandomized Controlled Trial evaluation of the low-tech to high tech fall prevention tools, we found significant reductions in both fall and related injuries after implementation in three healthcare system (Dykes et al. 2020).

B. Time and Motion Study Use Case Applied to Problem Analysis

Time and motion studies can be used to assess nursing workflow in the social context and environment. As such, this method can be leveraged in the problem analysis phase. This particular time and motion study use case is (Yen et al. 2016) presented to address common methodological limitations of time and motion studies described previously (see Sect. 10.4.A.2).

In this study researchers shadowed registered nurses (RNs) during the regular working shift and used the TimeCaT tool which is an open-source comprehensive electronic time capture tool that was developed to support time and motion studies (Lopetegui et al. 2012; TimeCaT 2015; Yen et al. 2020). The observations occurred in the general patient care areas including the nursing station, hallway, medication room, patient room, and supply areas. The typical 12-h nursing working shift was split into three time blocks: 7am−10:59am, 11am−2:59 pm, and 3−7 pm. The 4-h observation time block minimized the chance of unbalanced data if a 12-h working shift has a period of unusual heavy or light workload. In addition, to ensure the data quality the study implemented a three-phase data collection process, including (1) trial phase–generate and confirm observable nursing activities, (2) training phase–establish inter-observer reliability, and (3) observation phase–data collection with confidence. The trial and training phases help introduce the study and study personnel to nurse participants as well as other unit personnel. The prolonged engagement could also minimize the Hawthorn effect.

TimeCaT (Lopetegui et al. 2012; TimeCaT: 2015) a comprehensive electronic time capture tool was developed to support time and motion studies. TimeCaT records data in three activity dimensions: *communication*, *hands-on task*, and *location*. The *communication* dimension captures with whom nurses are interacting; *hands-on task* allows for recording of tasks that require nurses to physically touch the patient or care equipment required to perform a task (i.e. patient assessment); and the *location* variable allows capture of where nursing activities take place. This approach allows capture of information about the time spent on nursing activities as well as the phenomenon of multitasking in nursing practice. Figure 10.5 shows the sequence of nursing activities (nursing workflow) during a 4-h observation. The data collected provide opportunities to analyze nursing activities quantitatively, as well as qualitatively by visualizing nursing workflows that reveal the context of nursing activities (hands-on tasks with information of communication and location) (see Fig. 10.3). With similar approaches, future studies investigating nursing workflow changes before and after the implementation of a new health IT could discover the impact of health IT on workflow as well as identify environmental support needed for nurses.

C. **Data Science Use Cases Applied to Evaluation**

1. **Analytics of Nursing Data to Identify Healthcare Process Models**

We will describe work by Collins and colleagues (Collins et al. 2013, 2012; Collins and Vawdrey 2012) that uses analytics of nursing data to identify health care process models (HPMs) as an example of how data science methods can be used to evaluate health systems, including nursing documentation workflows, workarounds, and information silos. These HPMs are generated by EHR utilization data and embedded with information about clinical practice, can be applied to evaluation studies, and also used for predictive modeling that leverage HPMs as proxies of clinician concerns and decisions.

Evaluation of Heath IT systems can leverage analytics of usage data informed by clinical domain experts to identify and define Healthcare Process Models (HPM). Collins et al., have developed Healthcare Process Models of Clinical Concern (HPM-CC) which are generated from perceptions, interpretations, and recordings entered by clinicians (e.g., nurses, physicians), and are based on clinician decisions to observe and enter data in the EHR (Collins et al. 2013, 2012; Collins and Vawdrey 2012). These HPM-CCs are used to identify nursing documentation workflows that are associated with a nurses concern about risk for patient deterioration. These types of models demonstrate that EHR utilization patterns are rich in information that can

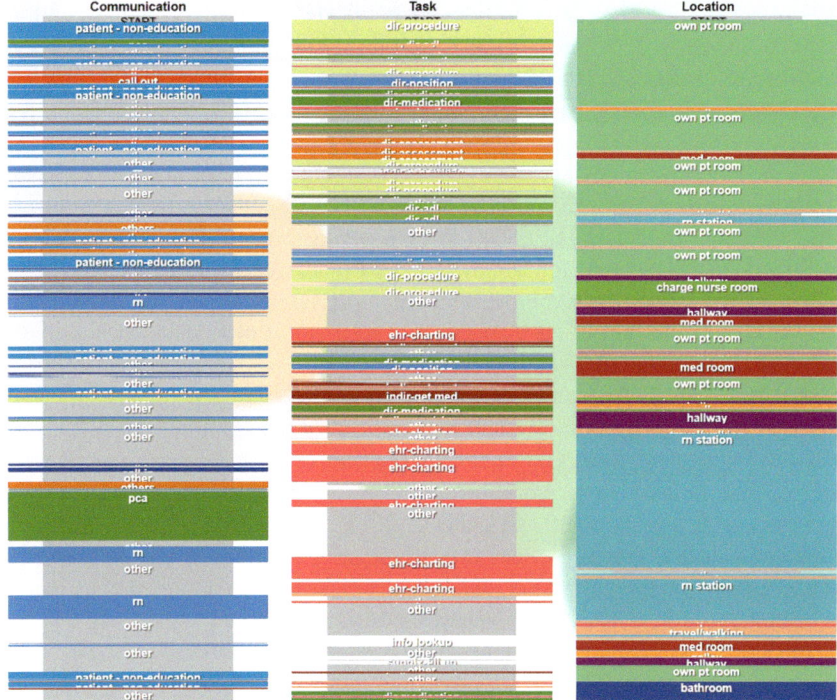

Fig. 10.5 Nursing workflow visualization

be used to understand and evaluate system design to support clinical care processes such as nursing surveillance activities and decrease information and communication silos (Hripcsak and Albers 2013). Collins and colleagues' data mining of nursing documentation workflows identified signals from annotations or comments placed in flowsheets that were associated with nursing surveillance patterns and patient outcomes (Collins et al. 2012). Triangulating those data with qualitative findings elucidated that nurses were utilizing free text comment fields as a documentation workaround to convey concern for a clinical change in patient state, and that these important data may be missed by other care team members (Collins et al. 2012).

2. **Standardized Clinical Data Element Reference Models**

Collaborative projects focused on defining standardized clinical data element reference models will be described to illustrate how they can both inform iterative optimization of system design and analytics of clinical data. These models define system implementation workflows and functionality that drive documentation practices, and ultimately data used for secondary analyses. We highlight the use of these models for the evaluation and optimization of nursing documentation within EHR systems.

Efficient documentation workflows often leverage EHR functionality that anticipate and facilitate clinicians in navigating to relevant modules within the EHR based on prior or current actions and selections, such as showing or hiding fields depending on prior data entered. When an EHR is well-designed, these documentation work-flows can be effective in increasing the efficiency and completeness of documentation. As discussed previously in this chapter, improvements in time efficiency is a primary outcome used to measure the successful implementation of a clinical system. Usage analytics from clinical systems can be used to quantify documentation burden by calculating data points recorded by nurses as a complementary method to obser-vational studies to understand nurses' documentation burden (Collins et al. 2018). EHR facilitated documentation workflows are particularly prevalent for nurses in the inpatient setting given the significant amount of patient assessment and intervention data documented in flowsheets by nurses (Penoyer et al. 2014). Secondary analysis of these data requires sufficient metadata to differentiate missing data from not appli-cable data. For example, information is needed to determine which fields: (1) were available in the nursing workflow and were completed (i.e., captured data), (2) were available in the nursing workflow but not completed (i.e., missing data), or (3) were not available in the nursing workflow and therefore were not completed (i.e., not applicable for a given patient) (Westra et al. 2015).

Westra and colleagues described these challenges in a study modeling flowsheet data for quality improvement and research, and presented lessons learned including an overall need for standards to represent flowsheet data (Westra et al. 2015). When nursing documentation reference models are data-driven, informed by best practices, validated by domain experts, and openly shared, they can serve to standardize nursing workflows, decrease nursing documentation burden, and further enable data science in nursing. For example, a validated Pain Reference Model implemented in a vendor EHR specified the data elements used to capture which pain scale was selected and used by a nurse, and was designed to explicitly capture pain score data in one field for all scores that used a scale of 0–10 to support reporting of pain scores across patients, settings, and time (Collins et al. 2017). A reference model that captures relevant EHR implementation specifications, such as cascading logic and documen-tation workflows, informs consistent design and reliable and accurate interpretation of data for secondary analysis while supporting efficient EHR navigation.

10.6   Discussion

Implementing new health IT is often disruptive. Studies to promote health IT imple-mentation have primarily focused on behavioral theories (Kukafka et al. 2003), such as technology acceptance model (Davis 1989), task-technology fit model (Goodhue and Thompson 1995), and diffusion of innovations (Rogers 1995). The measures of health IT implementation success primarily have relied on technology acceptance rate, usage, and clinical quality measures (Phichitchaisopa 2013; Venkatesh 2011; Patel et al. 2013; Steininger et al. 2014). In addition, health IT implementation is a process and it requires active participation of individuals and the organization. Understanding factors that address cultural differences and communication within and between clinical professions or departments are essential and should be understood in early phases of the system development life cycle. It has been reported that most health IT usability evaluation studies have been conducted in the implementation or post-implementation stage (Yen and Bakken 2012a; Ellsworth et al. 2017). Rather evaluation at all stages are useful and health IT vendors should conduct usability evaluation throughout the system development life cycle, including "in the lab" setting as well as larger scale process evaluations "in the wild" in clinical settings. Failure to address multi-level perspectives (individual, departmental or unit, organization) iteratively may cause the misalignment of expectations and goals, and result in workarounds and disruption in nursing practice.

Nevertheless, conducting sociotechnical evaluations iteratively or longitudinally is a challenge, due to a lack of agreement of sociotechnical research on definitions and guidance, causing both practical and conceptual interpretation problems (Cresswell and Sheikh 2014). Mixed-methods research with both qualitative and quantitative methods provides valuable multi-dimensional justification and data validation for reengineering changes in nursing workflow studies. Organizational culture and support, and how they affect nursing practice, are significant factors for health IT implementation success.

Overall patient outcomes are dependent on the complex relationship between the work activities and the systems used by the entire care team. To form a more relevant relationship between nursing activities, systems and processes, and patient outcomes, "nursing-sensitive" indicators were developed for both the inpatient and outpatient settings (Gallagher and Rowell 2003). These nursing sensitive indicators can be used to inform nursing documentation reference models that maximize the value of data points captured by nurses while minimizing unnecessary documentation burden, and can be used to incorporate nursing domain expertise into data science methods for evaluation of systems, as well as patient outcomes.

Despite activities described earlier in this chapter of nurse driven knowledge discovery using EHR data, there is still a lot to be discovered. From a nursing perspective, there still exist considerable knowledge gaps in learning health system analytics. To borrow a metaphor from Albers and colleagues (Albers et al. 2014), nursing practice and patient characteristics, including clinical outcomes, are not unified in the same way that engineers and physics are, even though nursing activities are integral to patient outcomes the same way that physics is crucial to building a bridge. The set of approaches needed to create this level of integration are both known and not known. Known approaches already in the literature, from other clinical contexts include more advanced natural language processing (Zhou et al. 2010), time series analysis (Albers et al. 2014 ; Hripcsak et al. 2015; Pivovarov et al. 2014a), automatic methods of analysis (Albers et al. 2014) and mitigating bias (Pivovarov et al. 2014b) in EHR related data. For example, Hripcsak et al. have developed deep models for understanding and characterizing the relationship between prescribers (i.e. physicians, nurse practitioners and physician's assistants), and associated patient outcomes (Hripcsak et al. 2016). Deep understanding of these types of relationships can inform innovative system design. Some of the still unknown methods includes ways of dynamically characterizing or phenotyping (Albers et al. 2014) nurses by their workflow and their patients' nurse-sensitive indicators to aid in knowledge discovery, prediction and evaluation. Additionally, implementing unique nurse identifiers to connect nursing care to clinical outcomes would aid this work (Sensmeier et al. 2020). Health systems engineering provides a flexible, yet targeted, framework to understand the impact of new systems on nursing and patient care throughout the system development life cycle and can be used to incorporate novel data-driven models that evaluate clinician-user profiles, documentation workflows, data capture, and associated outcomes to inform optimization and reengineering of clinical systems for continuous learning.

10.7   Conclusion

Health IT evaluation is complex and requires empirical studies to explore barriers and facilitators. It is critical to address the interdependent relationship between health IT and its social context where the health IT is implemented. Inattention to workflow assessment results in low health IT acceptance and workarounds (Blijleven et al. 2022; Sheehan and Bakken 2012). Usability evaluation guided by a framework (e.g., sociotechnical theory, stratified view of health IT evaluation model, or other framework) and observation approaches can assist in identifying problems in the interactive process and nursing workflow. Moreover, the use of a health systems engineering approach that leverages a range of methodologies (e.g., participatory design, usability evaluation, workflow observations, and documentation analytics methodologies) for development and redesign of applications promotes integration of health IT innovations within a system of systems.

In this chapter, we provide a series of examples that demonstrate the iterative nature of health IT evaluation. These examples highlight the complexity of nursing and patient care workflows and the significance of an iterative and multi-level approach to usability evaluation. This approach first identifies and resolves basic human–computer interaction issues before testing health IT systems in the context of clinical workflows, and then learning from EHR usage analytics. Evaluation of overall system effectiveness is conducted *after* usability and workflow issues are addressed.

However, this chapter also highlights the fact that even well-designed systems that adequately address sociotechnical dimensions as part of the development process, require continued attention to workflow during and after implementation. Post-implementation attention to end-users' concerns and feedback provides an opportunity for system enhancement and refinement, prevents workarounds, and maximizes the likelihood that the intended system benefits will be realized. Secondary analysis of EHR data after system implementation can provide important clues about the degree to which the system is built to capture data in the context of nursing documentation workflows and minimize silos, and the degree to which the reference model differentiates missing data from data that is not applicable for a given patient. This context is needed to achieve a learning health care system and can be realized if nursing domain experts work closely with data science experts throughout the system life cycle to contextualize clinical analyses and help to successfully convert data into knowledge. Nationally recognized safety and quality indicators can be used to provide useful and relevant clinical and process outcomes for continuous measurement and to support learning health system analytics to promote learning, reengineering, and safer care.

References

Abbey M, Chaboyer W, Mitchell M. Understanding the work of intensive care nurses: a time and motion study. Aust Crit Care. 2012;25(1):13–22. https://doi.org/10.1016/j.aucc.2011.08.002.

About Learning Health Systems. Accessed 7 November 2023. https://www.ahrq.gov/learning-health-systems/about.html

Abraham J, Kitsiou S, Meng A, Burton S, Vatani H, Kannampallil T. Effects of CPOE-based medication ordering on outcomes: an overview of systematic reviews. BMJ Qual Saf. 2020;29(10):1–2. https://doi.org/10.1136/bmjqs-2019-010436.

Ahn H, Garvan C, Lyon D. Pain and aggression in nursing home residents with Dementia: minimum data set 3.0 Analysis. Nurs Res. 2015 Jul-Aug;64(4):256–263. https://doi.org/10.1097/NNR.0000000000000099. PMID: 26126060

Albers DJ, Elhadad N, Tabak E, Perotte A, Hripcsak G. Dynamical phenotyping: using temporal analysis of clinically collected physiologic data to stratify populations. PLoS ONE. 2014;9(6). https://doi.org/10.1371/journal.pone.0096443

Ammenwerth E, Mansmann U, Iller C, Eichstadter R. Factors affecting and affected by user acceptance of computer-based nursing documentation: results of a two-year study. J Am Med Inform Assoc JAMIA. 2003;10(1):69–84.

Andersen P, Lindgaard AM, Prgomet M, Creswick N, Westbrook JI. Mobile and fixed computer use by doctors and nurses on hospital wards: multi-method study on the relationships between clinician role, clinical task, and device choice. J Med Internet Res. 2009;11(3): e32. https://doi.org/10.2196/jmir.1221.

Ash JS, Bates DW. Factors and forces affecting EHR system adoption: report of a 2004 ACMI discussion. J Am Med Inform Assoc JAMIA. 2005;12(1):8−12. M1684[pii].

Ball MJ, Lillis JC. Health information systems: challenges for the 21st century. AACN Adv Crit Care. 2000;11(3):386–95.

Ballermann MA, Shaw NT, Mayes DC, Gibney RT, Westbrook JI. Validation of the work observation method by activity timing (WOMBAT) method of conducting time-motion observations in critical care settings: an observational study. BMC Med Inf Decis Mak. 2011;11:32. https://doi.org/10.1186/1472-6947-11-32.

Bates DW. Using information technology to reduce rates of medication errors in hospitals. BMJ. 2000;320(7237):788–91.

Bates DW, Gawande AA. Improving safety with information technology. N Engl J Med. 2003;348(25):2526–34. https://doi.org/10.1056/NEJMsa020847[doi].

Bates DW, Leape LL, Cullen DJ, et al. Effect of computerized physician order entry and a team intervention on prevention of serious medication errors. JAMA. 1998;280(15):1311–6. https://doi.org/10.17226/9728[doi].

Bates DW, Kuperman GJ, Wang S, et al. Ten commandments for effective clinical decision support: making the practice of evidence-based medicine a reality. J Am Med Inform Assoc JAMIA. 2003;10(6):523–30. https://doi.org/10.1197/jamia.M1370[doi].

Bates DW, Levine DM, Salmasian H, et al. The safety of inpatient health care. N Engl J Med. 2023;388(2):142–53. https://doi.org/10.1056/NEJMsa2206117.

Benneyan JC, Bond C. Systems engineering approaches for improving reusable medical equipment reprocessing processes. Int J Innov Technol Manag. 2013;10(03):1340009.

Benneyan JC, Musdal H, Ceyhan ME, Shiner B, Watts BV. Specialty care single and multi-period location–allocation models within the veterans health administration. Socioecon Plann Sci. 2012;46(2):136–48.

Blijleven V, Hoxha F, Jaspers M. Workarounds in electronic health record systems and the revised sociotechnical electronic health record workaround analysis framework: scoping review. J Med Internet Res. 2022;24(3):e33046. https://doi.org/10.2196/33046.

Bodenheimer T, Sinsky C. From triple to quadruple aim: care of the patient requires care of the provider. Ann Fam Med. 2014;12(6):573–6.

Booch G, Rumbaugh J, Jacobson I. The unified modeling language user's guide. Addison-Wesley; 1998.

Bowles KH, Chittams J, Heil E, et al. Successful electronic implementation of discharge referral decision support has a positive impact on 30- and 60-day readmissions. Res Nurs Health. 2015;38(2):102–14. https://doi.org/10.1002/nur.21643.

Brennan PF, Bakken S. Nursing needs big data and big data needs nursing. J Nurs Scholarsh. 2015;47(5):477–84. https://doi.org/10.1111/jnu.12159.

Buis LR, Hirzel L, Turske SA, Des Jardins TR, Yarandi H, Bondurant P. Use of a text message program to raise type 2 diabetes risk awareness and promote health behavior change (part I): assessment of participant reach and adoption. J Med Internet Res. 2013;15(12): e281. https://doi.org/10.2196/jmir.2928.

Cho I, Park I, Kim E, Lee E, Bates DW. Using EHR data to predict hospital-acquired pressure ulcers: a prospective study of a Bayesian network model. Int J Med Inf. 2013;82(11):1059–67. https://doi.org/10.1016/j.ijmedinf.2013.06.012.

Cho I, Slight SP, Nanji KC, et al. The effect of provider characteristics on the responses to medication-related decision support alerts. Int J Med Inf. 2015;84(9):630–9. https://doi.org/10.1016/J.IJMEDINF.2015.04.006.

Christiansen TL, Lipsitz S, Scanlan M, et al. Patient activation related to fall prevention: a multi-site study. Jt Comm J Qual Patient Saf. 2020;46(3):129–35. https://doi.org/10.1016/j.jcjq.2019.11.010.

Clemmer TP. Computers in the ICU: where we started and where we are now. J Crit Care. 2004;19(4):201–07. S0883944104000838[pii].

Collins SA, Fred MR, Wilcox L, Vawdrey DK. Workarounds used by nurses to overcome design constraints of electronic health records. In: NI2012: proceedings of the 11th international congress on nursing informatics; 2012:93–97.

Collins SA, Cato K, Albers D, et al. Relationship between nursing documentation and patients' mortality. Am J Crit Care. 2013;22(4). https://doi.org/10.4037/ajcc2013426

Collins S, Bavuso K, Zuccotti G, Rocha RA. Lessons learned for collaborative clinical content development. Appl Clin Inf. 2013;4(2).

Collins S, Bavuso K, Swenson M, Suchecki C, Mar P, Rocha R. Evolution of an Implementation-Ready Interprofessional Pain Assessment Reference Model. In: AMIA annual symposium proceedings; 2017:10.

Collins S, Couture B, Kang MJ, et al. Quantifying and visualizing nursing flowsheet documentation burden in acute and critical care. In: AMIA Annu Symp Proc; 2018:under review.

Collins SA, Vawdrey DK. "Reading between the lines" of flowsheet data: nurses' optional documentation associated with cardiac arrest outcomes. Appl Nurs Res. 2012;25(4):251–7. https://doi.org/10.1016/j.apnr.2011.06.002.

Collins Sarah A. GEMPLCDMRRA. Prioritization and refinement of clinical data elements within EHR Systems. In: AMIA Annual Symposium Proceedings; 2016. p. 421–30.

Committee on Patient Safety, Technology. HI. Health IT and patient safety: building safer systems for better care; 2011.

Cresswell KM, Sheikh A. Undertaking sociotechnical evaluations of health information technologies. Inform Prim Care. 2014;21(2):78–83. https://doi.org/10.14236/jhi.v21i2.54.

Cusack CM, Hripcsak G, Bloomrosen M, et al. The future state of clinical data capture and documentation: a report from AMIA's 2011 policy meeting. J Am Med Inform Assoc. 2013;20(1):134–40. https://doi.org/10.1136/amiajnl-2012-001093.

Davis FD. Perceived usefulness, perceived ease of use, and user acceptance of information technology. MIS Q. 1989;13(3):318–40.

Delaney CW, Westra BL. USA nursing minimum data set (USA NMDS); 1991.

Delaney CW, Westra BL, Pruinelli L. Implementation guide for the nursing management minimum data set: NMMDS(c); 2015.

Detmer DE, Gettinger A. Essential electronic health record reforms for this decade. JAMA. 2023;329(21):1825–6. https://doi.org/10.1001/jama.2023.3961.

Doran D, Almost J. Nursing sensitive outcomes: the state of the science. Jones & Bartlett Learning; 2003.

Duckworth M, Adelman J, Belategui K, et al. Assessing the effectiveness of engaging patients and their families in the three-step fall prevention process across modalities of an evidence-based fall prevention toolkit: an implementation science study. J Med Internet Res. 2019;21(1):e10008. https://doi.org/10.2196/10008.

Dykes PC, Duckworth M, Cunningham S, et al. Pilot testing fall TIPS (tailoring interventions for patient safety): a patient-centered fall prevention toolkit. Jt Comm J Qual Patient Saf. 2017a;43(8):403–13. https://doi.org/10.1016/j.jcjq.2017.05.002.

Dykes PC, Rozenblum R, Dalal A, et al. Prospective evaluation of a multifaceted intervention to improve outcomes in intensive care: the promoting respect and ongoing safety through patient engagement communication and technology study. Crit Care Med. 2017b;45(8):e806–13. https://doi.org/10.1097/CCM.0000000000002449.

Dykes PC, Burns Z, Adelman J, et al. Evaluation of a patient-centered fall-prevention tool kit to reduce falls and injuries: a nonrandomized controlled trial. JAMA Netw Open. 2020;3(11): e2025889. https://doi.org/10.1001/jamanetworkopen.2020.25889.

Elganzouri ES, Standish CA, Androwich I. Medication administration time study (MATS): nursing staff performance of medication administration. J Nurs Adm. 2009;39(5):204–10. https://doi.org/10.1097/NNA.0b013e3181a23d6d.

Ellsworth MA, Dziadzko M, O'Horo JC, Farrell AM, Zhang J, Herasevich V. An appraisal of published usability evaluations of electronic health records via systematic review. J Am Med Inf Assoc. 2017;24(1):218–26. https://doi.org/10.1093/jamia/ocw046.

Fanjiang G, Grossman JH, Compton WD, Reid PP. Building a better delivery system: a new engineering/health care partnership. National Academies Press; 2005.

Flanagan ME, Saleem JJ, Millitello LG, Russ AL, Doebbeling BN. Paper- and computer-based workarounds to electronic health record use at three benchmark institutions. J Am Med Inform Assoc. 2013;20(e1):e59–66. https://doi.org/10.1136/amiajnl-2012-000982.

Foster EM, Hosking MR, Ziya S. A spoonful of math helps the medicine go down: an illustration of how healthcare can benefit from mathematical modeling and analysis. BMC Med Res Methodol. 2010;10(1):60.

Friedman C, Rubin J, Brown J, et al. Toward a science of learning systems: a research agenda for the high-functioning learning health system. J Am Med Inform Assoc. 2014;22(1):43–50. https://doi.org/10.1136/amiajnl-2014-002977.

Gallagher RM, Rowell PA. Claiming the future of nursing through nursing-sensitive quality indicators. Nurs Adm Q. 2003;27(4):273–84.

Gartemann J, Caffrey E, Hadker N, Crean S, Creed GM, Rausch C. Nurse workload in implementing a tight glycaemic control protocol in a UK hospital: a pilot time-in-motion study. Nurs Crit Care. 2012;17(6):279–84. https://doi.org/10.1111/j.1478-5153.2012.00506.x.

Gates PJ, Hardie RA, Raban MZ, Li L, Westbrook JI. How effective are electronic medication systems in reducing medication error rates and associated harm among hospital inpatients? a systematic review and meta-analysis. J Am Med Inform Assoc. 2021;28(1):167–76. https://doi.org/10.1093/jamia/ocaa230.

Goodhue DL, Thompson RL. Task-technology fit and individual-performance. MIS Q. 1995;19(2):213–36.

Goodman E, Kuniavsky M, Moed A, Goodman E. Observing the user experience: a practitioner's guide to user research. Morgan Kaufmann; 2012.

Grange ES, Neil EJ, Stoffel M, et al. Responding to COVID-19: the UW medicine information technology services experience. Appl Clin Inform. 2020;11(2):265–75. https://doi.org/10.1055/s-0040-1709715.

Halbesleben JRB, Wakefield DS, Wakefield BJ. Work-arounds in health care settings: literature review and research agenda. Health Care Manage Rev. 2008;33(1):2–12. https://doi.org/10.1097/01.HMR.0000304495.95522.ca.

Hayes N. Work-arounds and boundary crossing in a high tech optronics company: the role of co-operative workflow technologies. Comput Support Coop Work CSCW. 2000;9(3–4):435–55.

Health Level 7 International. Clinical Information Modeling Initiative—Clinical Information Modeling Initiative—Confluence [Internet]. [cited 2025 Feb 10]. Available from: https://confluence.hl7.org/spaces/CIMI/overview.

Hendrich A, Chow MP, Skierczynski BA, Lu Z. A 36-hospital time and motion study: how do medical-surgical nurses spend their time? Perm J. 2008;12(3):25–34. https://doi.org/10.1186/1472-6963-11-319.

Holtzblatt K, Beyer H. Contextual design: a customer-centered approach to systems designs. Academic Press, Inc; 1997.

Hoy D, Hardiker NR, McNicoll IT, Westwell P, Bryans A. Collaborative development of clinical templates as a national resource. Int J Med Inf. 2009;78(SUPPL. 1):95–100. https://doi.org/10.1016/j.ijmedinf.2008.06.003.

Hripcsak G, Albers DJ. Next-generation phenotyping of electronic health records. J Am Med Inform Assoc. 2013;20(1):117–21. https://doi.org/10.1136/amiajnl-2012-001145.

Hripcsak G, Albers DJ, Perotte A. Parameterizing time in electronic health record studies. J Am Med Inform Assoc JAMIA. 2015;22(4):794–804. https://doi.org/10.1093/jamia/ocu051.

Hripcsak G, Ryan PB, Duke JD, et al. Characterizing treatment pathways at scale using the OHDSI network. Proc Natl Acad Sci. 2016;113(27):7329–36. https://doi.org/10.1073/pnas.1510502113.

Hutton K, Ding Q, Wellman G. The effects of bar-coding technology on medication errors: a systematic literature review. J Patient Saf. 2021;17(3): e192. https://doi.org/10.1097/PTS.0000000000000366.

Hyun S, Johnson SB, Bakken S. Exploring the ability of natural language processing to extract data from nursing narratives. Comput Inform Nurs CIN. 2009;27(4):215e223. https://doi.org/10.1097/NCN.0b013e3181a91b58.

Ignatiadis I, Nandhakumar J. The effect of ERP system workarounds on organizational control: an interpretivist case study. Scand J Inf Syst. 2009;21(2):3.

Intermountain Healthcare. Clinical Element Model Browser. Published online 2015.

Institute of M. Preventing Medication Errors. In: Aspden P, Wolcott J, Bootman JL, Cronenwett LR, editors. The National Academies Press; 2007. https://doi.org/10.17226/11623

Institute of Medicine (IOM). To err is human: building a safer health system. In: Kohn LT, Corrigan JM, Donaldson MS, editors. National Academy Press; 1999.

Jaspers MW. A comparison of usability methods for testing interactive health technologies: methodological aspects and empirical evidence. Int J Med Inf. 2009;78(5):340–53. https://doi.org/10.1016/j.ijmedinf.2008.10.002.

Jaspers MWM, Steen T, van den Bos C, Geenen M. The think aloud method: a guide to user interface design. Int J Med Inf. 2004;73(11–12):781–95. https://doi.org/10.1016/j.ijmedinf.2004.08.003.

Johnson CM, Johnson TR, Zhang J. A user-centered framework for redesigning health care interfaces. J Biomed Inform. 2005;38(1):75–87.

Johnson CM, Johnston D, Crowle PK. EHR usability toolkit: A background report on usability and electronic health records. Rockv MD Agency Healthc Res Qual: Published online; 2011.

Kim Y, Park H. Development and validation of detailed clinical models for nursing problems in perinatal care. Appl Clin Inform. 2011;2(2):225–39. https://doi.org/10.4338/ACI-2011-01-RA-0007

Kontio E, Airola A, Pahikkala T, et al. Predicting patient acuity from electronic patient records. J Biomed Inform. 2014;51:35–40. https://doi.org/10.1016/j.jbi.2014.04.001.

Koopman P, Hoffman RR. Work-arounds, make-work, and kludges. IEEE Intell Syst. 2003;18(6):70–5. https://doi.org/10.1109/MIS.2003.1249172.

Koppel R, Metlay JP, Cohen A, et al. Role of computerized physician order entry systems in facilitating medication errors. JAMA. 2005;293(10):1197–203. 293/10/1197[pii].

Krippendorff K. Content analysis: an introduction to its methodology. Sage; 2012.

Kuhn KA, Giuse DA. From hospital information systems to health information systems-problems, challenges, perspectives. Yearb Med Inform. 2001;(1)(1):63–76. me01010063 [pii].

Kukafka R, Johnson SB, Linfante A, Allegrante JP. Grounding a new information technology implementation framework in behavioral science: a systematic analysis of the literature on IT use. J Biomed Inf. 2003;36(3):218–27.

Kushniruk AW, Patel VL. Cognitive and usability engineering methods for the evaluation of clinical information systems. J Biomed Inform. 2004;37(1):56–76.

Landman AB, Redden L, Neri P, et al. Using a medical simulation center as an electronic health record usability laboratory. J Am Med Inform Assoc. 2014;21(3):558–63.

Lee TT, Liu CY, Kuo YH, Mills ME, Fong JG, Hung C. Application of data mining to the identification of critical factors in patient falls using a web-based reporting system. Int J Med Inf. 2011;80(2):141–50. https://doi.org/10.1016/J.IJMEDINF.2010.10.009.

Lee TT, Lin KC, Mills ME, Kuo YH. Factors related to the prevention and management of pressure ulcers. CIN Comput Inform Nurs. 2012;30(9):489–95. https://doi.org/10.1097/NXN.0b013e3182573aec.

Leslie M, Paradis E, Gropper MA, Kitto S, Reeves S, Pronovost P. An ethnographic study of health information technology use in three intensive care units. Health Serv Res. 2017;52(4):1330–48. https://doi.org/10.1111/1475-6773.12466.

Lewis C. Using the "think aloud" method in cognitive interface design. IBM. 1982.

Lopetegui M, Yen PY, Lai AM, Embi PJ, Payne PR. Time capture tool (TimeCaT): development of a comprehensive application to support data capture for time motion studies. AMIA Annu Symp Proc. 2012;2012:596–605.

Machno A, Jannin P, Dameron O, Korb W, Scheuermann G, Meixensberger J. Ontology for assessment studies of human-computer-interaction in surgery. Artif Intell Med. 2015;63(2):73–84. https://doi.org/10.1016/j.artmed.2014.12.011.

Mathews SC, Pronovost PJ. The need for systems integration in health care. JAMA. 2011;305(9):934–5.

Merrill JA, Sheehan BM, Carley KM, Stetson PD. Transition networks in a cohort of patients with congestive heart failure. Appl Clin Inform. 2015;6(3):548–64. https://doi.org/10.4338/ACI-2015-02-RA-0021.

Modi S, Feldman SS. The value of electronic health records since the health information technology for economic and clinical health act: systematic review. JMIR Med Inform. 2022;10(9):e37283. https://doi.org/10.2196/37283.

Monsen KA, Farri O, McNaughton DB, Savik K. Problem stabilization. Appl Clin Inform. 2011;2(4):437–46. https://doi.org/10.4338/ACI-2011-06-RA-0038.

Monsen KA, Swanberg HL, Oancea SC, Westra BL. Exploring the value of clinical data standards to predict hospitalization of home care patients. Appl Clin Inform. 2012;3(4):419–36. https://doi.org/10.4338/ACI-2012-05-RA-0016.

Montalvo I. The national database of nursing quality indicatorsTM (NDNQI®). OJIN Online J Issues Nurs. 2007;12(3):112–214.

Moody LE, Slocumb E, Berg B, Jackson D. Electronic health records documentation in nursing: nurses' perceptions, attitudes, and preferences. Comput Inform Nurs CIN. 2004;22(6):337–44.

Moreno-Conde A, Moner D, Dimas W, et al. Clinical information modeling processes for semantic interoperability of electronic health records: systematic review and inductive analysis. J Am Med Inform Assoc. 2015;22(4):925–34. https://doi.org/10.1093/jamia/ocv008.

Niazkhani Z, Pirnejad H, Berg M, Aarts J. The impact of computerized provider order entry systems on inpatient clinical workflow: a literature review. J Am Med Inform Assoc JAMIA. 2009;16(4):539–49. https://doi.org/10.1197/jamia.M2419.

Olson CH, Dierich M, Adam T, Westra BL. Optimization of decision support tool using medication regimens to assess rehospitalization risks. Appl Clin Inform. 2014;5(3):773–88. https://doi.org/10.4338/ACI-2014-04-RA-0040.

Oniki TA, Zhuo N, Beebe CE, et al. Clinical element models in the SHARPn consortium. J Am Med Inform Assoc. 2016;23(2):248–56. https://doi.org/10.1093/jamia/ocv134.

openEHR Foundation. openEHR. Published online 2016.

Owens LD, Koch RW. Understanding quality patient care and the role of the practicing nurse. Nurs Clin North Am. 2015;50(1):33–43. https://doi.org/10.1016/j.cnur.2014.10.003.

Park HA, Min YH, Kim Y, Lee MK, Lee Y. Development of detailed clinical models for nursing assessments and nursing interventions. Healthc Inform Res. 2011;17(4):244–52. https://doi.org/10.4258/hir.2011.17.4.244.

Patel V, Jamoom E, Hsiao CJ, Furukawa MF, Buntin M. Variation in electronic health record adoption and readiness for meaningful use: 2008–2011. J Gen Intern Med. 2013;28(7):957–64. https://doi.org/10.1007/s11606-012-2324-x.

Peck JS, Gaehde SA, Nightingale DJ, et al. Generalizability of a simple approach for predicting hospital admission from an emergency department. Acad Emerg Med. 2013;20(11):1156–63.

Pedersen R, Wynn R, Ellingsen G. Semantic interoperable electronic patient records: the unfolding of consensus based archetypes. Stud Health Technol Inform. 2015;210:170–4.

Penoyer DA, Cortelyou-Ward KH, Noblin AM, et al. Use of electronic health record documentation by healthcare workers in an acute care hospital system. J Healthc Manag Am Coll Healthc Exec. 2014;59(2):130–44.

Phichitchaisopa Naenna TN. Factors affecting the adoption of healthcare information technology. EXCLI J. 2013; 12: 413−36.

Pinelle D, Gutwin C. Groupware walkthrough: adding context to groupware usability evaluation. In: Proc SIGCHI Conf hum factors comput syst. Published online. 2002:455–62. https://doi.org/10.1145/503376.503458

Pivovarov R, Albers DJ, Hripcsak G, Sepulveda JL, Elhadad N. Temporal trends of hemoglobin A1c testing. J Am Med Inform Assoc. 2014a;21(6):1038–44. https://doi.org/10.1136/amiajnl-2013-002592.

Pivovarov R, Albers DJ, Sepulveda JL, Elhadad N. Identifying and mitigating biases in EHR laboratory tests. J Biomed Inform. 2014b;51:24–34. https://doi.org/10.1016/J.JBI.2014.03.016.

Popejoy LL, Khalilia MA, Popescu M, et al. Quantifying care coordination using natural language processing and domain-specific ontology. J Am Med Inform Assoc. 2015;22(e1):e93-103. https://doi.org/10.1136/amiajnl-2014-002702.

Popovici I, Morita PP, Doran D, et al. Technological aspects of hospital communication challenges: an observational study. Int J Qual Health Care. 2015;27(3):183–8. https://doi.org/10.1093/intqhc/mzv016.

Pratt W, Reddy MC, McDonald DW, Tarczy-Hornoch P, Gennari JH. Incorporating ideas from computer-supported cooperative work. J Biomed Inf. 2004;37(2):128–37. https://doi.org/10.1016/j.jbi.2004.04.001.

Pronovost PJ, Bo-Linn GW. Preventing patient harms through systems of care. JAMA. 2012;308(8):769–70.

Qian S, Yu P, Hailey DM. The impact of electronic medication administration records in a residential aged care home. Int J Med Inf. 2015;84(11):966–73. https://doi.org/10.1016/j.ijmedinf.2015.08.002.

Qian S, Yu P, Hailey DM, Wang N. Factors influencing nursing time spent on administration of medication in an Australian residential aged care home. J Nurs Manag. 2016;24(3):427–34. https://doi.org/10.1111/jonm.12343.

Raju D, Su X, Patrician PA, Loan LA, McCarthy MS. Exploring factors associated with pressure ulcers: a data mining approach. Int J Nurs Stud. 2015;52(1):102–11. https://doi.org/10.1016/j.ijnurstu.2014.08.002.

Ranegger R, Hackl WO, Ammenwerth E. Development of the Austrian nursing minimum data set (NMDS-AT): the third delphi round, a quantitative online survey. Stud Health Technol Inform. 2015;212:73–80.

Read-Brown S, Sanders DS, Brown AS, et al. Time-motion analysis of clinical nursing documentation during implementation of an electronic operating room management system for ophthalmic surgery. AMIA Annu Symp Proc. 2013;2013:1195–204.

Robles J, Karnas J. The electronic medical record: shifting the paradigm. A conversation with Jane Robles and Joan Karnas. Interview by Beth Beaty. Creat Nurs. 2007;13(2):7–9.

Rogers EM. Diffusion of innovations. 5th ed. Free Press; 1995. citeulike-article-id:126680.

Rogers ML, Sockolow PS, Bowles KH, Hand KE, George J. Use of a human factors approach to uncover informatics needs of nurses in documentation of care. Int J Med Inf. 2013;82(11):1068–74. https://doi.org/10.1016/j.ijmedinf.2013.08.007.

Sakai Y, Yokono T, Mizokami Y, et al. Differences in the working pattern among wound, ostomy, and continence nurses with and without conducting the specified medical act: a multicenter time and motion study. BMC Nurs. 2016;15:69. https://doi.org/10.1186/s12912-016-0191-1.

Saleem JJ, Russ AL, Sanderson P, Johnson TR, Zhang J, Sittig DF. Current challenges and opportunities for better integration of human factors research with development of clinical information systems. Yearb Med Inf. 2009;2009:48–58.

Schumacher RM, Lowry SZ. NIST guide to the processes approach for improving the usability of electronic health records. Natl Inst Stand Technol: Published online; 2010.

Sensmeier J, MS, Androwich RBIM, et al. Demonstrating the value of nursing care through use of a unique nurse identifier. HIMSS. Published March 11, 2020. Accessed 30 January 2024. https://www.himss.org/resources/demonstrating-value-nursing-care-through-use-unique-nurse-identifier

Shaw RJ, Ferranti J. Patient-provider internet portals—patient outcomes and use. CIN Comput Inform Nurs. 2011;29(12):714–8. https://doi.org/10.1097/NCN.0b013e318224b597.

Sheehan B, Bakken S. Approaches to workflow analysis in healthcare settings. NI 2012 2012. 2012;2012:371.

Sittig DF, Singh H. A new sociotechnical model for studying health information technology in complex adaptive healthcare systems. Qual Saf Health Care. 2010;19(Suppl 3):i68–74. https://doi.org/10.1136/qshc.2010.042085.

Sittig DF, Wright A, Coiera E, et al. Current challenges in health information technology–related patient safety. Health Informatics J. 2020;26(1):181–9. https://doi.org/10.1177/1460458218814893.

Stead WW, Haynes RB, Fuller S, et al. Designing medical informatics research and library–resource projects to increase what is learned. J Am Med Inform Assoc. 1994;1(1):28–33.

Steininger K, Stiglbauer B, Baumgartner B, Engleder B. Factors explaining physicians' acceptance of electronic health records. In: 47th Hawaii international conference on system science. IEEE computer society; 2014.

Thate J, Rossetti SC, McDermott-Levy R, Moriarty H. Identifying best practices in electronic health record documentation to support interprofessional communication for the prevention of central line–associated bloodstream infections. Am J Infect Control. 2020a;48(2):124–31. https://doi.org/10.1016/j.ajic.2019.07.027.

Thate JA, Couture B, Schnock KO, Rossetti SC. Information needs and the use of documentation to support collaborative decision-making: implications for the reduction of central line–associated blood stream infections. CIN Comput Inform Nurs. 2020b; Publish Ahead of Print. https://doi.org/10.1097/CIN.0000000000000683.

TimeCaT: Time Capture Tool. 2015(April 30th).

Topaz M, Lai K, Dowding D, et al. Automated identification of wound information in clinical notes of patients with heart diseases: developing and validating a natural language processing application. Int J Nurs Stud. 2016;64:25–31. https://doi.org/10.1016/J.IJNURSTU.2016.09.013.

Topaz M, Radhakrishnan K, Blackley S, Lei V, Lai K, Zhou L. Studying associations between heart failure self-management and rehospitalizations using natural language processing. West J Nurs Res. 2017;39(1):147–65. https://doi.org/10.1177/0193945916668493.

Tuinman A, de Greef MH, Krijnen WP, Nieweg RM, Roodbol PF. Examining time use of dutch nursing staff in long-term institutional care: a time-motion study. J Am Med Dir Assoc. 2016;17(2):148–54. https://doi.org/10.1016/j.jamda.2015.09.002.

Usability.gov. Usability Testing: Improving the User Experience. Usability.gov. Published November 13, 2013. Accessed 7 August 2018. https://www.usability.gov/how-to-and-tools/methods/usability-testing.html

Usselman E, Borycki EM, Kushniruk AW. The evaluation of electronic perioperative nursing documentation using a cognitive walkthrough approach. Stud Health Technol Inf. 2015;208:331–6.

Venkatesh Sykes T, ZX V. Just what the doctor ordered" a revised UTAUT for EMR system adoption and use by doctors. In: Proceedings of the 44th Hawaii international conference on system sciences; 2011.

Werley HH, Devine EC, Zorn CR, Ryan P, Westra BL. The nursing minimum data set: abstraction tool for standardized, comparable, essential data. Am J Public Health. 1991;81(4):421–6.

Westbrook JI, Ampt A. Design, application and testing of the work observation method by activity timing (WOMBAT) to measure clinicians' patterns of work and communication. Int J Med Inf. 2009;78(Suppl 1):S25-33. https://doi.org/10.1016/j.ijmedinf.2008.09.003.

Westbrook JI, Braithwaite J, Iedema R, Coiera EW. Evaluating the impact of information communication technologies on complex organizational systems: a multi-disciplinary, multi-method framework. Stud Health Technol Inf. 2004;107(2):1323–7.

Westbrook JI, Braithwaite J, Georgiou A, et al. Multimethod evaluation of information and communication technologies in health in the context of wicked problems and sociotechnical theory. J Am Med Inform Assoc JAMIA. 2007a;14(6):746–55. https://doi.org/10.1197/jamia.M2462.

Westbrook JI, Ampt A, Williamson M, Nguyen K, Kearney L. Methods for measuring the impact of health information technologies on clinicians' patterns of work and communication. Stud Health Technol Inf. 2007b;129(Pt 2):1083–7.

Westbrook JI, Braithwaite J, Gibson K, et al. Use of information and communication technologies to support effective work practice innovation in the health sector: a multi-site study. BMC Health Serv Res. 2009;9:201. https://doi.org/10.1186/1472-6963-9-201.

Westbrook JI, Duffield C, Li L, Creswick NJ. How much time do nurses have for patients? a longitudinal study quantifying hospital nurses' patterns of task time distribution and interactions with health professionals. BMC Health Serv Res. 2011;11(1):319. https://doi.org/10.1186/1472-6963-11-319.

Westbrook JI, Li L, Georgiou A, Paoloni R, Cullen J. Impact of an electronic medication management system on hospital doctors' and nurses' work: a controlled pre–post, time and motion study. J Am Med Inform Assoc. 2013;20(6):1150–8. https://doi.org/10.1136/amiajnl-2012-001414.

Westra BL, Peterson JJ. Big data and perioperative nursing. AORN J. 2016;104(4):286–92. https://doi.org/10.1016/J.AORN.2016.07.009.

Westra BL, Sylvia M, Weinfurter EF, et al. Big data science: a literature review of nursing research exemplars. Nurs Outlook. 2017;65(5):549–61. https://doi.org/10.1016/J.OUTLOOK.2016.11.021.

Westra BL, Christie B, Johnson SG, et al. Modeling nursing flowsheet data for quality improvement and research. In: 25th summer institute in nursing informatics. University of Maryland School of Nursing; 2015.

Wharton C, Rieman J, Lewis C, Polson P. The cognitive walkthrough method: a practitioner's guide. In: Nielsen J, Mack RL, editors. Usability inspection methods. John Wiley & Sons; 1994.

What is workflow? | Digital Healthcare Research. Accessed January 22, 2024. https://digital.ahrq. gov/health-it-tools-and-resources/evaluation-resources/workflow-assessment-health-it-toolkit/ workflow

Williams CA. The nursing minimum data set: a major priority for public health nursing but not a panacea. Am J Public Health. 1991;81(4):413–4.

Wong D, Bonnici T, Knight J, Gerry S, Turton J, Watkinson P. A ward-based time study of paper and electronic documentation for recording vital sign observations. J Am Med Inf Assoc. 2017;24(4):717–21. https://doi.org/10.1093/jamia/ocw186.

Wright G, O'Mahony D, Kabuya C, Betts H, Odama A. Nurses behaviour pre and post the implementation of data capture using tablet computers in a rural clinic in South Africa. Stud Health Technol Inf. 2015;210:803–7.

Yen PY, Bakken S. Review of health information technology usability study methodologies. J Am Med Inform Assoc JAMIA. 2012b;19(3):413–22. https://doi.org/10.1136/amiajnl-2010-000020.

Yen PY, Kelley M, Lopetegui M, et al. Understanding and visualizing multitasking and task switching activities: a time motion study to capture nursing workflow. AMIA Annu Symp Proc. 2016;2016:1264–73.

Yen PY, Pearl N, Jethro C, et al. Nurses' stress associated with nursing activities and electronic health records: data triangulation from continuous stress monitoring, perceived workload, and a time motion study. AMIA Annu Symp Proc. 2020;2019:952–61.

Yen PY, Bakken S. Review of health information technology usability study methodologies. J Am Med Inf Assoc. 2012a; 19(3):413−22. amiajnl-2010-000020[pii]. https://doi.org/10.1136/ami ajnl-2010-000020.

Zhou LL, Plasek JMJM, Mahoney LMLM, et al. Using medical text extraction, reasoning and mapping system (MTERMS) to process medication information in outpatient clinical notes. AMIA Annu Symp Proc. 2010;2011:1639–48.

Chapter 11
Patient-Oriented Workflow Approach

Mustafa Ozkaynak, Siddarth Ponnala, and Nicole E. Werner

11.1 Introduction to the Patient-Oriented Workflow Approach

Existing research that focuses on designing, implementing, and assessing organizational interventions (such as information technology) in health care and improving care delivery have two important limitations: (1) care delivery is seen as a series of unrelated or independent (discrete) episodes (Elhauge 2010), and (2) the research focuses on individual care settings, predominantly formal health settings or daily-living environments, instead of the connections between settings. As a result, healthcare delivery (particularly chronic disease management) is often not examined in an integrated, holistic way, and organizational interventions to improve healthcare delivery across settings can create challenges impeding optimal design and implementation.

An integrated understanding of workflow across settings is important to inform the design of health information technology (HIT) to support improved health outcomes (Ozkaynak et al. 2016a; Werner et al. 2017). In general, workflow can be defined as "the flow of work through space and time" (Karsh 2009)—i.e. temporally organized activities that occur across settings. However, most workflow studies focus on limited boundaries, typically single settings such as emergency departments (EDs) (Fairbanks et al. 2007; Yen and Gorelick 2007), operating rooms (Kobayashi et al.

M. Ozkaynak (✉)
College of Nursing, University of Colorado-Denver, Denver, USA
e-mail: mustafa.ozkaynak@cuanschutz.edu

S. Ponnala
Saama Technologies, Chennai, India

N. E. Werner
Departments of Anesthesiology and Biomedical Informatics, School of Medicine, Vanderbilt University, Nashville, USA

© The Author(s), under exclusive license to Springer Nature Switzerland AG 2025
K. Zheng et al. (eds.), *Reengineering Clinical Workflow in the Digital and AI Era*,
Cognitive Informatics in Biomedicine and Healthcare,
https://doi.org/10.1007/978-3-031-82971-0_11

2005; Marjamaa et al. 2008), intensive care units (Malhotra et al. 2007), primary care settings (Unertl et al. 2009) or the workflows of individual clinician groups (physician's workflow, nurse's workflow) or individual care processes, such as barcode medication administration (Carayon et al. 2007), that take place in a single organizational context. Capturing workflow within a defined boundary or a single setting or role is less challenging methodologically. However, health care occurs beyond a single setting (Walker and Carayon 2009; Werner et al. 2016; Werner et al. 2018). Incomplete understanding of workflow across diverse settings may result in failure to adopt new technology, localization (lack of context awareness), and operational ineffectiveness (Walker and Carayon, 2009). For example, lack of adoption of personal health records by both clinicians and patients is likely if there is a gap between clinical workflow and patient's workflow at home (Tang et al. 2006). Extreme localization due to lack of understanding of workflow across diverse settings has been reported to be a barrier for health information exchange (Unertl et al. 2013; Ozkaynak and Brennan 2013). Suboptimal operational effectiveness related to coordination challenges can occur when the interaction of activities that take place across diverse settings is ignored, and when activities are studied in each setting separately rather than holistically (Abraham and Reddy 2010).

Although workflow is a useful concept, identifying appropriate system boundaries is needed for its full utilization (Xie et al. 2016). We argue that patient-oriented workflow is an appropriate approach to study workflow holistically (i.e. capturing all essential activities and other elements in the health care of the patient). Therefore, with patient-oriented workflow, system boundaries should be a meaningful consideration in this complex puzzle. Patient-oriented workflow re-conceptualized the concept of workflow so that it functions effectively in systems in multiple, diverse settings. In a healthcare context, this means decoupling workflow from the personnel who work in formal settings and coupling it, instead, to the patient (Ozkaynak et al. 2013), who is at the center of all work and who spans all settings, formal and informal.

The patient-oriented workflow approach allows us to re-define the system boundaries of healthcare activities (i.e., incorporating both clinical and daily-living environments). Identifying system boundaries precisely is critical to examining how the health care delivery systems function in its entirety (i.e., with all essential elements) (Xie et al., 2016; Karsh and Alper 2005). Studying workflow enables an understanding of how work elements (including information, resources, and influence) are organized. Workflow models can help explain patient interactions (Unertl et al. 2009) and reveal design directions for HIT that supports user performance (Yen and Bakken 2012).

A patient-oriented workflow approach focuses on the three essential elements of workflow: activities, roles, and sequence (Ozkaynak et al. 2013; Ozkaynak and Brennan 2013). We believe that a patient-oriented workflow model provides the "true flow of the work" perspective (Zheng et al. 2010) by including activities performed by the key players—patients, informal caregivers, "care partners" (Sarkar and Bates 2014), and clinicians—in the "coproduction of healthcare delivery" (Batalden et al. 2015). Patient-oriented workflow also captures the cooperative work that typically occurs across traditional organizational boundaries. In other words, the patient, rather than the clinician, drives the flow of work (Ozkaynak and Brennan 2013). This approach to workflow follows the patient "out the door" of the formal healthcare setting rather than stopping "at the door" {Zhang, 2022 #75}. It allows us to study workflow across healthcare environments by including all relevant activities in all settings.

Patient-oriented workflow focuses on actual episodes or instances, rather than "typical" cases. By examining many individual episodes, patterns and variations can be analyzed (Ozkaynak et al. 2015). For example, in a study of five ED sites, the pattern of unique interactions among disciplines in the ED, could be graphically mapped (Ozkaynak et al. 2015). Variations (in terms of how various activities are conducted in a sequence) in care received, as well as those providing the care, could be identified. These patterns and variations can then potentially be related to their effect on health outcomes. Recently developed workflow monitoring tools can facilitate data collection on patient-oriented workflow {Wu, 2022 #76}.

The holistic perspective that patient-oriented workflow provides, (Ozkaynak et al. 2016a; Ozkaynak et al. 2013) can inform the design and implementation of various interventions by: (1) accounting for multiple roles and their interrelated activities; (2) connoting continuity over time and between visits; (3) helping tailor care to patients' needs and preferences; and (4) capturing the relationships between patients and caregivers (Werner et al. 2018; Using Patient-Oriented Workflow to Develop a Holistic Understanding of Anticoagulation Management 2012).

11.1.1 Patient-Oriented Workflow Informs the Design of Health Information Technology (HIT)

HIT literature indicates that explicating workflow across settings is essential to obtaining desired results {Brennan and Casper 2015 #14; Kaufman et al. 2009 #15; Moen and Brennan 2005 #13; Ozkaynak, 2018 #3; Valdez, 2014 #16; Zhang, 2022 #75}. Un-nuanced workflow models may lead to reduced adoption of new technology (Tang et al., 2006), lack of awareness of external health information (Unertl et al. 2013), mistrust (Ozkaynak and Brennan 2013; Ross et al. 2010) and unintended consequences, such as medical error (Koppel et al. 2005) or coordination issues (Abraham and Reddy, 2010).

Development of HIT has traditionally focused either on clinical settings (e.g., electronic health records [EHR]) or on consumer use (e.g., home glucose devices). The design of most clinical information systems aims to effectively use clinical information such as laboratory results and/or radiological/other tests to formulate a diagnosis or guide treatment. Consumer HIT systems, on the other hand, are generally designed to provide information to patients for self-management at home. Therefore, existing HIT generally fits exclusively into a clinical-solution bucket or a consumer-solution bucket. Patient-oriented workflow can be an effective approach to bridge clinical and consumer HIT (Ozkaynak et al. 2018a) and inform a collaborative HIT design, which jointly optimizes clinical and consumer informatics technologies (Valdez et al. 2015).

As patient-oriented workflow eponymously focuses on the patient, it engenders a significant but undervalued healthcare-related work unit patient work (Werner et al. 2017; Valdez et al. 2014; Holden et al. 2015). Examination of patient work can help identify information/data needs across diverse settings (Coleman et al. 2004), and identify the gaps between activities in diverse settings (Ozkaynak et al. 2018a). Patient-oriented workflow can make technology more user-centered by getting the right information to the right people at the right time. These steps are essential for effective clinical decision support systems (CDSS) (Werner et al. 2017; Campbell 2013). For example, CDSS can support antimicrobial stewardship efforts in EDs effectively only if they can support decisions at multiple points of care (within overall care delivery) and at multiple physical locations (Ozkaynak et al. 2018a). Patient-oriented workflow can inform the development of CDSS by identifying these points and physical locations.

11.1.2 Patient-Oriented Workflow Informs Organizational Design

Workflow studies are common at various stages of organizational (re)design of healthcare institutions. An important objective of these workflow studies is to ensure that technical and social components (or subsystems) are congruent with each other and that together, they are congruent with the environment. Patient-oriented workflow, or patient-focused workflow (compared to traditional workflow methods), can potentially better inform organizational design by; (1) showing variability in how work is accomplished, (2) showing cooperation between involved parties, (3) identifying sources of problems, (4) facilitating communication and coordination, and (5) facilitating patient-centeredness.

Although some variability in healthcare work is inevitable lack of awareness of these variabilities in care can lead to poor outcomes. For example, treating patients with acute asthma with systemic corticosteroids within an hour of presenting to the ED significantly reduced admission rates, while administration of steroids later than 1 h after presenting to the ED may lead to poor outcomes (Rowe et al. 2001). Patient-oriented workflow can highlight the existence of inconsistencies during the delivery of care in health care settings {Ozkaynak, 2023 #77}. Likewise, in the setting of everyday living, a workflow pattern can capture inconsistencies in self-management. The patient-oriented workflow includes time-stamped information, enabling all relevant care-related activities to be closely examined. For example, Ozkaynak et al. (2015) studied patient-oriented workflow in 6077 asthma-related patient care episodes in five EDs. They demonstrated how variability in events and timing occurred for patients presenting to EDs with a similar diagnosis. The work also quantitated the workflow in various sites showing differences based on ED, patient acuity, and arrival mode (ambulance vs. walk-in). Electronic health records (EHR), barcoding technologies, and Radio Frequency Identification (RFID) technologies can allow researchers to make connections between the number and types of individuals who performed activities based on their background (education, experience etc.) to patient outcomes. Patient-oriented workflow can also show how various individuals perform various roles at different times throughout a patient episode.

Ability to identify problems at their source is an important organizational design objective (Clegg 2000). Effective organizations can capture and mitigate the problem as soon as they occur before it propagates over time across the entire organization. In the context of healthcare, these problems can be in the form of inefficiencies, safety concerns, quality of care issues, reduced access to care, low patient satisfaction, and high cost of care. Current EHRs and other technologies (e.g. barcoding, RFID) can successfully track and record workflow steps and patient outcomes at multiple points. By capturing patient episodes across diverse settings and associated activities, roles and temporal relationships to patient outcomes can allow for problem identification at their source. For example, if nursing assessment prolongs assessment of the patient by physician, a workflow targeting nursing activities alone would not reveal this barrier and the actual source of the problem. Patient-oriented workflow will both reflect the variety of challenges experienced by patients and providers and capture deviations from optimal care management.

Self-management is an increasingly important aspect of both chronic disease management and post-acute care (Wagner et al. 2001). Although the term "self-management" refers to health activities in daily-living environments, these activities are not generally created in the home. Self-management protocols are often created in formal, clinical healthcare settings. An important barrier to effective self-management is the disconnect with events in clinical settings (Nagelkerk et al. 2006; Rogers et al. 2005). Thus, workflow study can reveal inconsistencies between clinical and daily-living settings, and the way these inconsistencies lead to challenges and deviations optimal care delivery and health management.

In short, because the communication and coordination needs of contemporary healthcare delivery go beyond the boundaries of single settings {Coleman, 2004 #34; Zhang, 2022 #75}, understanding these needs will reveal problems and provide the basis from which to improve communication and coordination. Patient-oriented workflow helps identify these needs by focusing on the patient, operationalizing her or his needs, and identifying reasons for unmet needs.

11.1.3 Patient-Oriented Workflow Informs Implementation and Evaluation

To successfully implement HIT, it is essential to understand the workflow in which implementation is to be integrated. Without an accurate understanding of current roles and activities, the implementation of HIT in healthcare delivery may alter the workflow in an adverse way, resulting in unintended consequences (Carayon 2012; Carayon et al. 2007; Karsh et al. 2010). Moreover, congruency with workflow is also essential for the sustainability of the implementation {Ozkaynak, 2020 #78}. Because the focus of patient-oriented workflow is on the patient instead of the clinician, it can inform implementation practices across boundaries, personnel, and time (Werner et al. 2016). Implementation across boundaries is inevitable in some circumstances such as personal health records (Tang et al., 2006) and health information exchange initiatives (Unertl et al. 2013). Analysis of this type of workflow can highlight variations in practice and allow us to isolate an efficient or preferred workflow. For example, in the hospital, medication is typically administered by nurses, but when the patient leaves the hospital, the same task is performed by the patient or an informal caregiver. Clinician-centered workflow permits awareness of only of hospital-based workflow, leaving out critical implementation barriers that may be relevant in the home. The patient-oriented workflow allows us to take a holistic view of workflow as it occurs across work systems and informs whether or not the implementation of an organizational intervention (such as HIT) is suitable for a longitudinal process rather than discrete episode of care.

Patient-oriented workflow can also inform evaluation research. An important reason for unintended consequences of interventions in healthcare, is the complexity of healthcare systems (Sittig and Singh 2010). Interdependence between various settings (e.g., hospital, primary care clinic, home, workplace) requires inclusion of relevant settings and cross-setting connections for a comprehensive evaluation. Patient-oriented workflow takes the interdependence between settings into account and highlights the connections and/or problems with these connections.

11.1.4 Limitations of Patient-Oriented Workflow Approach

Despite the benefits of gaining an increased understanding of patient-oriented workflow, such models are challenging to develop. There are difficulties in conducting workflow studies in both formal and informal health settings (Holden et al. 2015). Methodological challenges include ensuring the reliability and validity of the collected data due to a high level of variability and complexity in health settings (Ozkaynak et al. 2018a; Chung et al. 2017). Theoretical challenges include the lack of comprehensive, robust conceptual frameworks that can be used to guide patient-oriented workflow studies (Ozkaynak et al. 2016b). Additionally, patient-oriented workflows involve a larger scope and more complex work phenomena. These workflows often rely on patient entry of data which may require technical literacy or written data input which often results in missing data. The home environment also will vary among individuals based on cultural, ethnic, and social factors etc. The inconsistencies across reported workflow studies have been attributed to the combination of these high levels of complexity as well as simplified modeling techniques (Zheng et al. 2011). More sophisticated modeling techniques are needed to address this escalated level of complexity. Lastly, patient-oriented workflow may not be an ideal approach to study various provider characteristics such as clinicians' fatigue or burden.

11.2   Approaches to Study Patient-Oriented Workflows

11.2.1   Qualitative Methods

Both qualitative and quantitative methods have been used to model and evaluate patient-oriented workflows (Ozkaynak et al. 2016a). Traditionally, workflow evaluation has consisted of in-depth (ethnographic-like) observations, interviews, and contextual inquiry that are leveraged to explicate individual workflows. These methods yield rich qualitative data that provides a depth of understanding to the multiple components of patient-oriented workflow (Ozkaynak et al. 2018a). However, several limitations are associated with this method. First, ethnographic work of this kind is resource intensive, often requiring time-consuming and costly data collection. Second, in-depth ethnography to explain workflows can be invasive and burdensome for study participants, requiring numerous prolonged interactions between study participants (clinicians and patients) and researchers. Third, as a result of the former limitations, sample sizes tend to be small and may lack representation of a broader context. Finally, qualitative methods yield descriptive findings that limit the ability to statistically associate workflow findings with outcomes.

Recent methods have been developed to quantify qualitative findings. For example, Epistemic Network Analysis (ENA) (Shaffer et al. 2016, 2009), a novel method of mixing qualitative and quantitative data, creates quantitative models of the qualitative data. ENA is a new analytical approach that combines principles from social network and discourse analysis, to identify and quantify connections among elements in coded data and represent them in dynamic network models (Shaffer et al. 2016, 2009; Gee 2014). A key feature of ENA is that it enables comparison of different networks, both visually and through summary statistics that reflect the weighted structure of connections. As such, ENA also provides a potential mechanism for quantifying workflow comparison.

ENA is based on an epistemic frame, which is a pattern of associations across knowledge, skills, and habits of mind along with other cognitive elements that characterize communities of practice. This data analysis method can be utilized to model interactions across work systems in healthcare delivery, and to better understand which cognitive patterns propagate through the patient journey. Woolridge et al., have used ENA to study task allocation communication in primary care teams (Wooldridge et al. 2018). Qualitative data were collected through 15 h of observations of a high performing primary care team that included a physician, nurse, medical assistant, and unit clerk in task allocation communication. ENA was employed to build a quantitate model of the observation data specifically to evaluate sender, receiver, and synchronicity impact of task acceptance. From this analysis, the researchers learned that physician and unit clerks were most efficient in allocating tasks. ENA can be employed in other applications across work systems to identify patterns of barriers and facilitators for desired work system outcomes.

11.2.2 Quantitative Methods

Recently, quantitative methods have been applied to study patient-oriented workflows (Ozkaynak and Brennan 2012, 2013; Ozkaynak et al. 2015; Chung et al. 2017). The quantitative data for patient-oriented workflow research includes structured observations and EHR data (e.g., patient charts and audit logs). Data typically includes time stamped activities and roles of individuals who conduct these activities. Quantitative methods, in particular temporal sequence analyses such as Markov modeling, provide a method of characterizing patient-oriented workflow in a way that allows for statistical comparisons (Ozkaynak et al. 2015). However, quantitative methods also have limitations; data from EHR needs to be validated in terms of completeness both within and across organizations (Dziadkowiec et al. 1201) and collecting the necessary quantitative data through field studies is resource-intensive.

The patient-oriented workflow approach in particular results in some unique challenges for data collection and analysis. Studying workflows as they occur across healthcare settings often requires data collection in a patient's home. In-home research typically limits researchers in the time they can spend in a house, the number of visits to a home, and may be restricted to a certain number of homes due to travel or cost limitations (Holden et al. 2015). Novel methodologies that engage patients in collecting data such as journaling (Ozkaynak et al. 2016b) and photovoice (Wang 1999; Woda et al. 2015) can help overcome this challenge. Additionally, crossing organizational boundaries pose challenges associated with getting buy-in from multiple organizations, clinicians, and patients, as well as accounting for procedural and environmental changes.

Taking a patient-oriented approach inherently broadens the scope of the analysis, increasing the complexity of the workflow. Variability due to this increased complexity can lend itself to challenges in ensuring the reliability and validity of the data (Ozkaynak et al. 2018a). Patient-oriented workflow is more likely to involve incompatible data sources and challenges in aggregating data, due to the study across diverse settings using actual individual episodes. Quantitative methods facilitate statistical analyses of workflows that allow for associations. However, the escalated level of complexity (e.g. involvement of multiple individuals (or entities) with activities at different levels of details, concurrency of activities and high level of variability across patient care episodes) can be problematic without thoughtful planning and resources such as statistics experts and other support personnel.

11.3   Case Studies

As mentioned above, the patient-oriented workflow approach has several applications in healthcare. To follow is a description of the application of the patient-oriented workflow, in four different care environments: EDs, daily-living environments, nursing homes, and skilled home health care.

11.3.1   Emergency Departments

The first author developed a preliminary version of a patient-oriented workflow in the context of EDs (Ozkaynak 2011). Although EDs represent a single setting, different roles are assumed in various sub-settings of EDs. Patient-oriented workflow can be used to identify cooperative work in EDs (Ozkaynak and Brennan 2012, 2013). Early stages of 108 patient care episodes were identified using structured observations in three EDs (Ozkaynak and Brennan 2012). Data were collected on time-stamped activities and roles of individuals who conduct these activities. Each episode was modeled as a workflow and included a sequence of activity-role pair. Data analysis yielded 96 different sequence patterns. Using data reduction techniques, such as multidimensional scaling and hierarchical cluster analysis, six patterns of care delivery were identified, differentiated primarily by whether the prescriber was a physician or midlevel clinician. Secondary differentiators included whether the patient arrived in the ED as walk-in or via ambulance, and in which ED patient care occurred. The high level of workflow variability reported in this study can inform the design of ED work systems. The variability in workflow could not have been captured using a strictly clinician-oriented approach (e.g. studying single type of clinician's workflow). The study concluded that work interventions should not limit EDs' flexibility to handle sequential variability in patient care.

In another study, patient-oriented workflow using EHR extracted data demonstrated factors that shape the workflow patterns and the relationship between workflow and patient outcomes (i.e. length of stay) (Ozkaynak et al. 2015). In this study, 6077 episodes for asthma patients were identified in five EDs in one calendar year. The data included time-stamped activity data. EHRs could track logs for many activities, the following activities were followed and used in the analysis; patient arrival, triage started, pain assessed, patient roomed, nurse/tech assigned, attending assigned, resident/fellow assigned, and patient departed from ED. Using Markov models and visual analytic techniques, patient-oriented workflow yielded workflow patterns for each of the five EDs by aggregating the sequence of activities for each episode. These patterns were correlated with length of stay. Moreover, the workflow displayed variations for different arrival modes, settings, and acuity levels. Clinician-oriented approaches on the other hand, would not have been linked to patient outcomes such as length of stay, as they are generally linked to clinician outcomes (e.g. spent time on various activities, clinician activity patterns) (Ozkaynak et al. 2018b).

Both of these ED studies identified workflow patterns and factors that resulted in these patterns. Identifying the factors and linking patterns to patient outcomes, allows the redesign of Eds systems that lead to better outcomes and discourage patterns that lead to worse outcomes.

As discussed previously, the patient-oriented workflow approach has been applied to study longitudinal processes of healthcare. Doutcheva et al. applied this method to study the workflow associated with older adults transitioning to the ED and then returning to their homes following hospital discharge (Doutcheva et al. 2017). Qualitative methods were used to identify: (1) the organizational boundaries crossed, (2) barrier/facilitator interactions across organizational boundaries, and (3) the patient work consequences that occur when patient work occurs across boundaries. Thirty-six semi-structured interviews were conducted with older adult patients who were discharged from a level 1 trauma center ED to their home. The goal of the interviews was to have patients describe their "patient journey" from their initial decision to go to the ED to their current state of care after being discharged home from the ED. Specifically, the SEIPS (Systems Engineering Initiative for Patient Safety) framework was used to guide the directed content analysis of the interview data to answer the research question described above (Carayon et al. 2006; Hsieh and Shannon 2005). Results revealed that patient work crossed several organizational boundaries including the home, hospital, primary care facility, pharmacy, and community organizations. Further, barrier/facilitator interactions across boundaries were connected to either positive or negative consequence for the patients from their perspective. In this study, the use of a patient-oriented workflow enabled the researchers to trace cross-boundary barriers, facilitators, and post-ED discharge patient consequences related to those barriers that would otherwise not have been identified had the focus only been on the clinical setting. The results highlight that ED transitions happen longitudinally, that is, beyond the care that occurs within the ED, and extend into the community. As a result, the process is vulnerable to variances in the different work systems. Currently, interventions to improve ED discharge and transitions from acute care settings to the home have focused on the discharge process that occurs in the clinical setting, leaving out the potential to identify and subsequently address downstream effects. Use of the patient-oriented workflow approach in this case allowed for the ability to identify many of the issues associated with transitions in healthcare that happen after the patient leaves the clinical setting. As a result, subsequent system redesign can focus on supporting patient work across system boundaries to ensure successful care transitions.

11.3.2 Daily-Living Environments

The patient-oriented workflow approach has been applied to understand performance barriers related self-management in the home environment. Holden et al. examined patient work among elderly chronic heart failure (CHF) patients in their homes

(Holden and Mickelson 2013). A sociotechnical system approach was used to understand patient work associated with self-care for patients with CHF and their caregivers, including therapy related knowledge, motivation, tools/technologies, barriers/ difficulties, strategies/resources, and social/ physical environment. Thematic analysis of interviews with patients and their caregivers revealed several patient-reported barriers in the patient work system. These barriers included physical limitations, knowledge gaps, medication complexity, side-effects, lack of or overdependence on aids, lack of indoor gyms, sodium-rich food culture and, stairs. Patient-oriented workflow allowed the researchers to expand the patient's work system beyond the clinical environment and identify challenges that may inhibit the delivery of quality care at home.

Management of anticoagulation treatment in daily-living settings has been studied using patient-oriented workflow (Ozkaynak et al. 2018a, 2016b). This approach allowed for identifying gaps between the clinical workflow and healthcare activities the setting of daily living. The term "gap" refers to a "break in continuity" between health-related activities across diverse settings. Gaps can disturb care delivery and lead to poor patient outcomes (Booth et al. 2013). These gaps can inform the design and implementation of gap-filling, collaborative health information technologies (HIT) (Valdez et al. 2014). Collaborative HITs can potentially allow patients to capture patient work (self-management practices, daily-living routines and context) (Ozkaynak et al. 2018a) and to share with their provider. Clinicians can then have a better understanding of patients' barriers and obstacles for self-management at home and community settings for patient-centered care to address management issues.

11.3.3   Nursing Homes

Nursing homes entail distinct workflows (Morrill et al. 2016) that comprise the numerous daily-living activities of residents and asynchronous communication between team members. This asynchrony occurs because, unlike hospital settings, some providers such as medical staff are often external to the facilities and thus not constantly. This situation results in enhanced roles for nurses and other caregivers in clinical decision-making (Lim et al. 2014). Nursing homes comprise differing levels of clinical or residential support for clients. Residents with high level clinical needs depend on staff and resources for care and assistance in activities of daily living. Staff work within their scopes of practice, guided by regulations i.e., formal rules and licensure responsibilities. In low-care hostel or nursing homes settings residents are relatively independent and require limited clinical services but have the support of services such as housekeeping and social engagement activities, and have access to staff nearby if required. Although each setting has their own dynamics, they need to coexist together and both residents and clinicians. Patient-oriented workflow can be an ideal approach for studying temporal organization of healthcare workflow, which lasts all day and interacts with the daily routines of residents. Workflow in nursing homes often crosses temporal (between shifts), organizational (e.g., hospital, lab, primary care, pharmacy) and institutional (clinical and daily-living) boundaries. Ignoring cross-boundary workflows in nursing homes can lead to safety and quality problems (Stokoe et al. 2016). Acknowledging cross-boundary workflows can lead to health IT and other interventions that ensure pertinent information (e.g. resident preferences, daily routines or medication list) is transferred across boundaries and is made available to the right people at right time.

11.3.4 Skilled Home Health Care

Another area where patient-oriented workflow has been applied is Skilled Home Health Care (SHHC), also known as community care services. SHHC is a formal, regulated program of care that provides a variety of skilled services such as nursing, physical therapy, speech therapy to patients in their home. Typical tasks involved in SHHC include wound care, physical therapy, and medication management, along with some housekeeping and social support activities. Werner and colleagues applied the patient-oriented workflow to understand medication management (MM) during transitions from hospitals to SHHC (Werner et al. 2017). Transitions in healthcare require the execution of several tasks distributed across multiple people, organizations, and time. Patient-oriented workflow allows researchers to study how processes are distributed across healthcare delivery settings through an analysis of interactions and emergent properties that would not have been possible at the task level. Werner and colleagues used interviews and observations with older adults, caregivers, and SHHC providers involved in care transitions from the hospital to SHHC (Werner et al. 2017). The study identified: (1) key attributes of the MM process through the transition from the hospital to SHCC, (2) emergent properties of MM across system boundaries and related barriers, and (3) patterns of barrier propagation through the transition processes. The patient-oriented workflow approach facilitated identification of barriers to the process specific to crossing organizational boundaries. Additionally, barriers identified in one system of care were traced throughout the hospital to SHCC care transition. Barrier propagation across organizational boundaries was associated with negative work system outcomes such as process delays like missed medication, as well as frustration and increased workload for the SHHC provider. The use of patient-oriented workflow allowed researchers to conceptualize care as a continuous process across systems rather than a discrete care episode. The results suggested that work systems need to be aligned to support critical care processes across transitions to reduce the potential for process breakdowns.

11.4 Conclusion

Although workflow analysis in general, and patient-oriented workflow analysis in particular, has inherent challenges and limitations, the potential benefits for both care delivery processes and HIT design/implementation far outweigh the potential disadvantages. To successfully redesign healthcare delivery, as well as design and implement HIT that can account for care across the entire patient journey, healthcare delivery must be examined as an integrated system of a longitudinal process rather than a cluster of discrete tasks/processes in isolated environments. Patient-oriented workflow can provide the needed integrated perspective.

References

Abraham J, Reddy MC. Challenges to inter-departmental coordination of patient transfers: a workflow perspective. Int J Med Inform. 2010;79(2):112–22. https://doi.org/10.1016/j.ijmedinf.2009.11.001.

Batalden M, Batalden P, Margolis P, et al. Coproduction of healthcare service. BMJ Qual Saf. 2015. https://doi.org/10.1136/bmjqs-2015-004315.

Booth AO, Lowis C, Dean M, Hunter SJ, McKinley MC. Diet and physical activity in the self-management of type 2 diabetes: barriers and facilitators identified by patients and health professionals. Prim Health Care Res Dev. 2013;14(3):293–306. https://doi.org/10.1017/S1463423612000412.

Brennan P, Casper G. Observing health in everyday living: ODLs and the care-between-the-care. Pers Ubiquit Comput. 2015;19(1):3–8. https://doi.org/10.1007/s00779-014-0805-0.

Campbell R. The five rights of clinical decision support: CDS tools helpful for meeting meaningful use. J AHIMA. 2013;84(10):42–7.

Carayon P, editor. Handbook of human factors and ergonomics in health care and patient safety. 2nd ed. Boca Raton, FL: CRC Press; 2012.

Carayon P, Schoofs Hundt A, Karsh BT, et al. Work system design for patient safety: the SEIPS model. Qual Saf Health Care. 2006;15 Suppl 1:i50–8. https://doi.org/10.1136/qshc.2005.015842.

Carayon P, Alvarado CJ, Hundt AS. Work design and patient safety. Theor Issues Ergon Sci. 2007;8(5):395–428. https://doi.org/10.1080/14639220701193157.

Carayon P, Wetterneck TB, Hundt AS, et al. Evaluation of nurse interaction with bar code medication administration technology in the work environment. J Patient Saf. 2007;3(1):34–42. https://doi.org/10.1097/PTS.0b013e3180319de7.

Chung J, Ozkaynak M, Demiris G. Examining daily activity routines of older adults using workflow. J Biomed Inform. 2017;71:82–90. https://doi.org/10.1016/j.jbi.2017.05.010.

Clegg CW. Sociotechnical principles for system design. Appl Ergon. 2000;31(5):463–77.

Coleman EA, Smith JD, Frank JC, Min SJ, Parry C, Kramer AM. Preparing patients and caregivers to participate in care delivered across settings: the Care Transitions Intervention. J Am Geriatr Soc. 2004;52(11):1817–25. https://doi.org/10.1111/j.1532-5415.2004.52504.x.

Doutcheva N, Shah MN, Borkenhagen A, et al. Process variances in older adults' care transitions from emergency department to home: process breakdown versus process resiliency. In: Proceedings of the human factors and ergonomics society annual meeting, vol. 61(1);2017. p. 565–66. https://doi.org/10.1177/1541931213601625.

Dziadkowiec O, Callahan T, Ozkaynak M, Reeder B, Welton J. Using a data quality framework to clean data extracted from the electronic health record: a case study. EGEMS (Wash DC). 2016;4(1):1201. https://doi.org/10.13063/2327-9214.1201.

Elhauge E. The fragmentation of U.S. health care: causes and solutions. New York: Oxford University Press;2010.

Fairbanks RJ, Bisantz AM, Sunm M. Emergency department communication links and patterns. Ann Emerg Med. 2007;50(4):396–406. https://doi.org/10.1016/j.annemergmed.2007.03.005.

Gee JP. An introduction to discourse analysis: theory and method. New York, NY: Routledge; 2014.

Holden RJ, Mickelson RS. Performance barriers among elderly chronic heart failure patients: an application of patient-engaged human factors and ergonomics. In: Proceedings of the human factors and ergonomics society annual meeting, vol. 57(1);2013. p. 758–62. https://doi.org/10.1177/1541931213571166.

Holden RJ, McDougald Scott AM, Hoonakker PL, Hundt AS, Carayon P. Data collection challenges in community settings: insights from two field studies of patients with chronic disease. Qual Life Res. 2015;24(5):1043–55. https://doi.org/10.1007/s11136-014-0780-y.

Holden RJ, Schubert CC, Mickelson RS. The patient work system: an analysis of self-care performance barriers among elderly heart failure patients and their informal caregivers. Appl Ergon. 2015;47:133–50. https://doi.org/10.1016/j.apergo.2014.09.009.

Hsieh HF, Shannon SE. Three approaches to qualitative content analysis. Qual Health Res. 2005;15(9):1277–88. https://doi.org/10.1177/1049732305276687.

Karsh B-T. Clinical practice improvement and redesign: how change in workflow can be supported by clinical decision support. Rockville, MD;2009.

Karsh B-T, Alper SJ. Work system analysis: the key to understanding health care systems. In: Henriksen K, Battles J, Marks E, Lewin D, editors. Advances in patient safety from research to implementation. Rockville, MD: AHRQ;2005.

Karsh BT, Weinger MB, Abbott PA, Wears RL. Health information technology: fallacies and sober realities. J Am Med Inform Assoc. 2010;17(6):617–23. https://doi.org/10.1136/jamia.2010.005637.

Kaufman DR, Pevzner J, Rodriguez M, et al. Understanding workflow in telehealth video visits: observations from the IDEATel project. J Biomed Inform. 2009;42(4):581–92. https://doi.org/10.1016/j.jbi.2009.03.012.

Kobayashi M, Fussell SR, Xiao Y, Seagull FJ. Work coordination, workflow, and workarounds in a medical context. CHI. Portland, OR: ACM Press;2005. p. 1561–64.

Koppel R, Metlay JP, Cohen A, et al. Role of computerized physician order entry systems in facilitating medication errors. JAMA. 2005;293(10):1197–203. https://doi.org/10.1001/jama.293.10.1197.

Lim CJ, Kwong MW, Stuart RL, et al. Antibiotic prescribing practice in residential aged care facilities–health care providers' perspectives. Med J Aust. 2014;201(2):98–102.

Malhotra S, Jordan D, Shortliffe E, Patel VL. Workflow modeling in critical care: piecing together your own puzzle. J Biomed Inform. 2007;40(2):81–92. https://doi.org/10.1016/j.jbi.2006.06.002.

Marjamaa RA, Torkki PM, Hirvensalo EJ, Kirvela OA. What is the best workflow for an operating room? A simulation study of five scenarios. Health Care Manag Sci. 2008;12(2):142–6.

Moen A, Brennan PF. Health@Home: the work of health information management in the household (HIMH): implications for consumer health informatics (CHI) innovations. J Am Med Inform Assoc. 2005;12(6):648–56. https://doi.org/10.1197/jamia.M1758.

Morrill HJ, Caffrey AR, Jump RL, Dosa D, LaPlante KL. Antimicrobial stewardship in long-term care facilities: a call to action. J Am Med Dir Assoc. 2016;17(2):183 e1–16. https://doi.org/10.1016/j.jamda.2015.11.013.

Nagelkerk J, Reick K, Meengs L. Perceived barriers and effective strategies to diabetes self-management. J Adv Nurs. 2006;54(2):151–8. https://doi.org/10.1111/j.1365-2648.2006.03799.x.

Ozkaynak M. Characterizing workflow in hospital emergency departments [Dissertation]. University of Wisconsin-Madison;2011.

Ozkaynak M, Unertl KM, Johnson SA, Brixey JJ, Haque SN. Clinical workflow analysis, process redesign, and quality improvement. In: Finnel J, Dixon B, editors. Clinical informatics study guide. New York: Springer International Publishing; 2016a. p. 135–61.

Ozkaynak M, Jones J, Weiss J, Klem P, Reeder B. A workflow framework for health management in daily living settings. Stud Health Technol Inform. 2016b;225:392–6.

Ozkaynak M, Valdez RS, Holden RJ, Weiss J. Infinicare framework for an integrated understanding of health-related activities in clinical and daily-living contexts. Health Syst. 2018a;7(1):66–78.

Ozkaynak M, Wu DTY, Hannah K, Dayan PS, Mistry RD. Examining workflow in a pediatric emergency department to develop a clinical decision support for an antimicrobial stewardship program. Appl Clin Inform. 2018b;9(2):248–60.

Ozkaynak M, Brennan PF. Characterizing patient care in hospital emergency departments. Health Syst. 2012;1(2):104–17. https://doi.org/10.1057/hs.2012.14.

Ozkaynak M, Brennan P. An observation tool for studying patient-oriented workflow in hospital emergency departments. Methods Inf Med. 2013;52(6):503–13. https://doi.org/10.3414/ME12-01-0079.

Ozkaynak M, Brennan PF. Revisiting sociotechnical systems in a case of unreported use of health information exchange system in three hospital emergency departments. J Eval Clin Pract. 2013;19(2):370–3. https://doi.org/10.1111/j.1365-2753.2012.01837.x.

Ozkaynak M, Dziadkowiec O, Mistry R, et al. Characterizing workflow for pediatric asthma patients in emergency departments using electronic health records. J Biomed Inform. 2015;57:386–98. https://doi.org/10.1016/j.jbi.2015.08.018.

Ozkaynak M, Brennan PF, Hanauer Da, et al. Patient-centered care requires a patient-oriented workflow model. J Am Med Inform Assoc: JAMIA. 2013;20(e1):e14–6. https://doi.org/10.1136/amiajnl-2013-001633.

Rogers A, Kennedy A, Nelson E, Robinson A. Uncovering the limits of patient-centeredness: implementing a self-management trial for chronic illness. Qual Health Res. 2005;15(2):224–39. https://doi.org/10.1177/1049732304272048.

Ross SE, Schilling LM, Fernald DH, Davidson AJ, West DR. Health information exchange in small-to-medium sized family medicine practices: motivators, barriers, and potential facilitators of adoption. Int J Med Inform. 2010;79(2):123–29. https://doi.org/10.1016/j.ijmedinf.2009.12.001%5B

Rowe BH, Spooner C, Ducharme F, Bretzlaff J, Bota G. Early emergency department treatment of acute asthma with systemic corticosteroids. Cochrane Database Syst Rev. 2001(1). https://doi.org/10.1002/14651858.CD002178.

Sarkar U, Bates DW. Care partners and online patient portals. JAMA. 2014;311(4):357–58. https://doi.org/10.1001/jama.2013.285825.

Shaffer DW, Hatfield D, Svarovsky G, et al. Epistemic network analysis: a prototype for 21st century assessment of learning. Int J Learn Media. 2009;1(2):33–53.

Shaffer DW, Collier W, Ruis AR. A tutorial on epistemic network analysis: analyzing the structure of connections in cognitive, social, and interaction data. J Learn Anal. 2016;3(3):9–45.

Sittig DF, Singh H. A new sociotechnical model for studying health information technology in complex adaptive healthcare systems. Qual Saf Health Care. 2010;19(Suppl 3):i68–i74. https://doi.org/10.1136/qshc.2010.042085.

Stokoe A, Hullick C, Higgins I, Hewitt J, Armitage D, O'Dea I. Caring for acutely unwell older residents in residential aged-care facilities: perspectives of staff and general practitioners. Australas J Ageing. 2016;35(2):127–32. https://doi.org/10.1111/ajag.12221.

Tang PC, Ash JS, Bates DW, Overhage JM, Sands DZ. Personal health records: definitions, benefits, and strategies for overcoming barriers to adoption. J Am Med Inform Assoc. 2006;13(2):121–6. https://doi.org/10.1197/jamia.M2025.

Unertl KM, Weinger MB, Johnson KB, Lorenzi NM. Describing and modeling workflow and information flow in chronic disease care. J Am Med Inform Assoc. 2009;16(6):826–36. https://doi.org/10.1197/jamia.M3000.

Unertl KM, Johnson KB, Gadd CS, Lorenzi NM. Bridging organizational divides in health care: an ecological view of health information exchange. JMIR Med Inform. 2013;1(1):e3. https://doi.org/10.2196/medinform.2510.

Using Patient-Oriented Workflow to Develop a Holistic Understanding of Anticoagulation Management. CHI workshop on bridging clinical and non-clinical health practices: opportunities and challenges;2012.

Valdez RS, Holden RJ, Novak LL, Veinot TC. Transforming consumer health informatics through a patient work framework: connecting patients to context. J Am Med Inform Assoc. 2014. https://doi.org/10.1136/amiajnl-2014-002826.

Valdez RS, Holden RJ, Novak LL, Veinot TC. Technical infrastructure implications of the patient work framework. J Am Med Inform Assoc. 2015;22(e1):e213–e15. https://doi.org/10.1093/jamia/ocu031.

Wagner EH, Austin BT, Davis C, Hindmarsh M, Schaefer J, Bonomi A. Improving chronic illness care: translating evidence into action. Health Aff (Millwood). 2001;20(6):64–78. https://doi.org/10.1377/hlthaff.20.6.64.

Walker JM, Carayon P. From tasks to processes: the case for changing health information technology to improve health care. Health Aff (Millwood). 2009;28(2):467–77. https://doi.org/10.1377/hlthaff.28.2.467.

Wang CC. Photovoice: a participatory action research strategy applied to women's health. J Womens Health. 1999;8(2):185–92.

Werner NE, Gurses AP, Leff B, Arbaje AI. Improving care transitions across healthcare settings through a human factors approach. J Healthc Qual. 2016;38(6):328–43. https://doi.org/10.1097/JHQ.0000000000000025.

Werner NE, Malkana S, Gurses AP, Leff B, Arbaje AI. Toward a process-level view of distributed healthcare tasks: Medication management as a case study. Appl Ergon 2017;65:255–68. https://doi.org/10.1016/j.apergo.2017.06.020.

Werner NE, Stanislawski B, Marx KA, et al. Getting what they need when they need it. Identifying barriers to information needs of family caregivers to manage dementia-related behavioral symptoms. Appl Clin Inform. 2017;8(1):191–205. https://doi.org/10.4338/ACI-2016-07-RA-0122.

Werner NE, Tong M, Borkenhagen A, Holden RJ. Performance-shaping factors affecting older adults' hospital-to-home transition success: a systems approach. Gerontologist. 2018. https://doi.org/10.1093/geront/gnx199.

Woda A, Belknap RA, Haglund K, Sebern M, Lawrence A. Factors influencing self-care behaviors of African Americans with heart failure: a photovoice project. Heart Lung 2015;44(1):33–8. https://doi.org/10.1016/j.hrtlng.2014.09.001.

Wooldridge AR, Carayon P, Shaffer DW, Eagan B. Quantifying the qualitative with epistemic network analysis: a human factors case study of task-allocation communication in a primary care team. IISE Trans Healthc Syst Eng 2018;8(1):72–82. https://doi.org/10.1080/24725579.2017.1418769.

Xie A, Gurses AP, Hundt AS, Steege L, Valdez RS, Werner NE. Conceptualizing sociotechnical system boundaries in healthcare settings: within and across teams, organizations, processes, and networks. In: Proceedings of the human factors and ergonomics society annual meeting, vol. 60(1);2016. p. 866–70. https://doi.org/10.1177/1541931213601198.

Yen PY, Bakken S. Review of health information technology usability study methodologies. J Am Med Inform Assoc. 2012;19(3):413–22. https://doi.org/10.1136/amiajnl-2010-000020.

Yen K, Gorelick MH. Strategies to improve flow in the pediatric emergency department. Pediatr Emerg Care. 2007;23(10):745–9; quiz 50-1. https://doi.org/10.1097/PEC.0b013e3181568efe.

Zheng K, Haftel HM, Hirschl RB, O'Reilly M, Hanauer DA. Quantifying the impact of health IT implementations on clinical workflow: a new methodological perspective. J Am Med Inform Assoc. 2010;17(4):454–61. https://doi.org/10.1136/jamia.2010.004440.

Zheng K, Guo MH, Hanauer DA. Using the time and motion method to study clinical work processes and workflow: methodological inconsistencies and a call for standardized research. J Am Med Inform Assoc. 2011;18(5):704–10. https://doi.org/10.1136/amiajnl-2011-000083.

Part III
Research Methods for Studying Clinical Workflow

Chapter 12
Computer-Based Tools for Recording Time and Motion Data for Assessing Clinical Workflow

Danny T. Y. Wu

Abstract Time and motion is a popularly used approach for quantifying clinical work processes and workflow. It has been generally considered the "gold standard" for conducting quantitative workflow studies because of the rich details it is able to reveal regarding workflow, and the accuracy of its measurements as compared to other competing methods such as self-reported questionnaires and work sampling. However, there are several methodological limitations that threaten the validity of time and motion studies. These include difficulties in assessing inter-observer reliability, difficulties for external observers to discern subtle activities by study participants, and difficulties in capturing multitasking. While completely eliminating these methodological limitations may not be possible, one way to mitigate their effects is to develop effective data capture tools to assist external observers in collecting high-quality time and motion data. Such tools need to be very easy to use, incorporate measures to reduce data entry inconsistencies and errors, and can be easily extended to accommodate new research questions and new empirical scenarios. In this chapter, we introduce four such tools developed by different research groups in the past ten years, namely Time Capture Tool (TimeCaT, 2012), Work Observation Method by Activity Timing (WOMBAT, 2008), CRISS TM Logger (1994), and T&M Data Collector (2015). The features of each of these tools are described, followed by a discussion of their pros and cons.

Keywords Workflow · Observation · Time and motion studies · Data collection · Mobile applications · Process assessment · Health care

D. T. Y. Wu (✉)
Department of Biostatistics, Health Informatics, and Data Sciences, University of Cincinnati College of Medicine, Cincinnati, USA
e-mail: wutz@ucmail.uc.edu

© The Author(s), under exclusive license to Springer Nature Switzerland AG 2025
K. Zheng et al. (eds.), *Reengineering Clinical Workflow in the Digital and AI Era*,
Cognitive Informatics in Biomedicine and Healthcare,
https://doi.org/10.1007/978-3-031-82971-0_12

233

12.1   Introduction

This chapter focuses on computer-based tools designed to facilitate field data collection for time and motion studies (TMS) conducted in healthcare settings. As a commonly used research method, TMS originated from industrial engineering with a goal to assess workers' time expenditure and physical movements when completing a task, a series of tasks, or distinct steps that constitute a task. In recent years, TMS have been widely adopted and frequently used to study clinical workflow, especially in the context of introduction of health information technology (IT) systems (Lopetegui et al. 2014). As of January 2024, a cursory search in PubMed[1] with the keywords ("time and motion study" OR "time motion study") yielded a total of 508 papers. More than 83% of them were published in and after year 2000.

TMS usually require a person (i.e., "external observer") to shadow clinicians' work to continuously record when, where, and what clinical tasks are performed. Since early 2000s, Several computer-based tools have been developed to facilitate time and motion data collection with features specifically designed to accommodate capture of complex workflow behaviors, such as multi-tier clinical task classifications and the ability to record multitasking and interruptions. In this chapter, we describe four such tools that have been used in multiple TMS-based research studies with established validity and generalizability. Our choice of these four tools, however, does not suggest they perform better than other competing tools available, or are more generalizable.

12.2   Time Capture Tool (TimeCaT)

The Time Capture Tool, or TimeCaT, was developed in 2012 with a focus on standardization, scalability, and dissemination. Its development began with a systematic review of the features and limitations of existing TMS tools at the time. Then, a pilot version of TimeCaT was created and tested through an empirical study conducted in an emergency medicine setting. User feedback was collected to inform refinement of the tool, leading toward a significantly modified version with improved usability and functionality. Lopetegui et al. (2012) provides more details on the history, design, and development process of TimeCaT (Lopetegui et al. 2012).

TimeCaT has a user-facing website available at http://www.timecat.org/. Its current version (v3.9) is capable of capturing multitasking and interruption events; and allows observers to correct data during the observation (Fig. 12.1). TimeCaT uses UNIX-based timestamps to calculate task duration to avoid discrepancies due to time zone difference. It also provides several dashboards for administrative and real-time data reporting purposes (Fig. 12.2). It is worth noting that TimeCaT uses visualization techniques to compare between observations to help researchers assess inter-rater reliability and discover patterns of differences (Fig. 12.3). One exemplary

---

[1] https://www.ncbi.nlm.nih.gov/pubmed

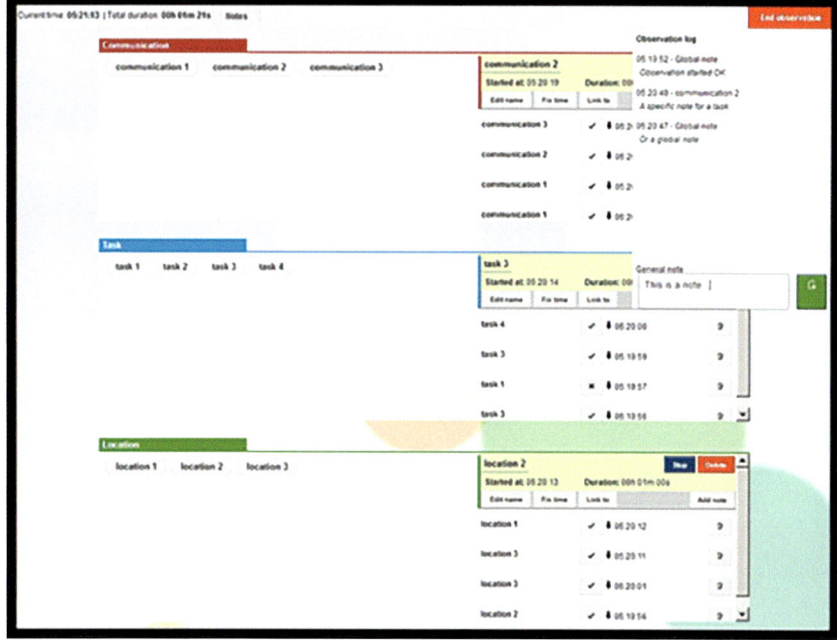

Fig. 12.1   TimeCaT: data capture and correction

study that used TimeCaT to quantify and visualize nursing clinical workflow was conducted by Yen et al. (2016).

12.3   Work Observation Method by Activity Timing (WOMBAT)

WOMBAT was developed in 2008 by Johanna Westbrook and her colleagues at the Macquarie University, Sydney, Australia. Its design objective is to create a digital tool for efficient, accurate, reliable, and detailed TMS data collection to effectively capture health professionals' work and communication patterns. WOMBAT is capable of recording clinical work activities in four dimensions, namely *What*, *Who*, *How*, and *Where*; in addition to *When* which is automatically captured as computer-recorded timestamps.

WOMBAT was initially developed on the Personal Digital Assistant (PDA) platform and was later migrated to Android. Tablets with larger screen sizes (7″ or 8″ at the minimum) are recommended for optimal experience when using WOMBAT as a field data collection tool. In addition to the Tablet-based app, WOMBAT provides a web front to manage the app as well as to analyze time and motion data collected. Figure 12.4 shows a screenshot of the app (left) and the web front (right), respectively.

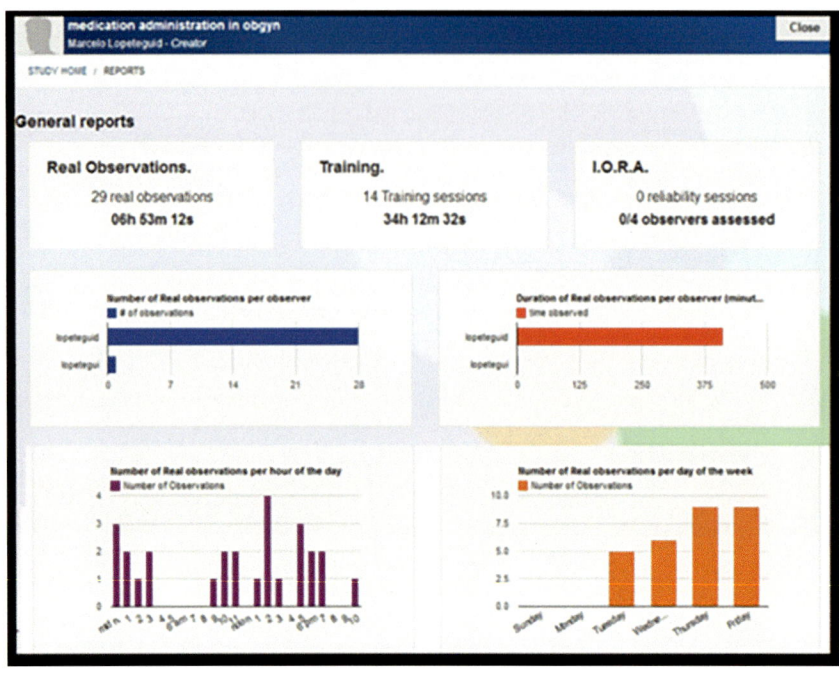

Fig. 12.2 TimeCaT: real-time data reporting dashboards

The initial version of WOMBAT was designed and evaluated through a nursing workflow study conducted by Westbrook and Ampt (2009) that involved four wards, 52 nurses, and 250 observation hours. The results of the study demonstrated that the nursing workflow data collected by WOMBAT accurately reflected known differences in clinical roles and tasks. WOMBAT was further validated in a study conducted in Canada in 2011 by Ballermann et al. (2011). This study observed clinicians' work in two intensive care units where a computerized clinical system was introduced. The study again demonstrated WOMBAT's utility in collecting high-quality workflow data to compare clinicians' time allocation before and after the system implementation. Since then, WOMBAT has been used in multiple TMS globally conducted by different research groups. A list of use cases of this tool can be found at http://aihi. mq.edu.au/content/wombat-case-studies.

The current version of WOMBAT can be accessed through its official website at https://aihi.mq.edu.au/project/wombat-work-observation-method-act ivity-timing. Of note, WOMBAT requires a license agreement for individual users. Once the license is obtained, WOMBAT can be used in any number of projects.

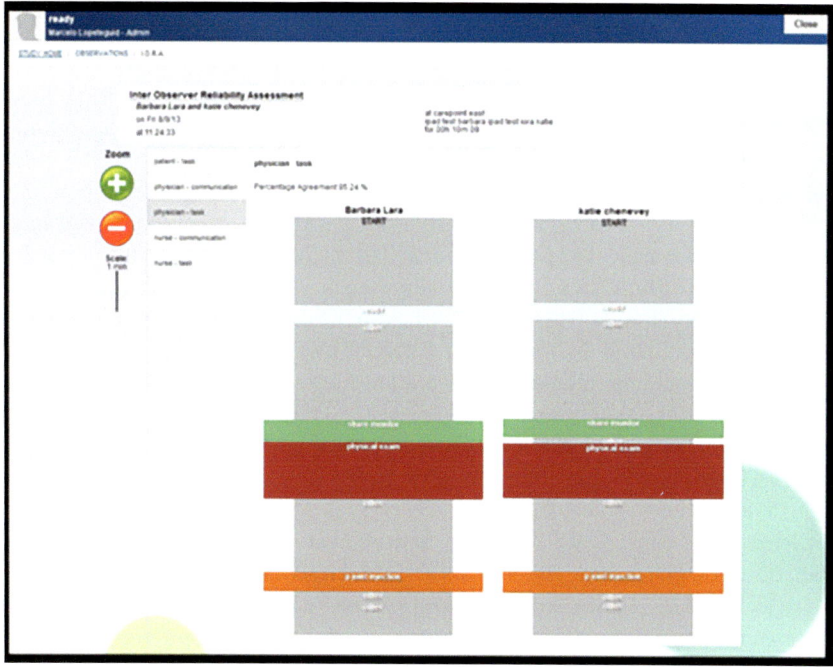

Fig. 12.3 TimeCaT: visual comparison to assist in evaluating inter-rater reliability

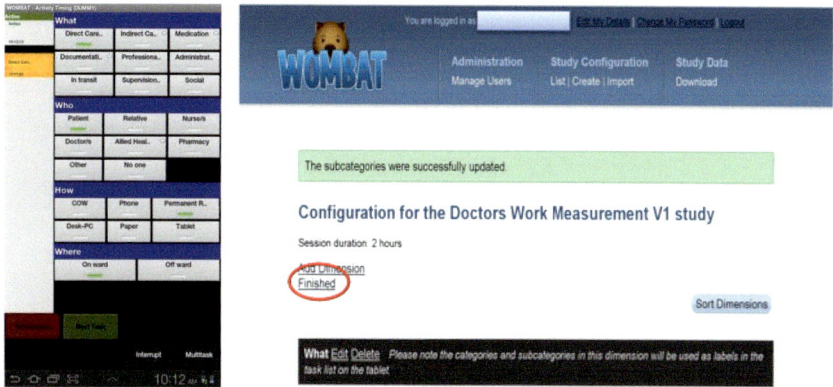

Fig. 12.4 Screenshots of WOMBAT Tablet (left) and web-based application (right) for data capture and tool administration, respectively

12.4 CRISS TM Logger

The CRISS TM logger was developed in 1994 by the Center for Research and Innovation in Systems Safety (CRISS) at Vanderbilt University to support a workflow and workload study in an anesthesiology setting (Driscoll et al. 2007). This study proposed an objective clinical task analysis methodology involving time-motion analysis, secondary task probing, and subjective workload assessment to evaluate anesthesiologist performance in operating rooms. The methodology was further refined to be applicable to other related clinical problems, such as drug and fluid administration in anesthesiology (Fraind et al. 2002). The researchers examined the reliability of this methodology and found that the interrater reliability on task durations was unsatisfactory due to the suboptimal capture of multitasking events, leading to a significant improvement of the functionality (Slagle et al. 2002). This tool has to date been used to support several workflow studies, especially in assessing the vigilance and workload in anesthesia care (Slagle and Weinger 2009; Fletcher et al. 2012; Slagle et al. 2018).

CRISS TM Logger is fully customizable and can be used for any domain and at any level of granularity. A screenshot of the customized task list and interface is provided in Fig. 12.5. CRISS TM Logger has been primarily used for patient safety applications and studies in operating rooms, intensive care units, and with hospitalists in internal medicine. Consultation with the CRISS researchers is strongly recommended to achieve optimal use of the tool. Requests to use CRISS TM Logger should be sent to criss_info@vumc.org. The use may be subject to a license fee.

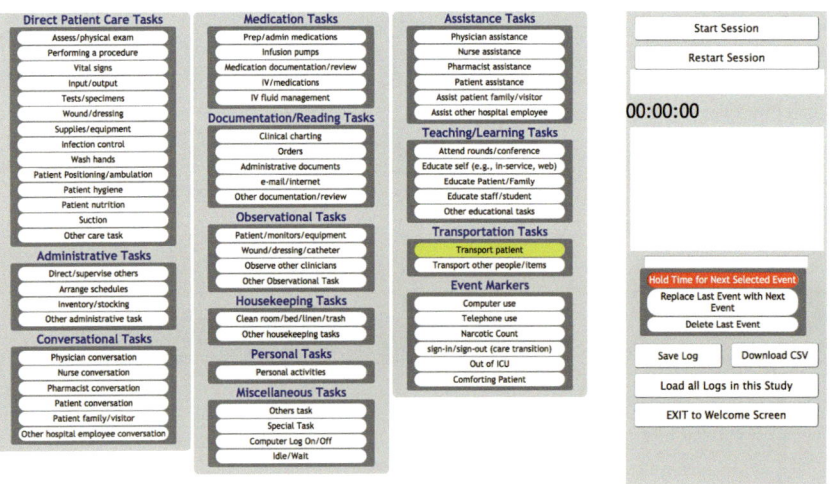

Fig. 12.5 A sample task list of CRISS TM Logger with a web-based application customizable to support data collection in time and motion studies

12.5   Time and Motion Data Collector

The Time and Motion Data Collector (the "TM Collector" hereafter) was developed in 2015 as part of a research project funded by the U.S. Agency of Healthcare Research and Quality (Zheng et al. 2015). The tool was designed to capture both discrete clinical activities based on customizable task taxonomies, as well as multitasking and interruptions.

The TM Collector incorporates carefully designed features to accommodate recording of multitasking and interruption events (Fig. 12.6). Tasks being performed simultaneously by the observee can be handled with two approaches depending on the use scenario. In the first approach, overlapped task durations because of multitasking are grouped into new "composite" activities. In the second approach, overlapped durations are split and attributed proportionally to each of the tasks being performed at the same time. Take two tasks, A and B, as an example. Assume task A lasted 10 s, task B lasted 15 s, and there was a 5-s overlap between them. Using the first approach, a new composite task A/B would be created so that it produces a new event sequence of A (5 s) to A/B (5 s) to B (10 s). When the second approach is applied, the overlapped portion would be split and attributed equally to activity A and B, resulting in a new event sequence of A (7.5 s) to B (12.5 s). This distinguishing is important when certain measures, such as how clinicians distribute their time across different clinical tasks, are computed.

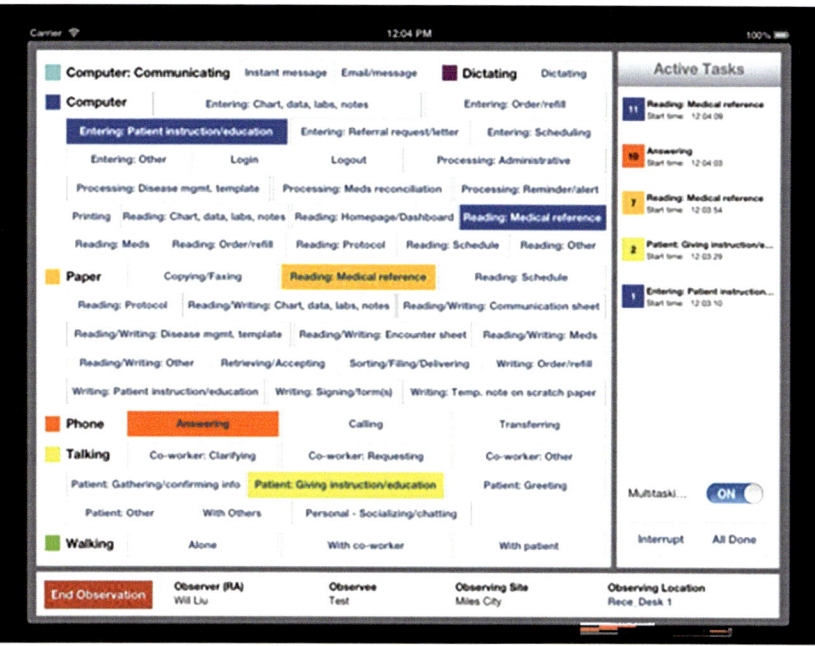

Fig. 12.6 Main data capture page of the T&M data collector

In addition to specifically developed features for accommodating the complex nature of clinical workflow, the TM Collector also has a web-based analytics platform for analyzing workflow data in real time using data mining and visualization techniques. Figure 12.7 shows the landing page of the analytics platform, which displays key descriptive statistics related to the duration of performance for each of the tasks or task groups. Users can then choose to conduct drill-down analyses at different levels. The platform also supports data analyses for *before-and-after* studies. Pre- and post-data can be separately uploaded, which will be automatically compared using common statistical procedures such as paired or unpaired t-test and chi-square test. The analytics platform also provides a variety of visualization options to help researchers discern patterns of potential interest from the visual representations of their data. Figures 12.8 and 12.9 exhibit two examples.

The TM Collector has been recently adopted by two researcher teams to conduct TMS outside its original development context, demonstrating its generalizability. In the first study, it was used to record workflow data in an emergency medicine setting at an academic medical center in the U.S. to inform the design of a computerized clinical decision-support system (Ozkaynak et al. 2018). In the second study, the tool was used to collect behavioral data on how bedside nurses used a mobile app in Geneva, Switzerland (Ehrler et al. 2018). A Clinical Workflow Analysis Tool (CWAT) was further developed using visual analytics principles to explore TM data in healthcare (Wu et al. 2022).

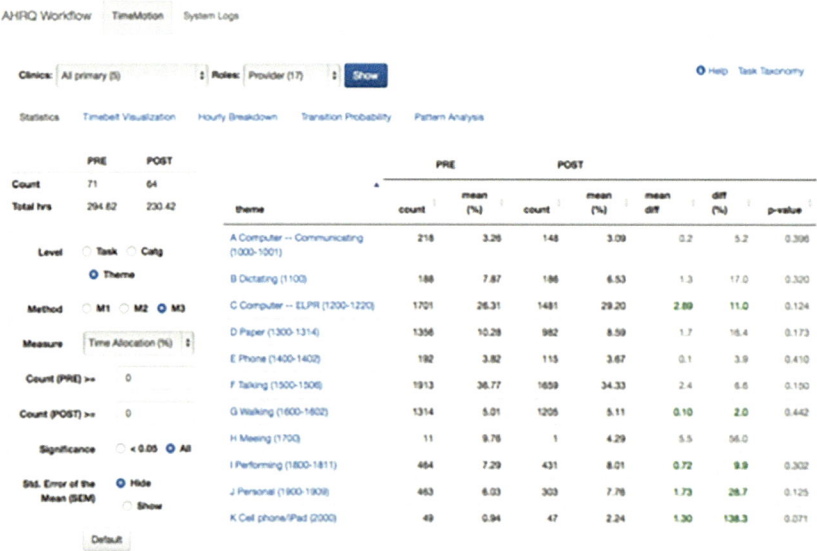

Fig. 12.7 Statistical summary of task allocation and continuous time on the analytics platform

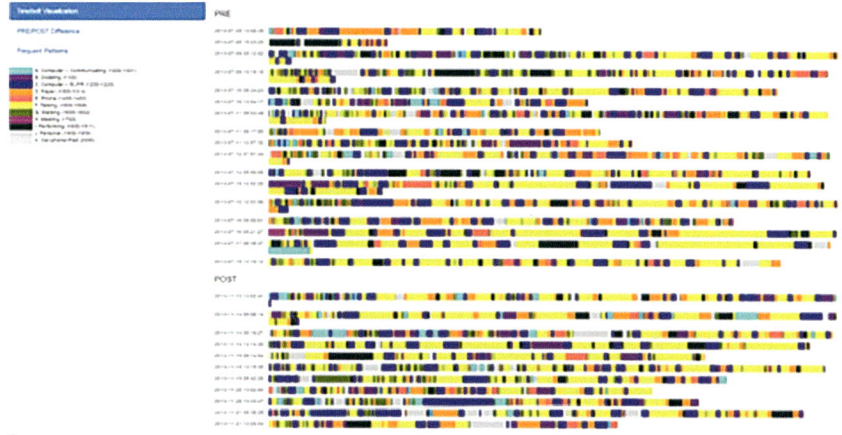

Fig. 12.8 Time-belt visualization on task sequences

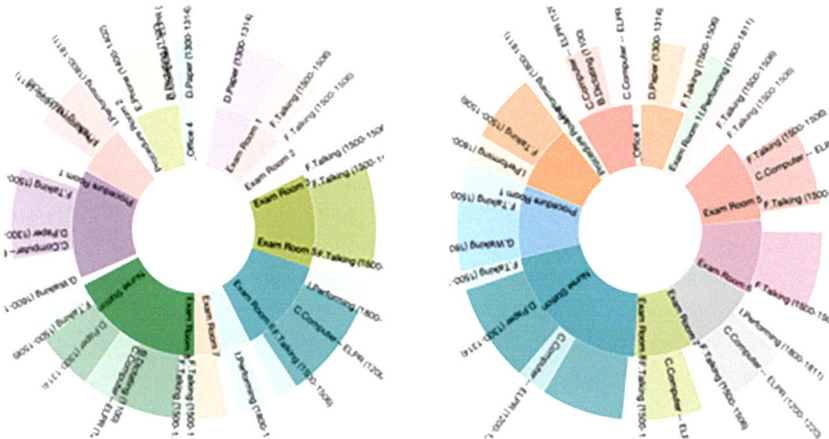

Fig. 12.9 Location-task analysis using a sunburst graph

12.6   Methodological Challenges and Potential Solutions

While TMS have been considered the "gold standard" approach for quantifying clinical workflow, it has its own limitations. First, collecting time and motion data requires a significant amount of resources, from hiring and training external observers to coordinating observation sessions with busy clinicians. Second, the quality of TMS data collected by human observers can be variable depending on each individual's capabilities and biases. For example, an observer might deem an activity unimportant, or not clinically related, and therefore did not record it; yet the activity might turn out to provide crucial information for answering some research questions down the road.

Moreover, the granularity of TM data and proper classification of activities require a thorough understanding of the clinical work being observed. This can be difficult for external observers who do not have relevant background. Further, TMS involving external observers is inherently intrusive. Study participants' behavior while being observed may deviate considerably from how they usually conduct their work.

Another critical limitation of TMS is that it is very difficult to compare results across different TMS studies due to the inconsistent methodologies they apply (e.g., how external observers are trained, how inter-observer reliability is assessed and calibrated, and whether the same observer is assigned to observe the same study participant across different study stages such as before and after an intervention is introduced). To address this issue, Zheng et al. developed a checklist called Suggested Time And Motion Procedures, or STAMP, based on a review of relevant TMS studies (Zheng et al. 2011). The STAMP list outlines 29 essential elements that need to be carefully considered in designing TMS and in reporting TMS-produced study results and research findings. These 29 elements are organized in eight key areas, including (1) intervention, (2) empirically setting, (3) research design, (4) task category, (5) observer, (6) subject, (7) data recording, and (8) data analysis.

Zheng et al. also provided a new perspective on how to analyze time and motion data. Specifically, they argued that the prevalent method that focuses on the "time expenditures" measure (e.g., how clinicians allocate their time across different tasks) is limited and can generate conflicting or misleading results. Alternatively, they argued workflow studies should focus on investigating the "flow of work" instead. Through an empirical study, they demonstrated that this could be achieved by introducing using new workflow measures and new analytical approaches, such as workflow fragmentation assessments, pattern recognition, and visualization. These new measures and new analytical methods could collectively contribute to uncovering the "hidden regularities" embedded in clinicians' work and workflow (Zheng et al. 2010). Among the proposed analytical methods, workflow fragmentation is particularly innovative. It is conceptually simple but can be very powerful to reflect the actual burden that clinicians experience. The workflow fragmentation assessment consists of two primary measures: (1) continuous time, and (2) frequency of task switching. The former is defined as "the average amount of time continuously spent on performing a single clinical activity," and the latter is defined as "the rate at which clinicians switch between tasks" (Zheng et al. 2010). These two measures are highly correlated. The shorter the continuous time is, the higher the task switching frequency is likely to be, and the more mental burden the clinicians may experience.

Acknowledgements The author of this chapter is grateful to Ms. Himaja Chintalapalli for her effort on copyediting.

References

Ballermann MA, Shaw NT, Mayes DC, Gibney RTN, Westbrook JI. Validation of the work observation method by activity timing (WOMBAT) method of conducting time-motion observations in critical care settings: an observational study. BMC Med Inform Decis Mak. 2011;11:32.

Driscoll WD, Columbia MA, Peterfreund RA. An observational study of anesthesia record completeness using an anesthesia information management system. Anesth Analg. 2007;104(6):1454–61, table of contents.

Ehrler F, Ducloux P, Wu D, Lovis C, Blondon K. Acceptance of a mobile application supporting Nurses workflow at patient bedside: Results from a pilot study. In 2018.

Fletcher KE, Visotcky AM, Slagle JM, Tarima S, Weinger MB, Schapira MM. The composition of intern work while on call. J Gen Intern Med. 2012;27(11):1432–7.

Fraind DB, Slagle JM, Tubbesing VA, Hughes SA, Weinger MB. Reengineering intravenous drug and fluid administration processes in the operating room: Step one: task analysis of existing processes. Anesthesiology. 2002;97(1):139–47.

Lopetegui M, Yen PY, Lai AM, Embi PJ, Payne PRO. Time Capture Tool (TimeCaT): development of a comprehensive application to support data capture for time motion studies. AMIA Annu Symp Proc AMIA Symp AMIA Symp. 2012;2012:596–605.

Lopetegui M, Yen PY, Lai A, Jeffries J, Embi P, Payne P. Time motion studies in healthcare: what are we talking about? J Biomed Inform. 2014;49:292–9.

Ozkaynak M, Wu DTY, Hannah K, Dayan PS, Mistry RD. Examining workflow in a pediatric emergency department to develop a clinical decision support for an antimicrobial stewardship program. Appl Clin Inform. 2018;9(2):248–60.

Slagle JM, Weinger MB. Effects of intraoperative reading on vigilance and workload during anesthesia care in an academic medical center. Anesthesiology. 2009;110(2):275–83.

Slagle J, Weinger MB, Dinh MTT, Brumer VV, Williams K. Assessment of the intrarater and interrater reliability of an established clinical task analysis methodology. Anesthesiology. 2002;96(5):1129–39.

Slagle JM, Porterfield ES, Lorinc AN, Afshartous D, Shotwell MS, Weinger MB. Prevalence of potentially distracting noncare activities and their effects on vigilance, workload, and nonroutine events during Anesthesia care. Anesthesiology. 2018;128(1):44–54.

Westbrook JI, Ampt A. Design, application and testing of the Work Observation Method by Activity Timing (WOMBAT) to measure clinicians' patterns of work and communication. Int J Med Inf. 2009;78(Suppl 1):S25-33.

Wu DTY, Shu D, Le K, Abbu R, Zheng K. Applying visual analytics to develop a clinical workflow analysis tool (CWAT) to explore time and motion data in healthcare. In: 2022 workshop on visual analytics in healthcare (VAHC) [Internet]. Washington, DC, USA: IEEE; 2022 [cited 2023 Nov 19]. p. 01–5. https://ieeexplore.ieee.org/document/10108522/

Yen PY, Kelley M, Lopetegui M, Rosado AL, Migliore EM, Chipps EM, et al. Understanding and visualizing multitasking and task switching activities: A time motion study to capture nursing workflow. AMIA Annu Symp Proc AMIA Symp. 2016;2016:1264–73.

Zheng K, Haftel HM, Hirschl RB, O'Reilly M, Hanauer DA. Quantifying the impact of health IT implementations on clinical workflow: A new methodological perspective. J Am Med Inform Assoc JAMIA. 2010;17(4):454–61.

Zheng K, Guo MH, Hanauer DA. Using the time and motion method to study clinical work processes and workflow: methodological inconsistencies and a call for standardized research. J Am Med Inform Assoc JAMIA. 2011;18(5):704–10.

Zheng, K, Ciemins, E, Lanham, H, Lindberg, C. Examining the relationship between health IT and ambulatory care workflow redesign. (Prepared by Billings Clinic under Contract No. 290–2010–0019I-1). AHRQ Publication No. 15–0058-EF. Rockville, MD: Agency for Healthcare Research and Quality; 2015.

Chapter 13
Understanding Clinical Workflow Through Direct Continuous Observation: Addressing the Unique Statistical Challenges

Scott R. Walter, William T. M. Dunsmuir, Magdalena Z. Raban, Johanna Westbrook, and Ling Li

13.1 Background

13.1.1 General Introduction

The nature of healthcare as a dynamic human process occurring within complex socio-technical systems means that there is no unique or standard way to examine its inner workings. Rather, a range of observational methods drawn from multiple disciplines have been used to study workflow in situ (McCurdie et al. 2017). A review of methods used to study and model workflow across different industries, including healthcare, identified qualitative approaches such as ethnographic observation and interviews along with quantitative methods, including structured or timed observations, and surveys (Unertl et al. 2010).

Analogous to timed observations, the term *time and motion* is applied in many studies of workflow in healthcare. This umbrella term encompasses a range of

S. R. Walter (✉)
National Institute for Health and Care Research, Applied Research Collaboration West (NIHR ARC West), University Hospitals Bristol and Weston NHS Foundation Trust, Bristol, UK
e-mail: scott.walter@bristol.ac.uk

Population Health Sciences, Bristol Medical School, University of Bristol, Bristol, UK

S. R. Walter · M. Z. Raban · J. Westbrook · L. Li
Centre for Health Systems and Safety Research, Australian Institute of Health Innovation, Faculty of Medicine and Health Sciences, Macquarie University, Sydney, Australia

W. T. M. Dunsmuir
Department of Statistics, School of Mathematics and Statistics, University of New South Wales, Sydney, Australia

© The Author(s), under exclusive license to Springer Nature Switzerland AG 2025
K. Zheng et al. (eds.), *Reengineering Clinical Workflow in the Digital and AI Era*, Cognitive Informatics in Biomedicine and Healthcare,
https://doi.org/10.1007/978-3-031-82971-0_13

245

methods and designs with the common feature of directly observing an individual's activities and recording aspects of that action, usually in a quantitative way. Zheng et al. (2011) reviewed time and motion studies used to assess the effect of interventions, especially technology-related interventions, on workflow in healthcare settings. From their synthesis, they developed the STAMP checklist (Suggested Time and Motion Procedures) to promote consistency in design, conduct and reporting of time and motion studies. Other authors have taken this theme further by reviewing the distinct methods used in healthcare under the banner of 'time and motion studies' (Lopetegui et al. 2014; Payne et al. 2019). The many variations they identified were categorized into three groups: (i) those involving external observers shadowing participants, (ii) those using information self-reported by participants, and (iii) those that employed automated data recording such as GPS devices or accelerometers. Of the first type, they identified a method employing continuous observation and coined the term *workflow time study* to describe it as a distinct but increasingly common approach (Lopetegui et al. 2014). This method constituted 26% of all time and motion studies reviewed, and over 60% of all studies that involved continuous observation by an external observer. Also, the proportion of studies employing continuous observation was noted to have increased over the review period. Of the studies using two of the more common workflow capture software programs (WOMBAT (Westbrook and Ampt 2009; https://www.mq.edu.au/research/research-centres-groups-and-facilities/healthy-people/centres/australian-institute-of-health-innovation/our-projects/wombat) and TimeCaT (Lopetegui et al. 2012; https://timecat.org/#articles-section)), there are close to 90 publications at the time of writing.

Although the workflow time study approach is one among many observational approaches, it offers many advantages over other quantitative methods, and its growing use in healthcare is a testament to this. This method itself involves observers shadowing individual clinicians and continuously recording time-stamped data about an individual's tasks and interactions (see Sect. 13.1.2 for more detail). Workflow time studies capture more of the fine-grained complexity of clinical work than methods such as work sampling, and the temporal continuity of the data forms the most complete record of an individual's workflow of any observational technique, barring audio-visual recording which is often not acceptable in a clinical environment. Workflow time studies have great potential to help us understand clinical work and workflow and can be applied to a diverse range of research questions and professional groups (Walter et al. 2015). This includes descriptive analyses that examine the way clinicians distribute their time between different tasks, between patients, between locations, and so on (Westbrook et al. 2008; Li et al. 2015; Richardson et al. 2016). It also supports assessment of the impact of interventions on workflow, such as the introduction of new technological systems, policies or practices (e.g. Georgiou et al. 2017). Furthermore, workflow time studies enable interrogation of more complex questions such as the way in which clinicians sequence, prioritize and interleave tasks. They can also examine associations between clinicians' work and safety-related outcomes, such as factors that contribute to errors of task omission and commission (e.g. Westbrook et al. 2018).

Capturing a more complete record of the complexity of workflow in healthcare settings is necessary to generate valid and relevant insights about everyday clinical work within a quantitative paradigm. However, this also introduces some unique methodological challenges in all aspects of the study process including design, data collection, analysis and interpretation of findings. Despite the importance of applying appropriate quantitative methods, methodology in the area is still evolving. While there has been increasing discussion around these challenges (Payne et al. 2019; Tanzini et al. 2019; Zheng et al. 2020), there is still a tendency for workflow time studies to apply conventional statistical methods to data that are inherently non-standard. This chapter examines the critical quantitative and statistical challenges with which workflow time studies are confronted, including reviewing methods applied in studies to date and suggestions for methodological improvements. Many of the aspects discussed in this chapter may also be relevant to the quantitative study of workflow more generally.

13.1.2 Defining Workflow Time Studies

The original definition of workflow time studies referred to those studies involving periods of continuous observation of a participant where "the observer records the occurrence and duration of unpredicted instances of tasks, producing a data schema of time-stamped tasks, which accounts for task fragmentation, interruptions and work variability" (Lopetegui et al. 2014). There are several features that distinguish this technique from other observational methods. First, the fact that observers continuously shadow participants sets it apart from approaches such as self-reporting of work activities (Ampt et al. 2007), work sampling or multimedia recording. Second, although carrying out detailed observations over extensive periods of time has parallels with ethnography, observers in workflow time studies apply predefined categories of task attributes at the time of observation, as distinct from ethnography where grouping of types of observed action into categories or themes occurs during the analysis phase (e.g. Malhotra et al. 2007). Third, the recording of time stamped intervals for each task generates data that represents a temporally complete record of the observed activity. In other words, at every time point during observation, action is assigned to one category or another, or, equivalently, no time in the workflow is unaccounted for. This contrasts with other methods where the observer may continuously shadow the participant but may only record data at certain times or on particular activities.

The data generated by workflow time studies is essentially a set of time intervals, each defined by a start and end time, and having any number of categorical attributes such as task type, location where the task was performed, with whom it was performed, and so on. Figure 13.1 provides a simple illustration of tasks plotted over time, in addition to one possible way to represent the raw data in a tabular form. The intervals can be contiguous where one task ends as another begins, as between tasks 1 and 2 in the figure; or they can overlap where two types of action occur in parallel (commonly called multitasking) as with tasks 2 and 3. When intervals represent fragmentation of tasks that are suspended due to interruptions and later resumed, this can be indicated with categorical labels, as shown by the 'interrupted by' column in the data table in Fig. 13.1. Some studies also augment with data from other sources such as patient load in the healthcare setting, self-reported measures or participant characteristics, in an effort to include factors at multiple system levels (see for example Westbrook et al. 2018).

The task attributes mentioned above are termed *dimensions*, each of which may have several *categories* (Westbrook and Ampt 2009). In workflow time studies, a dimension is an aspect of clinical work that is relevant to the research questions of a study. In the example in Fig. 13.1, 'type' is the main dimension which has categories 'A' and 'B'. In clinical settings, dimensions may be the type of task performed by the participant (usually the main dimension), the location where the task is performed, or with whom the participant interacts with while performing the task. In the language of quantitative analysis, dimensions can equivalently be thought of as categorical variables, and the categories represent all the potential values that a variable can take on. Table 13.1 illustrates two dimensions and their categories from a study of emergency doctors in Australia (Walter et al. 2017).

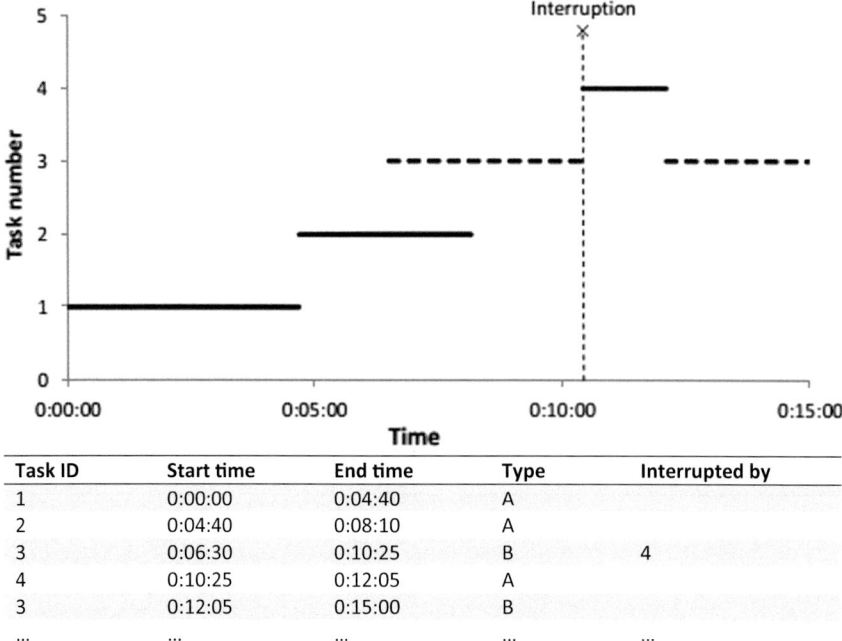

Task ID	Start time	End time	Type	Interrupted by
1	0:00:00	0:04:40	A	
2	0:04:40	0:08:10	A	
3	0:06:30	0:10:25	B	4
4	0:10:25	0:12:05	A	
3	0:12:05	0:15:00	B	
...	...	...	...	...

Fig. 13.1 Example of four tasks observed in a workflow time study, represented as intervals on a continuous timeline and as records in a data table

Table 13.1 Examples of dimensions and categories used in workflow time studies

Dimension	Category
Task type	Direct care
	Indirect care
	Documentation
	Clinical communication
	Management communication
	Social communication
	Prescribing
	Other
With Whom	Specialist (Consultant)
	Fellow (Registrar)
	Resident/intern
	Nurse
	Patient
	Relative
	Paramedic
	Other
	No one

Table 13.2 Sampling schedule used by Richardson et al. (2016) to study junior physicians working on day shifts over the weekend

Observation time	Saturday A	Sunday A	Saturday B	Sunday B
	Wk 1, 3, 5, 7, 9, 11, 13	Wk 1, 3, 5, 7, 9, 11, 13	Wk 2,4, 6, 8, 10, 12	Wk 2,4, 6, 8, 10, 12
0800–0950	Observing			Observing
0950–1140	Resting	Observing	Observing	Resting
1140–1330	Observing	Resting	Resting	Observing
1330–1520	Resting	Observing	Observing	Resting
1520–1710	Observing	Resting	Resting	Observing
1710–1900		Observing	Observing	

13.2 Sampling Strategies

The first major methodological challenge in conducting a workflow time study is how to approach data sampling. The sampling strategy naturally depends on the study design. As it is impractical to cover the sampling strategies for all possible workflow time study designs within this chapter, we limit our discussion to the following three major study types: (1) descriptive studies that provide a snapshot of the clinical work process, (2) intervention studies that assess change in workflow over time as a result of an intervention, and (3) association studies that aim to link aspects of clinical work to patient safety or quality of care outcomes.

One aspect of the sampling strategy that impacts all three study types is that there is a limit as to how much one observer can continuously observe without a break. However, much of health care, particularly critical care, occurs around the clock. Although in an ideal situation we may wish to observe all clinicians at all times throughout the study period, this is simply not practical. Thus, the data in workflow time studies are often collected across many separate observation sessions, wherein each session typically consists of a few hours of shadowing with a single participant. The data from these sessions are then combined to form a collection of workflow samples on multiple participants.

The nature of clinical work varies with time-related factors: time of day, day of the week, time of year, etc. (Walter et al. 2014) It also differs between clinician roles or seniority (Westbrook et al. 2010), and between the idiosyncrasies of individuals (Walter et al. 2014). Oversampling at certain times or among certain roles can therefore influence the study results, underscoring the need for an appropriate sampling strategy to avoid biases. Descriptive studies generally aim to generate a set of samples that, when combined, are representative of clinical work in a certain setting, among a particular professional group, or during a given period of the working day. For example, Arabadzhiyska et al. (2013) studied the work of resident physicians on night shifts (10 pm–8 am) on general hospital wards.

Generating a representative sample is usually accomplished by applying a time-based sampling scheme to collect approximately equal amounts of observation time balanced across known factors that may influence summary measures such as proportions and rates. To illustrate, the rate at which clinicians' work is interrupted is known to be higher for those who are more senior (Walter et al. 2017), during weekends (Richardson et al. 2016) and is related to workload (Weigl et al. 2012) which varies throughout the course of the day. If there is unintentional oversampling of senior clinicians, weekends or busy periods, it could then inflate the interruption rate to be observed. In contrast, balancing observation time across such factors provides an interruption rate estimate that is more representative of the 'average' workflow within the study population.

Such a sampling scheme was used by Richardson et al. (2016) who conducted a descriptive study of junior physicians working on day shifts during the weekend. The study population was from a single professional group of the same seniority; and a sampling scheme was developed to ensure balance in observation hours over time of day (between 8 am and 5 pm), day of the week (Saturday and Sunday) and also over the 13-week observation period (Table 13.2).

Another major source of variation in workflow is between individuals. A study of how clinicians in three hospital settings respond to interruptions found that significant variation between individuals persisted after adjusting for many task-level and temporal factors (Walter et al. 2014). Attempting to average individual differences by balancing (as shown in Table 13.2) would mean an unrealistically large increase in required sample size and hence observation time. For example, the Richardson et al. study had 16 participants, so to observe each of them, during every time of the day,

day of the weekend and week of the study period, it would require an increase of the total observation time from 132 h to more than two thousand hours. Randomisation offers a way to average out the effects of temporal factors and individual differences with a more realistic sample size. For each observation session the participant is randomly selected, as is the time of day, day of the week, and so on. Sessions can be assigned in this way until a sufficiently large sample is attained.

In practice, it is not always possible to implement either a balanced or randomised sampling scheme exactly as planned. Finding a certain participant at a particular time can be difficult, especially in a hospital setting where staff rosters change and clinicians swap shifts at the last minute. While it is important to have a sampling plan, it may be necessary to modify it over the course of the study period to compensate for imbalances introduced by unanticipated deviations from the schedule. If logistical constraints cause the final sample to be unbalanced, it is possible to adjust for this in the analysis phase using multivariable regression. For example, to calculate the interruption rate across task type categories (as in Table 13.1) when there has been oversampling of senior clinicians, Poisson regression could be applied with the main covariate as task type, but also including, say, time of day and participant seniority as additional variables. This does not preclude the need for a sampling plan, but rather provides a way to mitigate the effects of compromised implementation of the plan.

For studies assessing the impact of an intervention using a pre-post design, an additional consideration is to use a consistent sampling strategy for each time period. While studies of this type should ideally use a control group to capture any pre-post changes not attributable to the intervention, the controls may not necessarily capture pre-post differences due to sampling. For example, if senior clinicians are oversampled post-intervention for the intervention group, but not for the control group, then the intervention effect will be muddied with sampling effects, with no completely satisfactory way to separate them during the analysis.

For association studies, the sampling priority is somewhat different as the aim is not to generate representative summary measures of workflow, but to assess statistical associations between aspects of clinical work. Where descriptive studies use a sampling strategy based on observation time, association studies build sampling around the units of analysis (tasks, events, etc.). To examine associations in an observational study it is necessary to adjust for confounding factors (in the epidemiological parlance) to derive the least biased estimate of the association of interest, usually done through multivariable modelling. The variables generated by workflow time studies are typically categorical, so an important consideration is whether there will be sufficient outcome data in each category. Small numbers in certain categories may cause issues with model fitting, so it may be desirable to oversample certain times of day, certain professional groups, and so on, to avoid this issue. In a study by the authors (Walter et al. 2017) on physicians' response strategies for dealing with external prompts (i.e. interruptions), the original analysis plan involving both categorical outcome and covariates was not possible due to some outcome categories never occurring at the same time as certain covariate categories. This caused implausible or nonsensical model outputs for some variables even after collapsing of some categories, and an alternative analysis approach was necessary. Therefore, for association studies, the sampling strategy must necessarily be developed in parallel with dimensions and categories.

13.3 Inter-Observer Reliability

A fundamental aspect of generating high quality data from observations of clinical work is to ensure consistent application of dimensions and their categories between different observers. This is often called inter-rater reliability, a term taken from psychology, although in this context we use the term inter-*observer* reliability (IOR) since we are interested in observations as a more varied set of judgements, as opposed to ratings which tend to involve assigning a single value or category at a time. The fact that workflow data recorded at task-level have time stamps, involve temporal order and feature multiple categorical attributes makes it rather complex to compare between two or more observers who are following the same participant. To date, there has been persistent use of simple methods borrowed from other contexts that are not well suited for their purpose, and this is somewhat of an 'elephant in the room' in quantitative observational studies of clinical workflow.

A range of methods have been applied in workflow time studies to assess IOR and a review of these identified seven different approaches among the 27% of studies that provided some details of their IOR assessment (Lopetegui et al. 2013). The most common was Cohen's kappa, a well-known method used in psychology to quantify the level of agreement between two or more raters assigning units to a set of categories, such as assigning exam papers to either pass or fail (Cohen 1960). In workflow time studies this approach seems to be treated as somewhat of a gold standard, while at the same time most studies gloss over the details of its application to IOR assessment (Lopetegui et al. 2013). There are several issues with kappa, and other similar measures, that mean assessments of IOR are limited at best, and may even be misleading in that high kappa scores can be achieved even though significant observer differences are present.

The first main limitation is that for time-stamped and time-ordered tasks with multivariable attributes, identifying pairs of tasks from two observers that refer to the same observed action cannot be done with any certainty. Table 13.3 shows some example data from two observers shadowing the same physician. Task 2 recorded by the first observer lasted two and a half minutes, was of task type B, was performed with a nurse, and overlap with the next task for thirty seconds. In contrast, task 2 recorded by observer 2 lasted almost four minutes, was of type A, was performed with a nurse and overlapped with the next task for two minutes. Given the disagreement on several attributes, it is not possible to conclusively decide if task 2 for each observer refers to the same observed action, and to decide they *do* agree based on only some agreeing attributes introduces unreasonable assumptions, or even outright guessing.

The second main limitation is that most methods used for assessing IOR only apply to one variable at a time. This may be acceptable for descriptive studies reporting

Table 13.3 Example data from two hypothetical observers shadowing the same participant

Observer	Task ID	Start time	End time	Task type	Performed with Nurse
1	1	0:00:00	0:04:30	A	0
1	2	0:04:30	0:07:00	B	1
1	3	0:06:30	0:10:25	B	0
1	4	0:10:25	0:12:05	A	1
1	5	0:12:05	0:15:00	B	0
1	6	0:15:00	0:20:00	A	1
2	1	0:00:00	0:04:40	A	1
2	2	0:04:40	0:08:30	A	1
2	3	0:06:30	0:10:25	B	1
2	4	0:10:25	0:12:05	A	0
2	3	0:12:05	0:15:00	B	0
2	5	0:15:00	0:20:00	A	0

summary measures of individual variables but is likely inadequate for association studies involving multivariable analyses. In one of our prior studies (Walter et al. 2014), a reanalysis of the data collected from three hospital settings found significant observer effects in multivariable models despite high univariate IOR scores (Table 13.3).

13.3.1   Nonparametric Hypothesis Testing for IOR Assessment

In this chapter we look at two broad approaches to addressing these limitations. The first approach compares summary measures at an aggregated level using hypothesis tests. For example, the proportion of time spent performing direct care tasks could be compared between observers shadowing the same participant. This method ignores temporal order and thus does not require matching at either task or time window level, making it applicable only for descriptive studies where reliability at such an aggregate level is sufficient. This approach assumes that the data from different observers should be the same and that any observed difference in summary measures is due to observer effects. Rather than generating an IOR score, this method provides a p-value where we hope to find a non-significant (large) value indicating no evidence of a difference in time proportions for data collected by different observers (as in Westbrook et al. 2018).

Proportions of time are the most common measure in descriptive workflow time studies. However, since these are proportions of a continuous variable, they require unique methods (see Sect. 4.2.1 for more details). For this purpose, nonparametric resampling tests, specifically permutation tests, offer several advantages over conventional parametric options. Of the parametric tests, it is possible to aggregate the data into subgroups or clusters (e.g. by observation sessions) and to use a logistic transformation on the proportion for each subgroup. This is appropriate where the subgroups or clusters are fixed (Warton and Hui 2011). However, in workflow time studies, the choice of subgroups such as observation sessions or individual participants is not necessarily clear, and the outcome of the test may be influenced by this choice.

Permutation tests minimize the issues with distributional assumptions and sampling units. This approach involves reordering observer labels in the task-level data, cycling through all possible combinations and calculating the statistic of interest each time (such as the difference between proportions for two observers). These resampled values form the null distribution against which the actual difference can be compared. The proportion of null values more extreme than the 'true' difference provides the p-value. For large samples, the Monte Carlo permutation test uses many random shuffles of the labels to generate a p-value without having to calculate every possible label combination, thus reducing computation time. Good (2010) provides a comprehensive discussion of these methods. Applying a permutation test to the data in Table 3.3 to compare proportions of time spent on task types A and B and time spent working with a nurse yielded p-values of 0.61, 0.73 and 0.45, respectively. In other words, there was no evidence of a difference between observers in terms of time proportions.

13.3.2   Conventional IOR Measures Applied to Time Windows

The second approach addresses the time alignment issue by reformatting the task-level data into small time windows. This idea originated with Bakeman et al. (2009) who discussed applying Cohen's kappa in this way for timed-event sequential data, which is similar to workflow time study data. When comparing data from two observers shadowing the same participant, we can assume that during a given small time window they were observing the same activity, and this circumvents the issue with temporal alignment at the level of tasks described earlier in this section. Existing IOR methods, such as Cohen's kappa, can then be applied to the aligned time windows.

The time window approach then allows us to encompass the multivariable nature of data from workflow time studies. Janson and Olsson (2001) developed an IOR assessment method analogous to Cohen's kappa that is applicable to multivariable categorical data (pp. 282–283). When applied to two observers and one variable it is equivalent to Cohen's kappa, but can be generalised to any number of observers and variables. When applied to time windows, this is the best currently available single-score approach for IOR assessment in workflow time studies. It is represented by the Greek letter iota, ι (the letter before kappa).

Applying univariate kappa to the example data shown in Table 3.3 with time windows of one second (i.e. 1200 windows) we get scores of 0.57 for 'task type' and −0.45 for 'performed with nurse', indicating 'good' agreement for the former and moderate disagreement for the latter. If we apply Janson and Olsson's method to both variables, we get a score of $\iota = 0.04$. . This can easily be extended to include a third binary variable that represents multitasking (yes or no) in each time window. This has a univariate kappa score of 0.38, while the iota score for all three variables is 0.08.

The results for the 'task type' variable were consistent between the two methods, but were contradictory for the 'performed with nurse' variable. Also, the low agreement shown by the multivariable iota score did not concur with the high univariate kappa score for 'task type' alone. These results from the two general approaches highlight some key points about IOR assessment. First, the utility of any IOR measure must be considered relative to the analysis. The motivation behind assessing IOR is to identify and minimise observer biases in the data, however, IOR measures do not necessarily quantify the extent to which results are biased due to observer differences. For example, if there is good agreement on the overall proportions of individual categories between observers, but poor agreement at task level when multiple task attributes are considered together, then an analysis that aims to simply summarise proportions would not be biased by observed effects, while a multivariable regression model would be. A corollary of this issue is that IOR measures have limited comparability between studies, such that it only makes sense to compare IOR results when the IOR method *and* the analysis are the same.

Second, a high univariate IOR score, as is typically reported in workflow time studies, does not tell us much about agreement levels in the whole dataset. Unless the analysis only uses one variable, it is imperative to take a multivariable approach to IOR assessment and to pursue development of customised methods for workflow time studies. More generally, it is therefore important to move away from the idea that any existing approach as the gold standard for IOR assessment, to have more transparent reporting of IOR in workflow time studies, and to have more open discussions of the limitations of existing methods and how they can be improved. A related idea that also goes beyond univariate IOR scores is to assess multiple aspects of agreement (Lopetegui et al. 2013). An IOR tool developed by Guidi et al. uses one-second time windows to generate univariate IOR, a measure of correlation, and a sequence comparison index for individual variables as well as the multivariable iota score (Giudi et al. 2021).

A final consideration is that IOR is not the same as accuracy, as a high IOR score could simply mean two observers are both inaccurate in the same way. The lack of a true record of the observed activity necessitates assessment of IOR, but also makes it impossible to assess accuracy. While we would expect some correlation between IOR and accuracy, there will always be uncertainty about data accuracy that cannot be overcome by any IOR method.

13.3.3 Bootstrap Confidence Intervals for IOR Measures

IOR measures are reported in the form of a single value, analogous to a point esti-mate. IOR measures in workflow time studies are usually derived from samples of observation sessions where two observers were observing the same activity and then used to make inferences about the IOR of data from the entire study. Hence, like any other statistical measure, there is uncertainty around it when generalising to a wider population. It would be therefore important to report confidence intervals (CIs) for IOR measures. A simple solution to generating such intervals for IOR measures is via a bootstrapping approach, the simplest of which would resample the data many times with replacement, calculate the IOR measure each time and take the 2.5th and 97.5th percentiles as the bootstrap confidence limits.

13.4 Analysis

13.4.1 Summary Statistics

The descriptive studies discussed in this chapter use a range of measures to charac-terise observed workflow. Of these, we focus on the most commonly used measures: proportions of time, and rates of events per unit time.

Proportions of Time

Proportions of time are a key metric in workflow time studies, providing an indica-tion of how participants distribute their time across various activities, locations, or between the different people with whom they interact. They are a mainstay of descrip-tive studies but are also useful in intervention studies as an indicator of changes in work patterns. The summation of time intervals tends to be non-trivial, due to the presence of multitasking which creates overlap and hence multiple counting of time. While sums of time are not usually reported directly, they are part of the calculation of other frequently used measures such as proportions and rates.

Quantifying the uncertainty around estimated proportions in the form of CIs is important for interpreting results as discussed in the previous section. For proportions of countable units, such as people or events, constructing a CI is a well-trodden path described in most statistics textbooks: the CI for a binomial proportion. However, for proportions of time—a continuous measure—the binomial methods do not apply. Surprisingly, there is little methodology for calculating CIs for proportions of contin-uous variables. In the early 1980s Gilchrist (1982) noted the lack of discussion in the literature despite such proportions occurring frequently, and this is still the case more than 30 years later. Only a few papers to date have discussed analysis of continuous proportions using parametric assumptions (Warton and Hui 2011; Stephens 1982), but they do not directly tackle CIs. A simple modification of the CI for the mean of a normally distributed variable has often been used (Li et al. 2015; Arabadzhiyska et al. 2013), which is expressed in the following form:

$$\frac{T_c}{T} \pm z_{1-\alpha/2}\frac{s_c\sqrt{n_c}}{T}$$

where T_c is the time spent doing tasks from category c, T is the total observation time, s_c is the sample standard deviation of task times for category c, and n_c is the number of tasks in that category. In addition, $z_{1-\alpha/2}$ is the standard score from a normal distribution, for example for a 95% CI, this would have the value $z_{0.975} \approx 1.96$.

A drawback of this method is that what constitutes a task depends on the definitions of dimensions and categories and to some extent on interpretation of those definitions during observation. For example, if a task is completed in two fragments due to an interruption, should this be counted as one task or two? That is, choices regarding task definition affect the term n_c, , and hence the CI width is at the whim of these choices. Also, the normal assumption is only likely to be satisfied when samples of tasks (T_c) are at least 30, and in some cases it may generate values for the CI that are outside the plausible range, e.g. below zero or above one.

A natural alternative is to take a nonparametric approach, namely to use bootstrap CIs (as in Bellandi et al. 2018). This does not require parametric assumptions, which addresses the limitations just mentioned, making it an optimal choice for continuous proportions. DiCiccio and Efron (1996) offered a thorough discussion of the various approaches that can be used to construct bootstrap CIs. Below, we provide a brief description of the basic method.

For a dataset with n tasks, a random selection of n of these is drawn with replacement. Even though the new sample has the same number of tasks as the original data, it will not necessarily be the same dataset since the random selection *with replacement* means that in the new sample some tasks will appear multiple times while others may not appear at all. The proportion of interest for the resampled data is then calculated. This procedure is repeated many times to generate a large number of resampled proportions. The simplest way to generate an interval is to then take the 2.5th and 97.5th percentile of the resampled proportions (for a 95% CI) as the lower and upper limits of the confidence interval.

We use a simulation study to illustrate the utility of the bootstrap approach by comparing the normal approximation method to the simple bootstrap. We also apply the bias-corrected and accelerated (BC_a) bootstrap which accounts for asymmetry in the CI. A sample of tasks was drawn with time durations from either an exponential, gamma or normal distribution. A random subset of 5, 10 or 20% of tasks was selected to represent some category of interest. For that 'category' the proportion of time was calculated along with its CI according to the three methods. This was repeated 1000 times and the proportion of CIs containing the true value, the coverage probabilities, are shown in Table 13.4. By definition, a 95% CI should cover the true proportion

Table 13.4 Coverage probabilities for confidence intervals of proportions of time generated via three methods

Total tasks	'True' Proportion	Normal approximation			Simple bootstrap			BC_a bootstrap		
		Exp	Gamma	Normal	Exp	Gamma	Normal	Exp	Gamma	Normal
10	0.05	0.070	0.049	0.013	0.384	0.398	0.406	0.391	0.404	0.404
10	0.5	0.786	0.782	0.501	0.892	0.905	0.925	0.938	0.931	0.946
10	0.95	0.987	0.982	0.946	0.375	0.394	0.396	0.386	0.398	0.394
100	0.05	0.671	0.654	0.381	0.830	0.881	0.905	0.851	0.895	0.925
100	0.5	0.934	0.882	0.587	0.940	0.951	0.950	0.948	0.952	0.954
100	0.95	0.999	1.000	0.980	0.831	0.867	0.903	0.853	0.882	0.924
1000	0.05	0.830	0.732	0.452	0.933	0.947	0.942	0.946	0.950	0.945
1000	0.5	0.946	0.877	0.584	0.948	0.941	0.952	0.951	0.942	0.956
1000	0.95	1.000	1.000	0.993	0.926	0.927	0.948	0.931	0.939	0.949

95% of the time for a large number of repeated studies (or simulations in this case), so the expected coverage probability is then 0.95.

Both bootstrap approaches appear to perform better than the normal approximation method when the true proportion is near the lower boundary of the possible range of values (true proportion $\pi = 0.05$) or in the middle of the range ($\pi = 0.5$), especially for small and medium samples. The normal approximation performs particularly poorly for small proportions and small samples, with coverage probabilities less than 0.1. Towards the upper end of the range ($\pi = 0.95$), however, the normal approximation seems to perform better for small to medium samples, although proportions of this magnitude are rarely reported in the literature. Study samples are typically in the several thousands, and the results generated by the bootstrap method are consistently closer to the expected coverage probability of 0.95 for samples of that size. This suggests that the bootstrap CI is generally preferable to the normal approximation, which can be quite inaccurate. Further, the BC_a method consistently has slightly better coverage for all scenarios compared to the simple bootstrap and hence represents a better choice for calculating CIs of time proportions among the methods considered here (Table 13.4).

Rates of Events Per Unit Time

Discrete events occurring at different points in time are common in clinical work and can be easily captured in workflow time studies. The most common example is interruptions. Since the number of such events is proportional to the length of time observed, they are generally analysed as rates per unit time, such as interruptions per hour. This quantifies the intensity of events while being independent of the amount of observation time. Descriptive studies tend to report rates in this form along with their CIs (Li et al. 2015; Walter et al. 2017, 2014). A common and simple approach for generating CIs is to assume that event counts, λ, are drawn from a Poisson distribution and to then generate a normal approximation CI in the form of:

$$(\lambda \pm z_{1-\alpha/2}\sqrt{\lambda})/T$$

where T is the observation time. However, the Poisson assumption that the mean and variance are equal is not always met in workflow time study data and once again bootstrap CIs provide a more robust alternative.

We illustrate this through another set of simulations comparing the normal approximation method to both simple and BC_a bootstrap. This was done for task lengths drawn from two different distributions (exponential and normal), for small and large samples (n = 10 and n = 1000), for two different rates representing low and high rates relative to the typical range that appears in the literature on interruptions. We also simulated events to arrive according to either a Poisson or negative binomial distribution, where the former assumes that mean and variance are equal while the latter does not.

In the first part of Table 13.5, the simulated data satisfy the assumptions of all three methods and thus there is minimal difference between the three methods. The coverage probabilities are markedly lower for the small sample size scenarios, particularly when the underlying rate is also low. In the lower section of the table, the simulated events follow a negative binomial distribution. The differences in coverage between the three methods due to sample size and rate are similar, but a key difference can be seen for the scenario with large sample and high rate, in which the coverage for the normal approximation is lower than 0.95 while for the bootstrap method it is very close to the expected value of 0.95. This difference is amplified with increasing rate, such that for a rate of 300 events per hour the coverage for the normal approximation drops to 0.63 at best, compared to 0.96 for both bootstrap methods (data not shown in table). While the performance is comparable across most of the scenarios considered, the fact that the bootstrap approach is at least as good as, and in some cases clearly better than, the normal approximation method suggests that it may be considered a better choice to calculate CIs of rates.

13.4.2 Assessing Associations

Two Group Comparisons

Comparing outcomes between two groups is another common research goal in workflow time studies. For example, Richardson et al. (2016) (see Table 3 in that publication) compared both proportions of time and interruption rates between three studies of physicians, where each study used similar observational methodology and task definitions. Such comparisons in workflow time studies come with some important caveats, and some unique considerations are required for calculating significance.

Hypothesis testing was developed within the experimental paradigm in which factors extraneous to the effect of interest are controlled, such as randomly assigning

Table 13.5 Coverage probabilities for confidence intervals of rates per unit time generated via three methods

Total tasks	'True' rate[a]	'True' event distribution	Normal approximation		Simple bootstrap		BC_a bootstrap	
			Exp	Normal	Exp	Normal	Exp	Normal
10	3	Poisson	0.546	0.550	0.541	0.538	0.535	0.529
10	30	Poisson	0.919	0.921	0.868	0.904	0.865	0.903
1000	3	Poisson	0.939	0.960	0.940	0.961	0.938	0.961
1000	30	Poisson	0.932	0.948	0.930	0.944	0.933	0.944
10	3	NB[b]	0.533	0.567	0.529	0.561	0.521	0.553
10	30	NB	0.818	0.865	0.841	0.874	0.843	0.876
1000	3	NB	0.935	0.931	0.943	0.938	0.944	0.939
1000	30	NB	0.862	0.920	0.944	0.959	0.945	0.959

Notes
[a]Events per hour
[b]NB = negative binomial

subjects to one group or another. Any remaining difference in the outcome measure can then be attributed to the main effect. In other words, confounding is controlled through design. In observational studies of clinical work, this level of control is not possible, which means that the data represent a mixture of effects from many different factors, both known and unknown. When applying two group comparison tests to such data, it becomes difficult to definitively attribute the effect to any one factor. A study of physicians and nurses in surgical units (Bellandi et al. 2018) made such comparisons (adjusted for multiple testing), however, the authors appropriately refrained from attributing apparently significant differences to particular factors. Two-group comparisons in workflow time studies thus must be applied with caution.

As seen with calculating CIs, there is relatively little methodology for analysing proportions of continuous measures. The calculations for parametric hypothesis tests involve the sample size, which as seen several times in this chapter, can be open to interpretation. In the case of hypothesis testing, choices about what constitutes a task can then influence the sample size in the calculations and consequently level of significance, which could result in incorrect conclusions, whether unconsciously or not.

Following on from the hypothesis testing approach used to assess IOR in Sect. 13.3, a way around these issues is, once again, through nonparametric methods. Permutation tests, or their Monte Carlo variation (Good 2010), can not only be applied to comparisons of typical measures in workflow time studies such as proportions of time and rates per unit time, but also to comparing means and counts. Rather than resampling the data as in the bootstrap method, the permutation tests randomly shuffle the group labels and calculate the difference between groups for each shuffle, e.g. the difference between proportions. This generates a null distribution for the observed difference and a p-value can then be determined as the proportion of permuted differences larger than the observed difference.

Again, we use a simulation to illustrate the efficacy of this approach. Tasks with durations following an exponential distribution were generated for two separate groups. For each group, a certain proportion of tasks (the 'true' proportion) were assigned to the category of interest and the difference between the group-level proportions of time for that category was calculated. The Monte Carlo permutation test was then applied to derive a p-value for the observed difference. This process was repeated 1,000 times, from which the proportion of significant results was obtained using $\alpha = 0.05$. When there is a true difference, this proportion represents the power of the test. For a fixed proportion ($p1$) in the first group, the proportion in the second group ($p2$) was varied through a range of values and the power calculated each time as described above. This was done for $p1 = 0.05$ and $p1 = 0.2$, , and also for sample sizes of 100 tasks (50 per group) and 1000 tasks (500 per group).

Figure 13.2 shows the estimated power for these four scenarios. Both plots show that power increases with greater true difference between groups and that this increase is more rapid for higher proportions (dotted lines for $p1 = 0.2$ versus solid lines for $p1 = 0.05$), and for larger samples (plot **b** versus plot **a**). The two groups were simulated to have equal sample size. In additional simulations, it was found that keeping the same total sample size but allowing imbalance in group size reduced the power. The grey lines indicate power curves for the difference between two independent binomial proportions generated using the G*Power program (Faul et al. 2007). While there is clear similarity, the power for the simulated permutation tests (black lines) are systematically lower. Nevertheless, the fact that they are in the same region and that the permutation test is applicable to proportions of continuous variables while binomial proportion methods are not, supports the permutation test as a reasonable choice for comparing proportions of time in workflow time studies.

An alternative testing approach, as outlined in Sect. 13.3, is to aggregate the data into subgroups. A proportion can be calculated for each subgroup, then the set

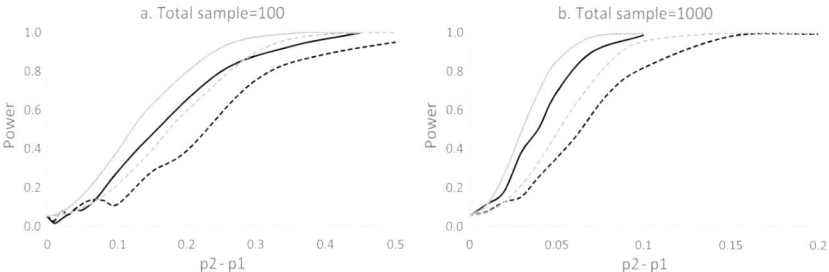

Fig. 13.2 Simulated power of the Monte Carlo permutation test to detect difference between two proportions of a continuous variable, for **a** a total sample of 100 tasks and **b** a total sample of 1000 tasks. The solid black line represents $p1 = 0.05$; the dashed black line represents $p1 = 0.2$. The computed power for equivalent differences in binomial proportions is shown as grey lines for reference

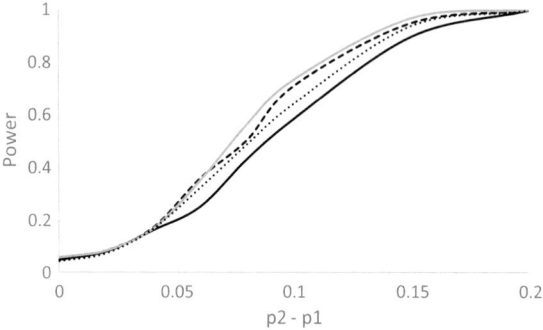

Fig. 13.3 Simulated power for t-tests applied to subgroups-level proportions for 50 subgroups of 10 tasks each (solid black line), 10 subgroups of 50 tasks each (dashed black line), and 6 subgroups of 8 or 9 tasks (dotted black line). The total sample of tasks was 1,000 (500 per group), the underlying proportion of the group 1 was $p_1 = 0.2$ and proportions for group 2 ranged from 0.2 to 0.4. The power for a permutation test is shown for comparison (solid grey line)

of subgroup-level proportions can be analysed as continuous data, using methods such as t-tests or linear regression. We assessed this approach through simulation and compared it to permutation testing. To replicate a two-group comparison, we simulated 500 tasks per group (with exponentially distributed task duration) and divided the task in each group into either 10 subgroups of 50 tasks each, 50 subgroups of 10 tasks each, or six subgroups of eight or nine tasks each. In one group the underlying proportion of interest was set at 20% and for the other group this varied between 20 and 40%, that is, the difference between groups ranged from 0 to 20%. A t-test was applied to the subgroup-level proportions and the whole process was repeated 1000 times to obtain power estimates for the range of group differences.

The results of these simulations are shown in Fig. 13.3 where the power curves for t-tests applied at different levels of subgroup aggregation are relatively similar (all black lines). Although having fewer subgroups reduces the effective sample size of the tests, this seems to be counteracted by a proportional decrease in variance. The somewhat surprising result of which is that the power is not greatly affected by the level of aggregation. The grey line in the plot shows the power for the permutation testing approach. This is consistently as good or better than t-tests applied to aggregated data. The choice of units over which to aggregate data (e.g. observation sessions, clinicians, etc.) is not necessarily obvious in workflow time studies. Combined with the fact that permutation tests are at least as powerful, then once again a nonparametric approach is the better option.

Multivariable Analyses

There are many ways to apply multivariable methods in workflow time studies. Indeed, there is a strong case to make that most association studies should take a multivariable approach to better understand the factors operating at multiple system levels and minimise the bias in particular effects by adjusting for other influential factors. We have discussed general considerations of multivariable analysis in workflow time studies in our previous work (Walter et al. 2015).

Multivariable analysis of continuous proportions of time has the potential to address important questions in workflow time studies, such as determining the factors associated with how long participants spend on particular activities. However, this approach has rarely been applied in workflow time studies. In the field of ecology, where continuous proportions are more common, a parametric regression approach has been proposed (Douma and Weedon 2019), namely, beta regression for one task type, such that time is divided into two proportions spent either doing that task or not doing that task. Dirichlet regression can be used for multiple task types, where time is divided between multiple different task categories analogous to multinomial proportions.

There are several ways to apply nonparametric methods to multivariable analyses. First, when fitting garden variety parametric models, such as linear regression, it is possible to use bootstrapping to determine the significance of the model estimates or to generate CIs for the estimates. This is essentially an extension of what we have discussed earlier regarding CIs and hypothesis tests, and similarly this may be an appropriate alternative when the data do not satisfy parametric model assumptions, as is often the case.

Second, there is a wide range of nonparametric multivariable modelling techniques that do not rely on assumptions about the distributional form (normal, Poisson, etc.) of the data or about the relationships between dependent and independent variables. Some can be used as explanatory models, such as generalised additive models or spline regression, that can describe non-linear associations. In the study of prescribing errors among ED physicians, Westbrook et al. (2018) found no evidence of an effect of time of day (categorised into two-hour blocks) on error rates using a Poisson regression model. However, Fig. 13.4 shows that fitting a nonparametric model (LOESS smoother) reveals a significant and distinctly non-linear relationship. Another explanatory approach is the classification tree, a version of which was used by Walter et al. (2017). In that study, discussed at the end of Sect. 13.2, the lack of data in certain categories necessitated a change from the original analysis plan. The alternative analysis used was a nonparametric model called a conditional inference tree, which iteratively splits the data into groups such that each group has a distinct outcome profile. Finally, in the area of predictive nonparametric models there is now a vast and growing collection of methods, such as Bayesian networks and random forests, that would be applicable to answering appropriately framed research questions in workflow time studies.

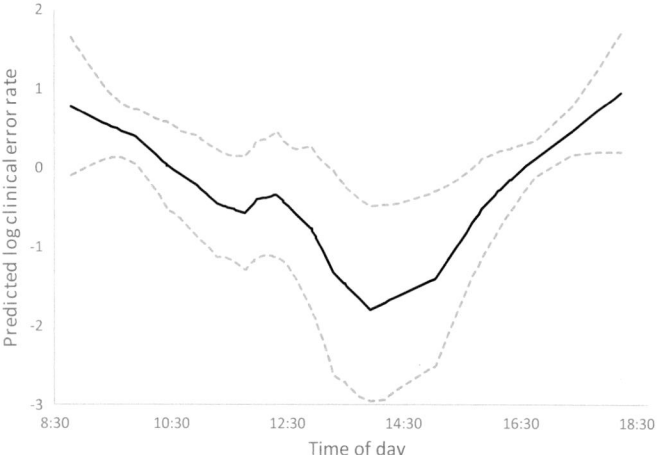

Fig. 13.4 Nonparametric estimate (LOESS smoother) of the relationship between time of day and clinical prescribing errors. The black line represents the predicted clinical prescribing error rate on the log scale and the dotted grey lines are the 95% confidence limits. This smoothing component for time of day had a p-value of 0.014

13.5   Discussion

Workflow time studies are an important type of research for generating knowledge about both the functioning of clinical work and workflow at a fine-grained level, and about the workflow-related factors that influence patient safety and quality of care. The data generated by such studies, and likely other types of time and motion studies, are not always amenable to conventional statistical methods. In this chapter we have highlighted some of the non-standard aspects of the data and offered alternative approaches that draw heavily from the family of nonparametric analysis techniques.

This chapter is somewhat technical, and it may be tempting for readers to form the impression that workflow time studies are overly complicated. The basic concept of these studies is, in fact, straightforward, but the complexity largely comes from the contexts in which they are applied. Clinical work is undeniably complex, and to understand its inner workings and interrelationships we must embrace that complexity into study design and data analyses, challenging as it may be. To design studies and analyses that fit within conventional approaches is to essentially shy away from or ignore those challenges. The methodological discourse in this chapter takes some steps towards tackling the intricacies of conducting quantitative studies of clinical work but is intended as a starting point for ongoing discussions rather than a definitive account of best practices.

Some recent studies have begun to employ more sophisticated methods such as multilevel models (Walter et al. 2014; Grundgeiger et al. 2010), transition state models (Carayon et al. 2015; Myers and Parikh, 2019), and nonparametric models

(Walter et al. 2017). However, explicit discussion of quantitative methodology appropriate for workflow time studies remains relatively rare. As we have highlighted in this chapter, there is an imperative to develop innovative approaches even for fundamental analyses such as IOR assessment, confidence intervals and hypothesis tests. Improving both our understanding of clinical workflow and the integrity of the workflow time study literature will require ongoing methodological innovation.

References

Ampt A, Westbrook JI, Creswick N, Mallock N. A comparison of self-reported and observational work sampling techniques for measuring time in nursing tasks. J Health Serv Res Pol. 2007;12(1):18–24.

Arabadzhiyska PN, Baysari MT, Walter SR, Day RO, Westbrook JI. Shedding light on junior doctors' work practices after hours. Internal Med J. 2013;43(12):1321–6.

Bakeman R, Quera V, Gnisci A. Observer agreement for timed-event sequential data: a comparison of time-based and event-based algorithms. Behav Res Methods. 2009;41(1):137–47.

Bellandi T, Cerri A, Carreras G, Walter SR, Mengozzi C, Albolino S, et al. Interruptions and multitasking in surgery: a multicentre observational study of the daily work patterns of doctors and nurses. Ergonomics. 2018;61:40–7.

Carayon P, Wetterneck TB, Alyousefa B. Impact of electronic health record technology on the work and workflow of physicians in the intensive care unit. Int J Med Inform. 2015;84:578–94.

Cohen J. A coefficient of agreement for nominal scales. Educ Psychol Meas. 1960;20(1):37–46.

DiCiccio TJ, Efron B. Bootstrap confidence intervals. Stat Sci. 1996;11(3):189–228.

Douma JC, Weedon JT. Analysing continuous proportions in ecology and evolution: a practical introduction to beta and Dirichlet regression. Methods Ecol Evol. 2019;10:1412–30.

Faul F, Erdfelder E, Lang AG, Buchner A. G*Power 3: a flexible statistical power analysis program for the social, behavioral, and biomedical sciences. Behav Res Methods. 2007;39:175–91.

Georgiou A, McCaughey EJ, Tariq A, Walter SR, Li J, Callen J, et al. What is the impact of an electronic test result acknowledgement system on Emergency Department physicians' work processes? A mixed-method pre-post observational study. Int J Med Inform. 2017;99:29–36.

Gilchrist R. An analysis of continuous proportions. In: Caussinus H, Ettinger P, Tomassone R, editors. COMPSTAT 1982 5th Symposium held at Toulouse. Heidelberg: Physica;1982.

Giudi S, Tanzini M, Westbrook JI. IORapp: an R tool for inter-observer reliability assessment of time and motion data. In: European Conference on Cognitive Ergonomics 2021 (ECCE 2021), April 26–29, 2021, Siena, Italy. New York, NY, USA: ACM;2021.

Good PI. Permutation, parametric and bootstrap tests of hypotheses. 3rd ed. New York: Springer; 2010.

Grundgeiger T, Sanderson P, Venkatesh B, MacDougall HG. Interruption management in the intensive care unit: predicting resumption times and assessing distributed support. J Exp Psych Appl. 2010;16(4):317–34.

https://timecat.org/#articles-section.

https://www.mq.edu.au/research/research-centres-groups-and-facilities/healthy-people/centres/australian-institute-of-health-innovation/our-projects/wombat.

Janson H, Olsson U. A measure of agreement for interval or nominal multivariate observations. Educ Psychol Meas. 2001;61(2):277–89.

Li L, Hains I, Hordern T, Milliss D, Raper R, Westbrook JI. What do ICU doctors do? A multisite time and motion study of the clinical work patterns of registrars. Crit Care Resusc. 2015;17:159–66.

Lopetegui M, Yen PY, Lai A, Jeffries J, Embi P, Payne P. Time and motion studies in healthcare: What are we talking about? J Biomed Inform. 2014;49:292–9.

Lopetegui M, Yen P-Y, Lai AM, Embi PJ, Payne PRO. Time Capture Tool (TimeCaT): development of a comprehensive application to support data capture for Time Motion Studies. In: AMIA Annual Symposium Proceedings, vol. 2012. American Medical Informatics Association;2012, p. 596.

Lopetegui MA, Bai S, Yen P-Y, Lai A, Embi P, Payne PRO. Inter-observer reliability assessments in time motion studies: the foundation for meaningful clinical workflow analysis. In: AMIA Annual Symposium Proceedings 2013;889–96.

Malhotra S, Jordan D, Shortliffe E, Patel VL. Workflow modeling in critical care: piecing together your own puzzle. J Biomed Inform. 2007;40(2):81–92.

McCurdie T, Sanderson P, Aitken LM. Traditions of research into interruptions in healthcare: a conceptual review. Int J Nurs Stud. 2017;66:23–36.

Myers RA, Parikh PJ. Nurses' work with interruptions: an objective model for testing interventions. Health Care Manag Sci. 2019;22(1):1–15. https://doi.org/10.1007/s10729-017-9417-3.

Payne P, Lopetegui M, Yu S. A review of clinical workflow studies and methods. In: Zheng K, Westbrook J, Kannampallil T, Patel V, editors. Cognitive informatics: reengineering clinical workflow for safer and more efficient care health informatics. Cham: Springer;2019.

Richardson LC, Lehnbom EC, Baysari MT, Walter SR, Day RO, Westbrook JI. A time and motion study of junior doctor work patterns on the weekend: a potential contributor to the weekend effect? Int Med J. 2016;46(7):819–25.

Stephens MA. Use of the von Mises distribution to analyse continuous proportions. Biometrika. 1982;69(1):197–203.

Tanzini M, Westbrook JI, Guidi S, Sunderland N, Prgomet M. Measuring clinical workflow to improve quality and safety. Textbook of patient safety and clinical risk management, 2019;393–402.

Unertl KM, Novak LM, Johnson KB, Lorenzi NM. Traversing the many paths of workflow research: developing a conceptual framework of workflow terminology through a systematic literature review. J Am Med Inform Assoc. 2010;17:265–73.

Walter SR, Li L, Dunsmuir WTM, Westbrook JI. Managing competing demands through task-switching and multitasking: a multi-setting observational study of 200 clinicians over 1000 hours. BMJ Qual Saf. 2014;23:231–41.

Walter SR, Dunsmuir WTM, Westbrook JI. Studying interruptions and multitasking in situ: the untapped potential of quantitative observational studies. Int J Hum Comput Stud. 2015;79:118–25.

Walter SR, Raban MZ, Dunsmuir WTM, Douglas HE, Westbrook JI. Emergency doctors' strategies to manage competing workload demands in an interruptive environment: an observational workflow time study. Appl Ergon. 2017;58:454–60.

Warton DI, Hui FKC. The arcsine is asinine: the analysis of proportions in ecology. Ecology. 2011;92(1):3–10.

Weigl M, Muller A, Vincent C, Angerer P, Sevdalis N. The association of workflow interruptions and hospital doctors' workload: a prospective observational study. BMJ Qual Saf. 2012;21:399–407.

Westbrook JI, Ampt A. Design, application and testing of the work observation method by activity timing (WOMBAT) to measure clinicians' patterns of work and communication. Int J Med Inform. 2009;78S:S25–33.

Westbrook JI, Ampt A, Kearney L, Rob MI. All in a day's work: an observational study to quantify how and with whom doctors on hospital wards spend their time. Med J Aust. 2008;188:506–9.

Westbrook JI, Coiera E, Dunsmuir WTM, Brown BM, Kelk N, Paoloni R, Tran C. The impact of interruptions on clinical task completion. Qual Saf Health Care. 2010;19:284–9.

Westbrook JI, Raban M, Walter SR, Douglas HE. Task errors by emergency physicians are associated with interruptions, multitasking, fatigue and working memory capacity: a prospective, direct observation study. BMJ Qual Saf. 2018;27:655–663. https://doi.org/10.1136/bmjqs-2017-007333.

Zheng K, Guo MH, Hanauer DA. Using the time and motion method to study clinical work processes and workflow: methodological inconsistencies and a call for standardized research. J Am Med Inform Assoc. 2011;18:704–10.

Zheng K, Ratwani RM, Adler-Milstein J. Studying workflow and workarounds in electronic health record–supported work to improve health system performance. Ann Internal Med. 2020; 172(11_Supplement):S116-22.

Chapter 14
Clinical Workflow and Human Factors

Aaron Zachary Hettinger, Emilie M. Roth, Rollin J. Fairbanks, and Ann M. Bisantz

14.1   Introduction to Human Factors Engineering

Human factors engineering is a well-established scientific discipline that studies the functional capabilities and limitations of humans in order to design and optimize systems, processes and technology to reliably obtain a desired outcome (Lee et al. 2017). It incorporates principles and methods from disciplines such as industrial systems engineering, cognitive psychology, and computer science to analyze and model human-system interactions and to support system designs which meet quantifiable needs of the users and which support work in ways that are effective, efficient, and safe.

Human factors engineering has had a major influence on the design of systems and workflows in a wide range of safety critical industries including nuclear power, military and defense, and aviation. By understanding human capabilities, limitations, and common pathways for error, systems can be designed to prevent errors and—importantly—mitigate their effects, thus reducing harm to users and others who may be affected. In health care, the benefits of human factors engineering design approach extend to keeping patients free from error-based harm, to improving care through more efficient and effective workflows, to protecting staff members from fatigue and injury. Human factors engineering is particularly important in the successful integration of new technology into an existing work system. Recent examples include

A. Z. Hettinger (✉) · R. J. Fairbanks
MedStar Health Research Institute, Columbia, MD, USA
e-mail: Aaron.Z.Hettinger@Medstar.net

Georgetown University School of Medicine, Washington, DC, USA

E. M. Roth
Roth Cognitive Engineering, Stanford, CA, USA

A. M. Bisantz
University at Buffalo, Buffalo, NY, USA

© The Author(s), under exclusive license to Springer Nature Switzerland AG 2025
K. Zheng et al. (eds.), *Reengineering Clinical Workflow in the Digital and AI Era*,
Cognitive Informatics in Biomedicine and Healthcare,
https://doi.org/10.1007/978-3-031-82971-0_14

the use of drones in military and civilian applications and the emergence of self-driving cars that may share the road with human-driven cars. In each case human factors methods and principles are being applied to analyze the implications for the humans in the system, and to design effective user interfaces and workflows to enhance overall safety of operations (Casner et al. 2016; Roth and Pritchett 2018).

An important strength of human factors engineering is the focus on a broader context within which a system workflow or device operates (Carayon 2006). This includes describing specific physical, cognitive, and perceptual capabilities and limitations of the populations of system users involved; understanding and formally modeling the purposes and tasks being performed; mapping task requirements to human-system capabilities; and considering relevant aspects of the physical environment and work situations in which the system will be deployed. For example, a portable intravenous pump undergoing testing may work flawlessly in a simulated environment with experienced intensive care unit nurses, however that same pump may present significant hazard when an alarm goes off at home with a patient that misplaced their reading glasses.

This chapter introduces core concepts and methods from the discipline of human factors and describes how they can be applied to the study and improvement of clinical workflow. We begin by presenting a set of core human factors concepts (or human factors 'lenses') that are important to adopt when trying to identify sources of problems and opportunities for improvement to healthcare-related workflows. This is followed by a description of specific human factors methods that can be used to analyze and improve workflow.

Human factors engineering is an important consideration as we think about human strengths and limitations of introducing a new technology like AI into everyday life. How will the trust or lack of trust play into integration? What are the backups in place if an AI model breaks down? What are the safeguards in place to prevent patient harm from occurring? A similar struggle has been playing out with the mainstream use of automotive driver assistance technologies. The hand off between automated driver assistance technologies and drivers can be associated with collisions (Biever et al. 2020). Misunderstandings of the capabilities of the systems (e.g. not being ready to take over) and poor transitions between car and driver control when the environment exceeds the systems capabilities are two common scenarios that will need to be addressed when incorporating AI into healthcare, among others.

14.2 Applying Human Factors Lenses to Workflow Analysis and Design

When considering the application of human factors to the healthcare environment including health IT systems it is important to have a context within which to work. The following core Human Factors concepts and theoretical perspectives will aid the reader in applying a human factors lens when analyzing or trying to identify improvements to specific workflows and situations. These include situations where healthcare organizations may be trying to understand the factors that are contributing to performance problems or errors and how they can be mitigated; as well as situations where organizations are trying to develop and/or introduce new health IT and monitor and manage its impact on performance and satisfaction. There can be many points where there is value in adopting a 'human factors lens'—early in the process when requirements for a health IT system are being defined, during design in determining whether the system being developed will work as imagined, and after implementation, to understand and address human performance problems that emerge (e.g., near misses, adverse events, productivity bottlenecks).

14.2.1 Supporting 'Work as Done' Versus 'Work as Imagined'

A core precept of human factors is that it is important to begin any analysis or design project by studying how work is actually done, in all its messiness. Too often there is a significant gap between the way in which leaders believe the work is performed at the front line, and the way in which it actually occurs. Some authors refer to this as the different between 'work as imagined' and 'work as done' (Hollnagel et al. 2015; Braithwaite et al. 2017). Clinical work is fundamentally collaborative, involving multitasking, frequent interruptions, time-pressure, and incomplete, ambiguous, time-lagged information. Problems arise when there is a disconnect between the realities of the work 'as done' and the assumptions underlying the Health IT system (i.e., work as imagined). A case in point is decision-support tools where the implicit assumption is often that of a single decision-maker deciding at a particular point in time, with the all the information in hand. This contrasts with the demands of actual work practice, with the result that such tools are less likely to be adopted in real clinical settings. (Wears and Berg 2005).

The rapid adoption of electronic health records in the United States since the Health Information Technology for Economic and Clinical Health Act (HITECH) in 2009 has introduced technology with variable degrees of success and unintended consequences (Bernstam et al. 2009). Often problems arise because of a mismatch between the implicit model of the work inherent in health IT and the actual complexities of the clinical work environment. As Wears and Berg (2005) put it, the problem is not one of 'not developing the systems right' but rather of 'not developing the right systems'.

Good design and implementation needs to go beyond a narrow focus on the technology to be implemented. A sociotechnical lens is required that includes examining the characteristics of the organization to be supported (the people, values, norms, and culture), the technical environment in which the new system is to be inserted (the equipment, processes, procedures, and physical facilities), and the work demands and complexities that healthcare practitioners face. Only through this type of broad perspective will the gap between work as imagined and work as done be narrowed.

This perspective will be critical in the integration of AI in the healthcare space. As individuals and electronic health record (EHR) vendors and third parties seek to integrate the technology into clinical workflow there is often a lack of understanding of how the tool will be used across the care continuum across different settings and specialties. For example, AI has been implemented to replace human scribes in the clinical setting. This technology promises to reduce costs, improve efficiency and improve accuracy of clinical documentation. However they are limited by the complexity of clinician-patient interactions in places like the emergency department and intensive care units versus a 1:1 office visit that follows a consistent pattern. Furthermore, as the scribes transition to digital assistants that can help in placing orders, referrals and diagnostic testing there is a host of potential new hazards similar to when healthcare transitioned from paper to electronic records. While some problems, like legibility of written notes and orders improved significantly, there were new hazards of physicians selecting the wrong orders due to sort order or poorly design user interfaces (Wright et al. 2015). The transition from dry erase boards to electronic tracking boards/EHRs in the emergency department (ED) to track patients during their course of stay in the ED encountered similar issues of solving some hazards while introducing new systematic hazards, many of which were unanticipated but could have been predicted by human factors engineering review of the environment during the development phase of the technology (Fairbanks et al. 2008).

14.2.2 Addressing Context Independent Versus Context Dependent Design Elements

One of the significant challenges when introducing technology into any complex environment is addressing both its usability and usefulness. Usability is defined as how intuitive a tool is, how easy it is to learn and to use by the intended user. In contrast, usefulness refers to the extent to which the device, technology or workflow provides meaningful improvement in performance by the intended user under anticipated working conditions. To highlight the differences between usability and usefulness, one can imagine a new application within the EHR is tested in a lab and found to be intuitive to use with few errors by the user (usability). But when used by nurses in the emergency department who are frequently interrupted and multitasking across many patients the application becomes burdensome to enter data and found to have limited usefulness in the clinical environment due to missing critical information from other parts of the EHR.

Usability is generally affected by context independent features of a design often framed as design "heuristics" including making system status visible, providing meaningful and rapid feedback, maintaining consistency in indications and actions, using language and labels, and supporting error recovery (Nielsen 1995). These design principles are largely independent of the content and context of the interface or device being investigated. A recent human factors review of electronic medical record and electronic health record systems found that there were extensive usability issues (Zahabi et al. 2015a). These authors noted that these often resulted from a lack of application of standard human factors usability guidelines including: using simple natural dialogue, speaking the user's language, minimizing memory load; providing feedback and good error messages; maintaining consistency in design and error prevention (Molich and Nielsen 1990).

Human factors engineering provides extensive guidelines for identifying and correcting these 'context-independent' aspects of design. There are well established rules and guidelines that have been agreed upon for decades in the human factors and associated literature regardless of the application, from medical device to electronic airplane dashboard. For example, yellow text on a white background provides less contrast than black text and will be more difficult for the user to interpret. In addition, providing a list of choices on a display that are only separated by one pixel is more likely to lead a user to make an accidental selection if they are distracted or slip. While the rush to implement health IT systems may not followed many of these guidelines, the incorporation of User-Centered Design principles and human factors engineers in the design and certification of EHRs in the United States has begun to standardize the approach and remove these basic design errors that can lead to patient harm (Tolley et al. 2017).

In contrast to usability, usefulness of a health IT system is based on context-dependent design considerations that rely on an understanding of the purposes of system implementation, user goals, and context of use (Hettinger et al. 2015). For example, when placing an electronic order for a patient, providers frequently need to refer to previous laboratory values to make the most appropriate choice. A well-designed computerized provider order entry (CPOE) system would not only allow the user to view previous orders while placing a new order, but may make specific values more salient based on the current order selections. For example, a radiology test with intravenous contrast requires normal kidney function to prevent serious adverse events. Relying on the provider to remember the results of prior tests of kidney function or requiring them to navigate away from the ordering screen and potentially get distracted on another task will lead to the predictable error of ordering the wrong test or a delay in care. It would be preferable to display prior kidney function values on the screen used to order radiology tests.

Context dependent design is much more challenging and requires in-depth study of the users and their workflow in the environment where the work will be performed. This entails anticipating the needs of the users based on the context of use and making it easier for users to make the correct decision or action. Effective design requires consideration of both context independent and context-dependent aspects, and an interactive process that allows both usability and usefulness in context to be assessed.

The introduction of AI into healthcare and the large amount of computer processing power behind the tools have the potential to drive innovation. Historically it was very expensive to study context dependent design, frequently it entailed direct observation of subjects in simulated or real practice with analysis of qualitative and quantitative data produced from the observations. Now with the storage of large amounts of user interaction data and the outputs of everyday clinical practice being recorded in the EHR there is potential to use AI models to better understand clinical practice and potential hazards by learning based on these secondary markers in the EHR. However, the initial large language models (LLMs) available to the public are trained on non-clinical data sources. Later healthcare specific models, both commercial and open-source, are trained on healthcare claims and EHR data, yet concerns remain regarding the use of LLMs in healthcare given their limitations (Harrer 2023). It is important to note that prior to the development of LLMs there have been clinical decision aids leveraging machine learning and natural language processing that are at a more mature stage of development yet human-interface design considerations remain important. Implementation with these limitations in mind will be critical to the safe and effective introduction of AI into clinical workflow if the wrong models are applied to the right clinical situation, the best case scenario would be that clinicians identify completely inaccurate model outputs, while the worst case scenario is that the models provide plausibly accurate information that introduces systematic bias and/or hazards but goes undetected. As a result, in 2023 the US federal government called for the monitoring of safe and effective implementation of AI in healthcare (https://www.whitehouse.gov/briefing-room/presidential-actions/2023/10/30/executive-order-on-the-safe-secure-and-tru stworthy-development-and-use-of-artificial-intelligence/). There are also a number of organizations that are looking at supporting this partnership between healthcare organizations, third parties and the government.

14.2.3 Engineering for Resilience

Resilience Engineering offers a complementary human factors lens through which to examine clinical workflow (Fairbanks et al. 2014). Instead of focusing on the rare errors and failure modes, it encourages examining the adaptive behavior of individuals in the everyday context that keep things from going wrong, and how these behaviors can be better supported and more widely adopted (Braithwaite et al. 2015).

The basic premise of Resilience Engineering is that healthcare is a very complex process that presents multiple challenges. The different policies, procedures, patients, staff members and other various components interact in such a manner that there are often unanticipated outcomes when trying to change clinical workflow and that no one individual in the system has a clear understanding of all the components and how they interact with each other. However, humans are incredibly adaptable and often serve to hold the system together. For example, if a particular component in the system is not working correctly, e.g. the CT scanner stops working, then it is the humans that will develop the work arounds to get other testing, transfer patients to a facility that has the necessary equipment or delay the testing in those patients that have less time sensitive conditions until the equipment is working again. Without humans, the brittle interconnected system of electronic orders and medical equipment would grind to a halt until the equipment could be repaired, causing potential serious delays in acutely ill patients.

Resilience Engineering seeks to learn from the positive everyday behaviors of the humans in the system that keep the system going and prevent harm. In effect, instead of focusing only on the rare cases of errors and system breakdowns, it asks why more errors aren't happening and what can be done through better designs and workflows to enhance positive behaviors across users and not just the individuals that are anticipating the hazards through previous experience and institutional knowledge (Braithwaite et al. 2015).

The use of machine learning and large sets of electronic health record data can now allow informaticists and researchers to better understand typical workflow as performed by front line healthcare professionals and the true rate of positive everyday behaviors when things go well, rather than waiting for hazards and harm to occur.

14.2.4 Guiding the Co-evolution of Technology and Work Practice

A core Human Factors precept with extensive empirical support is that when new technology is introduced it inevitably changes work practice, sometimes in unanticipated ways. People adapt to the new health IT and learn to use it in ways that were not necessarily envisioned by the system developers. These new and unanticipated uses can in turn trigger a need for new technology development. This dynamic cycle of technology development and user adaptation has been referred to as the task-artifact cycle, to emphasize that how tasks are performed and the artifacts that support them co-evolve over time (Carroll and Rosson 1992; Carroll and Campbell 1998). This implies a need to continue to track the impact of a new health IT system after it is introduced to identify emerging practices and changing needs.

New technology cannot simply be 'dropped' into a work context. Rather, its impacts on the larger work context and organization needs to be tracked and unanticipated reverberations need to be recognized and addressed (Woods 2002). As Wears and Berg (2005) noted, the introduction of new health IT cannot be thought of in isolation, but rather as part of the larger context of organizational change. This includes recognizing that there will be a period of exploration and mutual learning involving users and system developers (Wears and Berg 2005). New workflows will emerge and additional support needs will be identified. This in turn will trigger new design cycles—be it through changes in training, workflow or design changes to the IT system. For example, the patient tracking boards (i.e., dry erase white boards) in emergency departments (EDs) originally were developed independently across organizations by the front line users. For example research by Bisantz et al. (2010) noted that with the transition to electronic information systems (EDIS) that attending physician workflow with resident physicians and students was no longer supported. Specifically, the method by which case presentation, attending exam and final note had been tracked on the dry-erase board with a series of colors and symbols was no longer supported (Bisantz et al. 2010a). Attending physicians adapted by using paper notes kept in the pocket to track this information (new 'home grown' artifact). Because the information was no longer publicly displayed, residents and nurses were not able to maintain awareness of where the attending physician was in their workflow. An unintended consequence was that patients were sometimes discharged before the attending physician evaluation and plan was complete. This task-artifact loop spurred EHR design changes. More recent EHRs used in clinical practice have been observed using these findings to incorporate the tracking of resident/attending workflow and note status in a more comprehensive manner.

When planning for the use of artificial intelligence tools in healthcare it is important to determine the specific AI tools to be implemented in the right environment with an optimal level of training and support. Implementation could include the use of historic machine learning, machine vision, natural language processing and more recent developments like large language models. Implementing tools out of sync with clinical needs or not optimized to the right circumstances could lead to suboptimal outcomes. For example, the integration of AI tools, like machine vision in radiology, can help improve the detection of clinical findings (Thrall et al. 2018). However, this assistance can lead to several challenges. First it may be helpful in some clinicians more than others, second, it could make it more difficult to address false positives and false negative findings, finally it may lead to an increased number of incidental findings that are not clinically relevant and that would have previously gone undetected.

14.2.5 Adopting a Patient Safety Transformational (PST) Prevention Model

Human factors approaches are intended to anticipate and prevent or mitigate the use errors before they can occur and cause potential harm. The Patient Safety Transformational Prevention (PST) model in healthcare can be used to proactively address unsafe systems. This is analogous to the primary/secondary/tertiary prevention model that has been used in cardiovascular care. The PST model distinguishes primary prevention—prevention before the hazard occurs; secondary prevention—prevention after the hazard occurs but before the patient is harmed; and tertiary prevention—prevention after the harm event has occurred but during the critical time that an intervention could improve a patient's outcome. The aim is to design for primary prevention whenever possible, followed by secondary, and then tertiary prevention.

Cardiovascular care for patients has undergone major changes since the 1950s when researchers were just starting to understand the link between heart disease and risk factors that we now take for granted like diabetes, hypertension and hypercholes-terolemia (Dawber et al. 1951). As a result of this improved depth of understanding and new methods for diagnostic testing, medicine went from a model of waiting for patients to have heart attacks to actively trying to prevent cardiovascular disease through life style modification (primary prevention) and aggressive management of chronic disease (secondary prevention). While there is still significant effort in tertiary prevention, reducing the long term impact of the heart attack once it occurs through rapid cardiac angioplasty and bypass surgery, there is considerable effort to prevent the patient from ever needing those dramatic efforts.

In stark contrast to changes made in cardiovascular disease, healthcare safety and operations often focus on the critical events that demonstrate breakdowns and try to improve their systems from one adverse event to the next. Using processes like Root Cause Analysis (RCA) often lead to brief analysis of adverse events that culminate in short term fixes such as disciplining those involved and training the other team members to vigilant instead of implementing sustainable and effective changes to the clinical workflow of the front-line staff (Hettinger et al. 2013). By taking a similar primary/secondary/tertiary prevention approach as that taken in cardiovascular care, the hazard under investigation may be designed out of the system. For example, a surgical department investigates a retained piece of medical equipment despite performing a surgical count of equipment and a post-operative x-ray at the comple-tion of the case. In an effort to prevent future cases the organization decides to apply the PST prevention concept instead of a traditional model of referring the involved staff to their respective peer review committees and sending a memo to staff to be more vigilant. Under the PST model investigation they do not run the risk of prema-ture closure and discover multiple pieces of surgical equipment that are not visible on x-ray and develop a plan to replace them, removing them from circulation in the operating rooms (primary prevention). Furthermore, they investigate technology that will allow wireless scanning and counting of surgical equipment to remove a foreign body before the end of surgery (secondary prevention). Finally, after reviewing clin-ical data they determine that most retained foreign body cases are in surgical cases that are either long duration or complex with many pieces of equipment. Finally, the team develops a clinical workflow so that these cases are pre-operatively identified as high risk and streamline a process for getting post-operative x-rays looking for foreign bodies before the patient leaves the operating room (tertiary prevention).

The PST prevention model can be embraced in the health IT system develop-ment process, before any adverse event has occurred. For example, the use of robust user centered design processes during the formative development period is likely to prevent many hazards from making it into the system (primary prevention) or catch the hazards during usability testing with representative end-users (secondary preven-tion). The use of EHR safety surveillance during the post implementation period for health IT system can then catch hazard and harm events where the contribution of the health IT system may be unrecognized (tertiary prevention). One of the benefits of human factors approaches is that it provides methods to catch and correct problems during different phases of design and implementation – before there is opportunity for harm. Without designing for primary, secondary and tertiary prevention in clinical workflow, individual healthcare providers are destined to make the same errors over and over again.

As the adoption of AI continues to increase special attention should be applied to primary and secondary reporting. For example, primary prevention would include the testing of AI before use in the clinical environment. This could include clinically appropriate use cases being developed and tested in by researchers and third parties while developing the AI models. The research team has done this with success when testing the usability and safety of EHRs (https://www.pewtrusts.org/-/media/assets/2018/08/healthit_safe_use_of_ehrs_report.pdf; Ratwani et al. 2018). Secondary prevention, could include hazard reporting of "hallucinations" (erroneous text not supported by reference text) from a generative AI. In addition to recommending proactive reporting by clinical staff, reviewing edits to text generated by clinical staff or help desk tickets mentioning AI could also be evaluated for near misses and hazardous situations.

14.3 Human Factors Methods for Analyzing and Improving Workflow

Evaluating, designing and optimizing clinical workflow is a critical part of providing safe and effective care to patients. The section above presented some core human factors concepts that are intended to provide guiding perspectives when trying to identify sources of problems and opportunities for improvement to healthcare-related workflow. A common thread across the multiple lenses presented is the need to understand the broader context of work, the complexities that can arise, and the cognitive and collaborative demands they impose, when trying to understand or improve workflow. This includes cases where an organization is trying to understand why problems or errors are occurring and develop mitigations. As well as cases where an organization is trying to design new health IT or insert new systems developed by vendors so as to improve performance.

In this section we provide brief descriptions of some core human factors methods that can be used to analyze the context of work and the impact of new technologies on work. These include methods that can be used early in the analysis process when one is trying to understand sources of performance problems and define requirements for more effective support, methods that can be used during design when a team is trying to determine whether the health IT system being developed will work as imagined, and methods that can be used after a system is implemented to understand and address human performance problems that are identified (e.g., near misses, adverse events, productivity bottlenecks). As we introduce each method we will highlight the types of analyses and stages of technology design and introduction for which they are best suited. We will also briefly describe their strength and limitations. A specific focus will be applied to the implementation and surveillance of artificial intelligence systems.

The review of human factors methods provided below is necessarily selective. We focus on methods for uncovering information about workflow and the context of work, particularly the cognitive and collaborative demands of work that can lead to performance problems, as well methods for evaluating and guiding the design new health IT systems as part of the development cycle. Broader surveys of human factors methods and more in-depth descriptions of the methods described below can be found in the literature (Bisantz et al. 2015; Bisantz and Roth 2008; Hettinger et al. 2017; Lee et al. 2013; Lowry et al. 2014; Stanton et al. 2017).

It is important to note for the reader that while each of the methods are covered individually below, in practice researchers will use a combination of methods to obtain a richer picture of the workflow of interest and the broader context in which it is imbedded than would be possible with any single method. For example researchers will often combine interviews and focus groups with observational studies (Militello et al. 2014) as well as with artifact analysis (Xiao et al. 2010).

These methods can be effectively used by multiple types of organizations and stake-holders and tailored to the scope, size, and budget of the project. This includes technology vendors who may be trying to develop and upgrade health IT systems for applications across multiple hospitals, clinical organizations (e.g. ambulatory clinics, hospitals, larger healthcare systems) that might be trying to roll-out and manage new health IT systems to minimize error, and improve performance, satisfaction and safety, as well as individual healthcare researchers or leaders who may be trying to examine sources of problems or errors and identify appropriate solutions. Despite the recent popularity and adoption of artificial intelligence tools like large language models and machine vision in healthcare, these methods still hold significant relevance in understanding the work as performed by clinical staff and the potential risks associated with adopting new technology was well as understanding the positive impact of the tools.

14.3.1   Interviews and Focus Groups

Interviews and focus groups are among the most common methods for learning about workflow and obstacles to effective performance (Bisantz et al. 2015). They are particularly useful during the early stage of information gathering to get an overview of the ideal workflow and obtain multiple perspectives on challenges and barriers to effective performance that may result in a disconnect between work as imagined and work as done. Interviews and focus groups can also assist in tertiary prevention when analyzing an adverse event that has occurred and safety experts are attempting to assess the severity of hazard for future patients and the potential frequency with which they may occur.

Interviews using human factors methodologies frequently employ a semi-structured format to ensure that key topics (e.g., previously identified key pieces of a workflow or known work-arounds) are discussed, while remaining flexible enough for the interviewer to discover new information and allow the participant to guide the discussion based on their experience with the process, system and culture. This facilitates learning the true work as performed versus work as imagined discussed previously. As one example, McDonald et al. used a semi-structured interview approach to map the clinical workflow for high-risk patient monitoring at 5 specialty clinics (pulmonary medicine, breast cancer, gastroenterology, urology and otolaryngology). Based on the interviews they were able to identify (1) the steps that were most critical, time-intensive, and risky from a patient-safety perspective; (2) critical data elements needed for effective monitoring of high-risk patients; and (3) candidate technical and organizational interventions to address the identified workflow vulnerabilities (McDonald et al. 2017).

Focus groups also employ semi-structured interview questions but allow the participants to clarify and build upon each other's comments, enabling a richer, more nuanced, construction of the workflow. A critical decision is whether to mix individuals from different backgrounds (e.g., different job positions; experience levels; status in the organization) in one focus group. An important consideration is to ensure that everyone feels free to express themselves openly. One example where this concern came up is in a focus group conducted seeking to understand communication patterns between nurses and physicians (Benda et al. 2016). In this study, separate focus groups with nurses, residents and attending physicians were chosen because of anticipation of different perspectives based on both roles and experience level between and among nurses and physicians. Indeed during focus group interviews residents and attending physicians expressed very different views. Attending physicians were more likely to discuss the importance of two-way communication and listening to nurses as their eyes and ears within the ED. In turn nurses talked about strategies for guiding less experienced residents, given the formal hierarchy relationship.

Interviews and focus groups, in general, require less expertise and time to conduct than some of the following methods. However, lack of appropriate preparation for both techniques are likely to result in less helpful data collected. Further, focus groups often require two moderators—one to conduct the focus group and one to record the discussions. The use of audio and/or video recording devices can help reduce the number of personnel used but require a significant amount of resources to turn the recordings into usable data. Audio/video recordings can also negatively impact the participant's willingness to share more controversial views and observations.

Interviews and focus groups can specifically be used to understand current comfort level of clinical staff with AI as well as their current experience. Both before and after AI systems are in place, the use of focus groups and semi-structured interviews can identify themes in reasons for lack of trust, slow adoption or identified safety hazards if AI tools are not well integrated into clinical workflow. For example, generative AI responding to patient portal messages may cause additional work for staff that may hinder adoption of the tool. Similar challenges have been observed with the adoption of electronic prescriptions where clinical practices that historically integrated administrative staff and clinicians to help route refill or change requests from pharmacies. EHRs may lack the appropriate workflow and permissions in an EHR for administrative staff to assist when they would have historically helped an ordering provider with ensuring written scripts were routed to correct pharmacies.

14.3.2   Critical Decision Method

One of the most powerful methods for learning about the demands in the environment and the strategies that people have developed for coping with them is to ask them to describe a specific past challenging situation they personally experienced and how they handled it (Flanagan 1954). The critical decision method (CDM) is a widely used structured interview technique that builds on this approach (Klein et al. 1989). It was initially developed to understand the decision making process of firefighters when making rapid decisions with limited access to information that could have life-threatening consequences. It consists of a trained individual in the method conducting a structured interview with a single participant, typically an expert in the workflow under consideration. The method involves having the individual go through the incident in progressively deeper passes to understand the decisions that were made, the information that was used and alternative events that could have occurred and how they were avoided (Crandall et al. 2006).

CDM has been used in multiple high-risk settings, including urban and wild land firefighting, military command and control, and software engineering. It has been extensively used in health care, including to study the perceptual cues used by experienced neonatal intensive care unit nurses; Crandall and Getchell-Reiter (1993) and to compare the strategies employed by physicians of different levels of expertise for early recognition of sepsis (Patterson et al. 2016). The results have been used to propose improvements to workflow, new forms of decision-support, and new training.

More recently a variant of CDM has been developed as a means to identify resilient behavior and workflows by healthcare providers. For example, Hegde and colleagues are developing a lesson-sharing tool called Resilience Engineering Tool to Improve Patient Safety (RETIPS) based on CDM interviews of nurses and physicians that focus on examples of resilient behavior (Hegde et al. 2014, 2015). The intent was to collect a corpus of cases that demonstrate how people adapt in everyday clinical work to perform effectively and avoid harm to patients under challenging conditions as a means of generating safety lessons.

While CDM is powerful method for collecting information on workflow challenges and the adaptive strategies that individuals develop in response, it has some limitations. In particular it requires significant training and expertise to conduct CDM interviews. Often CDM interviews are conducted by trained human factors consultants and there are short-courses offered in the methodology. In addition there have been efforts to adapt the methodology to on-line questionnaires (Hegde and Jackson 2017).

CDM interviews may be able to provide powerful insights into how experience and non-experienced clinicians handle integrated AI tools. For example, an experienced radiologist may over trust an AI tool and miss false negative reads whereas a less experienced physician may struggle with disagreeing with a read (false positive) from a machine vision tool. Using the CDM approach could help understand the decision making process of both experienced and less experienced clinicians and improve the interface of the associated tools. E.g. presenting AI confidence levels or intentionally having simulated cases in the workflow, similar to how the transportation and safety administration monitors agents who screen luggage for their ability to detect simulated banned items (Department of Homeland Security 2025).

14.3.3 Observations

One of the most useful human factors techniques for studying workflow is to conduct observations in the actual work context or in a close analogue such as a high fidelity simulator (Roth and Patterson 2000). Observing individuals and teams working in their work environment allows the analyst to document the range of complexities that arise that challenge workflow and the various adaptations and work arounds that individuals have developed to cope with demands, overcome obstacles, fill in gaps and otherwise contribute to the overall safety of the system (or not).

Observational studies involve having one or more observers unobtrusively shadow individuals as they go about their work. The goal is to observe the activities and communications that occur without getting in the way, serving as a source of distraction, or otherwise influencing the behavior of the individuals being observed. The observer typically records their observations in real time either in free form or using a predefined set of coding categories (Bisantz et al. 2015). These are then analyzed after the fact using qualitative grounded theory methods and/or quantitative methods (e.g., recording and analyzing the frequency of different types of occurrences).

Often the observational team will include a behavioral scientist (e.g., a human factors specialist) with knowledge and skill in observational methods, and a second individual with knowledge and expertise in the domain of practice being observed (e.g., a physician or a nurse in studies of health care environments). For example, a study examining workflow challenges in complex surgeries had a two-person observation team in the operating room that included a practicing surgeon and a human factors specialist (Christian et al. 2006). The surgeon could draw on their surgical knowledge to interpret what was observed while the human factors specialist could draw on their cross-domain knowledge of human performance drivers and systems challenges to point to patterns of behavior and systems problems whose significance might not be recognized by the surgeon. Both took notes in real-time during the surgery being observed which were then combined to obtain a more complete and accurate description of what took place.

Whenever feasible, observations are coupled with opportunistic interviews that occur during periods of low workload or at the end of a shift. This allows for the subject to answer clarifying questions or provide elaborations or confirmations of what was observed without interfering with the work. In some cases, if the environment allows, the sessions are audio or video recorded for later review and analysis. For example, a study examining inter-operative deviations in care had video-recordings made of 10 high acuity operations. These were then transcribed and analyzed by a multidisciplinary team consisting of surgeons and human factors specialists (Hu et al. 2012). This resulted in more complete data capture than would be possible when relying solely on real-time observations. In another study, Tiferes et al. used video- and audio-recordings of robotic assisted surgeries to code and characterize verbal and non-verbal communication among members of the surgical team (Tiferes et al. 2018).

Observational studies are useful early in an investigation when trying to understand the work as actually done (as opposed to the work as imagined). This includes situations where human performance problems have been identified and there is a need to understand why they are occurring and what can be done to reduce the problem. One good example was an observational study that was conducted to understand the 'counting protocol' used by nurses to keep track of surgical objects (needles, sponges, instruments) during operations in order to reduce the risk of leaving a foreign object in the patient (Dierks et al. 2004). Hospital leadership wanted to understand why surgical objects were sometimes left in patients in spite of having the counting protocol. The observational study showed that the counting protocol was difficult to perform and documented multiple factors that contributed to challenges in maintaining an accurate count (e.g., incomplete surgical kits; shift changes in the middle of surgery; differences in counting conventions across nurses). Further it showed that the counting protocol itself had unanticipated negative consequences that in some cases compromised patient safety. Complications in the count, which occurred in six of the nine observed surgeries, triggered activities to reconcile the source of the inconsistency. This drew attention away from the ongoing surgery, resulting in delays and additional risk to the patient. The study led to numerous recommendations for improving performance ranging from increasing standardization to eliminating the count through use of new technologies for keeping track of surgical objects.

Observational studies are also useful after a new system is put in place to understand the impact of the new system on practitioner workflow. This includes tracking whether the system is being used in the manner envisioned by the developers, whether it is having the positive effects anticipated, and whether any new issues are emerging. For example, an observational study was conducted to understand use of Electronic Health Record (EHR) systems in primary care outpatient clinics (Flanagan et al. 2013). The study identified mismatches between the EHR system designs and the demands of outpatient settings that led to a variety of work arounds (some paper-based and some computer-based) intended to improve efficiency and support memory and awareness of the healthcare practitioners. These pointed to limitations of the EHRs that contributed to their lack of use and opportunities for improvement. Another study examined the impact of the introduction of EHRs on nurse-physician verbal communication in emergency departments (Benda et al. 2017). The goal was to understand the content and pattern of physician-nurse communication given the availability of

EHRs. Among other things the study identified the situations where verbal communication continued to be needed in spite of the availability of the information in the EHR. For example, verbal communication was used to draw the attention of the provider to important patient status information that might otherwise not be salient, as well as to confirm that the provider was aware of the information. The results pointed to opportunities to improve EHR systems.

Observational studies have also been used to examine the impact of new technology such as surgical robots, on operating room workflow, teamwork and patient safety. For example, observational studies have been used to document workflow disruptions in robotic surgeries, the factors contributing to them and the impact on safety (Catchpole et al. 2018). Catchpole and colleagues observed 89 robotic surgeries and documented 4229 flow disruptions, defined as deviations from the natural progression of the operation. The researchers found that flow disruptions rates due to problems in communication and coordination were comparable to those for other types of surgeries. In contrast flow disruption rates due to equipment problems (e.g. improper insertion of the camera; fogging of the endoscope) were much higher pointing to opportunities to improve performance through changes in training, equipment or workflow.

Observational methods have also been used to explore verbal and non-verbal aspects of team communication in robotic surgery where the surgeon sits at a robot console away from direct view of the patient on the operating table (Tiferes et al. 2016). The authors documented numerous types of verbal and non-verbal interaction between the surgeon and the physician assistants located by the patient. This included use of the robotic tool itself as a means of non-verbal communication (e.g., positioning and zooming the camera to draw the attention of the physician assistant to a particular location). This last example illustrates how new technology results in new adaptations and uses unanticipated by the system developers. The authors pointed to how the results could be leveraged to design more effective team training for robotic surgeries.

While observational studies are a powerful tool for understanding the actual demands of work, they have some limitations. First they are time and labor intensive, both in terms of the time required to conduct the study and the time required to analyze the results. Second, they require expertise in performing observational studies. Their success depends on the skills of the observers and the representativeness of the sample of observations (Roth and Patterson 2000). Third, there is a potential that the presence of the observer to impact the workflow or get biased results, for example if the individuals being observed are concerned that they are being evaluated or that they may be reported if they deviate from prescribed policies and procedures. Finally, while the approach is useful for studying every day work, it is not suitable for studying rare events that by definition would be unlikely to be observed during any particular observation period.

The use of observational studies for the study of AI in clinical workflow could take several strategies. For example, observational studies of radiologists at their workstations using machine vision products to assist with image interpretation or clinicians using generative AI to summarize office visit encounters. Primary care doctors using AI to respond to patient messages may require in clinical or after hours observations to understand the impact of the tools and the level scrutiny of summative or generative activities. For example, how long does a clinician spend reading a clinical note that was the result of a summative AI digital scribe? If the clinician is unsure of the content or feels like content is missing, can they access recordings or a transcript of the meeting to clarify findings. In addition, during an observation the research team could review how well the clinician integrates non-verbalized findings in their note, e.g. smells, observed behavior and physical exam findings that would be missing unless verbalized by the clinician during the patient visit. Furthermore, what happens if the recording does not happen in real-time and needs to be reviewed later in the day or after hours, does that reduce the accuracy of the note or contribute significantly to delays in documentation.

14.3.4 Artifact Analysis

One of the best ways to gain insights into how work is actually performed and the requirements for more effective support is to examine the tools ('artifacts') currently in use (Xiao 2005). Artifacts include formal aids provided and sanctioned by the institution such as procedures and checklists (e.g., formal OR checklists) as well as 'home grown' artifacts that practitioners have developed on their own initiative to support their own work (Xiao et al. 2009).

'Home-grown' artifacts developed by practitioners can highlight mismatches between the formal systems in place and the requirements of the work (Bisantz et al. 2010a; Xiao 2005). They provide a window on the cognitive and collaborative aspects of work that need to be supported and the information needed to effectively support work. Artifacts can be simple, low tech, items such as 'sticky-notes' and paper-based 'cheat sheets' (also sometimes called 'brain sheets') that practitioners routinely use to support memory and situation awareness. Increasingly one also finds highly sophisticated computer-based visualizations and decision aids developed by computer-savvy practitioners to facilitate their own work (Xiao et al. 2009). For example, Roth and colleagues examined work practice in a military airlift organization (Roth et al. 2006). They documented a variety of new computer-based visualizations; local databases; and decision-aids that were developed as 'home-grown' artifacts to compensate for limitations of the formal computer-systems in place.

Analysis of participant-developed artifacts can provide a rich source of information to guide design of new health IT. For example, Bauer, Guerlain & Brown studied the use of paper-based patient flow sheets in pediatric intensive care (Bauer et al. 2006). Positive features identified included that it was portable, that it supported easy comparison of information and that it allowed for free-form annotation. Based on these observations the researchers were able to specify important functions that electronic systems should continue to support including the need to allow for flexible rather than sequential data entry; the need to allow users to optionally leave data fields unfilled; and the need to support unstructured annotations. At the same time the researchers were able to identify ways that an electronic system could improve on the paper flow sheets, including automatic calculations that were done manually with the paper form.

Similarly, Gurses, Xiao and Hu studied the paper-based clipboard created by nurse coordinators to compensate for inadequate support of the formal hospital information system (Gurses et al. 2009). Nurse coordinators painstakingly created clipboards that synthesized and reorganized information obtained from multiple disparate sources to better support their fast-paced work demands. The authors recommended modifications to the hospital information system to allow users to create and print tailored single page views that could provide 'at a glance' summaries of key information.

One of the most studied home-grown artifacts in healthcare is the dry erase white board (Wears et al. 2007a; Bisantz et al. 2010b; Pennathur et al. 2009; Patterson et al. 2010; Xiao et al. 2007). Dry-erase status boards arose spontaneously and became ubiquitous in the ED in the mid 1980s as a means to track patients (Wears et al. 2007a). Dry erase status boards have largely been replaced by electronic systems, however, as mentioned above, not all of the functions supported by the dry-erase status board were successfully transferred to the electronic versions. While the electronic versions support basic information exchange functions (e.g., patient demographics; location; caregiver assignments), they are less effective at directing attention, maintaining awareness of provider workflow status, and coordinating work across providers (Bisantz et al. 2010b; Pennathur et al. 2007). For example, as mentioned earlier, attending and resident physicians used hand drawn symbols to track (and allow others to see) their patient specific workflow status with the dry erase status board but this was not supported with the electronic version. Similarly, with the dry-erase status board it was possible to provide information about the overall ED (e.g., where a resident or attending physician was in their evaluation) and to annotate and track aspects of medical care by making annotations outside the matrix structure (e.g., notes at the top, lines along the side). This flexibility was no longer supported by the electronic versions.

Comparison of dry-erase status boards and electronic versions led Bisantz et al. to draw several conclusions and recommendations (Bisantz et al. 2010b). Most importantly, it is not sufficient to reproduce the literal format of an existing technology. Mimicking the matrix format and basic information of the dry-erase status boards failed to support the variety of cognitive and collaborative functions that the dry-erase status boards supported. System developers need to gain a deeper understanding of the demands of the work, how existing artifacts support work and where they fall short in order to develop a firm foundation for new health IT design. In particular, the fact that dry-erase boards are highly flexible, easy to tailor, and easy to simply walk up to and input information of any kind without having to first log in, and without being limited with respect to what can be entered and where it can go, turned out to be critical elements contributing to their success (Wears et al. 2007b). The results of the analyses provided the foundation for a more extensive project to design and evaluate improved display concepts for ED status displays (Guarrera et al. 2015).

Artifact analysis provides an important window on the multiple, often subtle, demands of work. As such it is a valuable tool for health IT developers trying to gather user support requirements. Its primary limitation is the risk of adapting too literally superficial aspects of the artifact (e.g., the particular format used; the specific bits of information included) without fully appreciating all of its functionality and the full range of cognitive and collaborative support it provides. This risk can be mitigated by coupling artifact analysis with other human factors techniques such as work practice observations and practitioner interviews to obtain a richer understanding of the demands of the work environment, how the artifact supports work, and limitations of the artifact that can be overcome through effective use of new technology (e.g., automating computations, synthesizing information).

As clinical workflow becomes increasingly digitized there may be fewer and fewer artifacts outside of the EHR. However there continue to be instances of circumstances where clinicians rely on paper-based artifacts or even electronic artifacts outside of the EHR. This could include note taking on paper to facilitate rapid patient hand off, reviewing paper notes from external facilities that are not able to transmit electronically and even handheld guides and note cards with frequently called numbers, protocols or reference guides. It is possible that future AI tools customized to the environment and appropriately tested could provide ready access to information. For example, asking an AI digital assistant "What is the number for the vascular surgery team?" or even "Call the vascular surgery team" as well as "What is the best antibiotic for X infection given a penicillin allergy, local resistance patterns and this patient's recent diagnostic testing, including recent bacterial cultures?". Even if asked "What is the best antibiotic for X infection given a penicillin allergy?" the model should be tested to make sure that it incorporates local resistance patterns and patient level factors while stating those were taking into consideration. Direct observation of clinicians using the tool in situ and in simulation will provide important findings to aid in the safe adoption of the technology.

14.3.5 Work Oriented Evaluations

Health IT systems are often plagued with usability problems that make them difficult to use adding to inefficiency and potential for error (Zahabi et al. 2015b). Of even greater concern, they may not provide effective support for the cognitive and collaborative work of the healthcare providers. One way to overcome this problem is to encourage multiple work-oriented evaluation cycles as part of the system design process.

Traditionally a distinction has been made between two types of user evaluations: *formative evaluation* and *summative evaluation* (Neilsen 1994). Formative evaluations are designed to provide feedback with respect to what aspects of the system design work well and which can be improved—that is they are intended to be learning opportunities. There are a variety of approaches to formative evaluation ranging from fast and relatively low-cost heuristic evaluations that consist of structured reviews by usability experts, to more formal usability tests that bring in representative users to exercise the system. Usability tests typically collect both performance data (e.g., number of key strokes, time to complete a task, errors) and user feedback data (e.g., via structured questionnaires). *Summative evaluations* are designed to provide an overall assessment of the system. They are typically conducted at the completion of a system development process to establish that the system meets pre-defined evaluation criteria.

A work-centered evaluation is an example of a usability test approach that is work-oriented (Truxler et al. 2012; Roth et al. 2010). The focus is on insuring that the health IT supports the cognitive and collaborative work of the healthcare practitioners. Work-centered evaluations are designed to be *diagnostic*. They are intended to not only provide an overall assessment of the usability and usefulness the health IT system, but to also provide detailed a detailed assessment of: (1) which cognitive and collaborative activities the health IT supports well and which less so; (2) which features of the health IT system are useful to the health practitioners and which less so; and (3) which features of the health IT are easy to use (usable) and which less so. These provide important information to guide health IT design course correction.

Work-centered evaluations couple elements of both formative and summative evaluations (Roth et al. 2010). From a summative perspective the aim is to evaluate the design against a predefined set of *cognitive performance support objectives* that the system is designed to meet (Clark et al. 2017). For example a cognitive performance support objective might be 'identify hold-ups in the care of an individual patient'. Work-centered evaluations include explicit metrics to establish whether these cognitive performance support objectives have been met. These metrics include performance on test cases that are representative of the cognitive and collaborative challenges that arise in that work context that the health IT is intended to support. For example, if a health IT system is to support 'identifying hold-ups in the care of an individual patient' then one or more of the test cases would involve recognizing that there is a 'hold up' preventing progress in the flow of care of a particular patient and being able to identify what that hold up was (e.g., the attending is waiting to hear back from a consulting physician). Work-centered evaluations also collect direct user feedback on whether that cognitive performance support objective has been met. This feedback is typically obtained via rating questions on a final questionnaire that is administered after all test cases have been completed. For example, the test participant might be asked to rate on a nine-point scale whether they feel that the health IT effectively supports 'Identify hold-ups in the care of an individual patient'.

Work-centered evaluations also include a *formative* evaluation aspect—an opportunity to discover need for additional improvement. The evaluations are designed to catch any usability problems that need to be addressed prior to final implementation. This is accomplished by identifying any confusions, difficulties or usability errors that test participants make during the test cases portion of the evaluation, as well as via usability rating questions included on the final questionnaire. Work-centered evaluations are also designed to probe for additional work demands not previously identified that may signal new cognitive performance support requirements and propel further design innovation. Previously unrecognized work demands and additional cognitive performance support requirements are typically elicited via open-ended questions on the final questionnaire as well as via end of session verbal debriefs. This includes explicitly asking participants to consider situations beyond the ones sampled in test cases, and indicate any ones they feel the health IT might not handle well, as well as any situations where the health IT would be particularly helpful.

A work-centered approach was used to evaluate an Emergency Department information System (EDIS) prototype designed to support awareness of the overall ED state and flow of patients through the ED, patient care, staff workload, and available resources (Clark et al. 2017). Participants performed patient planning and orientation tasks using the EDIS displays. They then rated the ability of the EDIS to support the work-oriented cognitive needs of emergency clinical staff that were identified as part of the cognitive analysis that drove the system design (i.e., the cognitive performance support requirements). The questionnaire employed a 9-point rating scale with '9' indicating 'extremely effective'. Example cognitive performance support questions include ability to 'Identify bottlenecks or holdups preventing overall patient flow through ED''; 'Maintain awareness of overall acuity of patients waiting and currently being treated'; and 'Provide support for prioritizing your tasks'. The participants also rated the usability, usefulness, and predicted frequency of use of specific system components.

Overall mean ratings were positive (i.e., mean above 5) for cognitive performance support objectives, usability, usefulness, and frequency of use, indicating that the EDIS prototype would provide effective cognitive support for emergency medicine staff. At the same time, the evaluation generated diagnostic information regarding which aspects of the EDIS displays were most useful, where there were issues in usability, and the extent to which the displays supported the cognitive work of different types of providers. For example, in some cases mean usefulness scores were significantly higher than mean usability scores (e.g., for the waiting room and patient progress displays) suggesting that while waiting room and patient progress information is useful to ED staff members, the information could be displayed better.

The study also illustrated the diagnostic power of cognitive performance support oriented questions. For example, the question 'provide support for prioritizing your tasks' received significantly lower mean ratings (5.9 on a 9-point scale) than many other of the questions (all with mean ratings above 7). This result made sense because while the researchers identified the need to support individual task prioritization as an important requirement for the ultimate full system, this particular cognitive task was beyond the design goals of the prototype being tested. The evaluation also revealed that nurse and physician provider roles had significantly different perceptions of the usability and usefulness of certain EDIS components, suggesting that they have different information needs while working.

In summary key elements of work-centered evaluations include: (1) An explicit articulation and test of the *cognitive performance support requirements* underlying the aiding system that are used to guide the selection of test cases and test measures; (2) test participants that are representative of the target user population; (3) test cases that reflect the range of cognitive and collaborative complexity that arises in the work context; and (4) multi-faceted assessment measures, including objective measures of performance as well as a final user-feedback questionnaire that addresses usability and usefulness of the aiding system. A main strength of the approach is its work-oriented focus. A primary limitation is that it can be resource intensive to design, implement, and analyze.

Work-centered evaluations in regards to AI integration in clinical workflow will be an important approach to ensuring that AI tools provide meaningful improvement in clinical needs as well as addressing the cognitive needs of the user. For example, if an AI model will be used to assist in diagnostic testing and generating differential diagnoses for a patient, it must be able to operate with the same limited information that clinicians may have when a patient presents to an emergency department. Training an AI model on retrospective data and then attempting to use it prospectively in the care of patients may significantly reduce it's utility. For example, some mortality predictive scores require tests or measurements that may not be available for 24 hours, like urine output or urine creatinine levels, and would not be available at the time of a patient's initial presentation to the emergency department. Furthermore, with the current excitement of AI there is a potential that AI tools get applied to circumstances where they add no or marginal improvements in performance but introduce added cost, complexity and potential risk.

14.3.6 Task Analysis

There are a variety of human factors task analysis methods used to formally describe work activities. These methods decompose work in terms of goals, tasks, and subtasks. Requirements for successful task completion are identified, including knowledge or skills, equipment, or information needs, and opportunities for error or other performance limiting factors are made explicit. The granularity of decomposition depends on the needs of analysis, and can range from high-level activities (e.g., "order medication") to keystroke or mouse-click level actions. In some cases, time estimates are associated with activities in order to predict task completion times.

Hierarchical Task Analysis (HTA) is a common task analysis method that begins by decomposing task goals, hierarchically, into subtasks and actions (Kirwan and Ainsworth 1992; Stanton and Karwowski 2001). A distinguishing feature of HTA is the articulation of plans, which describe the manner in which subtasks and activities are executed. For instances, activities can be performed sequentially, subject to if–then or branching conditions, or performed iteratively until some stopping condition is met. Each node that has been decomposed into lower level actions is provided with a plan. The HTA method therefore supports a description of activity in a way that is reflective of predictable situational conditions or more flexible choice of strategy.

The family of GOMS task analytic methods (task Goals, Operators or actions, Methods or sequences of actions, and Selection rules to choose the appropriate Method) includes operators that describe cognitive, perceptual, and motor actions at the keystroke level of detail along with the times associated with the operators. GOMS models can be used to model predictable sequences of actions, including interactions with health IT systems such as electronic health records (John and Kieras

1996). Models can be used to compare task times across different systems (during procurement) or to understand impacts of operational change. A number of architectures influenced by GOMS have been implemented which support computational modeling of human activities (Byrne et al. 2009).

Data necessary to complete task analyses (regardless of form) comes primarily from observation or interviews to allow the work tasks, performance indicators, and support requirements to be identified. Task times can be obtained through measurement, and in some cases (e.g., perceptual, cognitive, or keystroke level GOMS operators) from the published literature. Results for task analyses can be used in design (i.e., to insure critical information is present, to identify and mitigate likely sources of error, to understand when activities exceed perceptual capabilities), in system procurement (i.e., to compare times or skill requirements for critical activities), and in training (i.e., to document required knowledge and skills). For example, hierarchical task analysis was used to compare interactions across two different drug infusion pumps in order to predict potential user errors (Chung et al. 2003). Importantly, however, task analyses are limited by the degree to which tasks are predictable a priori, and therefore are best applied to well-defined, repeated tasks (e.g., entering a medication order) rather than complex higher level tasks (e.g., diagnostic decision-making). Such complex work activities should be analyzed using other methods, such as the critical decision methods (described above) and related cognitive task analysis techniques (Bisantz and Roth 2008).

The adoption of AI in clinical workflow has the potential to dramatically disrupt traditional tasks for clinical staff. For example, the complex cognitive task of reviewing a patient's chart and all the potentially siloed information both within the EHR as well as potentially external in health information exchange systems could be dramatically reduced with a summative AI model. However that summative model could filter out important information that a specific clinician may find helpful. Would the AI model include a patient's occupation in every summary? What if the patient works with chemicals as a housekeeper, scientist or mortician where a chemical exposure may be pertinent? Would the model be accurate enough to include that level of potential environmental exposure or would that signal be missed unless another clinician made special note of it. However, the current state of clinical care dictates that a clinician only has a set amount of time that they have to spread across review of historic data while also actively caring for the patient. There is a high likelihood that a clinician would not catch errors or important omissions in the clinical note. One study found error rates of 7% after using electronic dictation software without the use of AI (Zhou et al. 2018). Anticipating errors and omissions studied in different modalities will be critical for safe and efficient use of the tools.

14.3.7   Cognitive Informatics Techniques

The development of cognitive informatics presents new opportunities to interface with human factors engineering principles. Whereas many of the previously mentioned methods and techniques can be challenging to gather data on more than 10–20 participants, the use of cognitive informatics can allow for observations across thousands of users and millions of interactions. Cognitive informatics goes beyond just measuring clicks and mouse movements, but seeks to both identify and understand the circumstances of a particular action or outcome across large numbers of users. Adelman et. al. were able to identify instances of where medical providers ordered a test on a wrong patient by creating algorithms based on provider workflow (Adelman et al. 2013). The authors were able to significantly reduce the incidence of these errors by having ordering providers re-identify their patients with each order. Follow up work by Green et al. was able to replicate the work, but noted that the change in workflow increased workflow duration by 4.1–4.9 seconds per order. A reduction in wrong patient orders of almost 25% was sustained at two years after the implementation (Green et al. 2015). Yet further analysis of their implementation, extrapolated across the national healthcare system would require 400 additional full time emergency physicians and 900,000 extra hours of checking to make sure that the order is placed on the correct patient (Wears 2015). While the intervention is effective, future research is needed to better understand the human factors engineering principles behind why users order on the wrong patient. It could due to patient names on the screens being next to each other, interruptions, or errors in the health IT systems that route users to the wrong patient despite making the correct selection or some combination of other causes. Each of these require different interventions and improvements to the EHR workflow to design the errors out of the system. For this problem and many others, the use of cognitive informatics with human factors engineering is critical to identifying the underlying reasons for the errors and inefficiencies, and to help prioritize the most frequent and potentially catastrophic events from impacting our patients and clinicians.

Cognitive informatics techniques are particularly well suited for the systematic study of AI tools. As mentioned above, understanding not only the adoption of the tools but provider interventions on AI generated content will be critical to have in place to refine those algorithms. In addition, the rapid pace of AI models will require equally nimble analytics that are both human-centered and able to leverage data generated by the human–computer interactions to understand subtle findings that may otherwise go unnoticed or lead to harm events that seem sporadic but are linked by the AI models and tools in place. For example, machine vision tools have been shown to be comparable to radiologist in certain circumstances (Ahn et al. 2022). However they may lack the context of the patient present in the EHR or clinical correlation that a physician may communicate to the radiologist via conversation/phone/text. In addition clinical medicine changes so quickly that it may be difficult to keep the models on top of the latest developments without keeping a human-in-the-loop. For example, a FDA approved medication was found to be associated with abnormal brain imaging that could appear similar to a stroke that would necessitate blood thinning medications associated with high risk for life threatening complications (Cogswell et al. 2022). A machine vision AI tool could potentially misread a diagnostic image without knowing the patient was on the new medication and without the training in the model on the rare event to distinguish between stroke and artifact from the medication.

14.4 Conclusion

This chapter provided an introduction to human factors perspectives and methods with insights into the value of human factors when considering the integration of AI in clinical workflow. Key methods include semi-structured interviews and focus groups, critical incident analyses, observational methods, artifact analyses and cognitive informatics approaches. Multiple health care examples of applications of these methods were provided to illustrate the power of studying work as practiced to identify sources of complexity that create risk as well as adaptive behavior of healthcare providers that contribute to system resilience and enhance safety. The examples also illustrated how human factors methods can be leveraged to identify opportunities for improvement whether through training to disseminate and reinforce effective strategies or through technology enhancements. A key point is the need to include multiple opportunities to collect information on the usability and usefulness of new technologies throughout the development process, up to and including fielding of systems in the actual work environment.

An important point to stress is that the human factors methods are appropriate for use by multiple types of organizations and stake-holders, and can be and tailored to the scope, size, and budget of the project. This includes technology vendors who may be trying to develop and upgrade health IT systems for applications across multiple hospitals. Clinical organizations (e.g. ambulatory clinics, hospitals, larger healthcare systems) may use these methods to roll-out and manage new health IT systems to minimize error, and improve performance, satisfaction and safety. Finally, individual healthcare researchers or leaders may find value in using human factors methods to examine sources of problems or errors and identify appropriate solutions. As the rate of technology adoption and complexity increase these methods are even more relevant as we seek to integrate the best aspects of artificial intelligence into clinical workflow. It will be critical for all stakeholder to study and mitigate both known and unknown hazards while improving the care of patients.

References

Adelman JS, Kalkut GE, Schechter CB, Weiss JM, Berger MA, Reissman SH, Cohen HW, Lorenzen SJ, Burack DA, Southern WN. Understanding and preventing wrong-patient electronic orders: a randomized controlled trial. JAMIA 2013;20:305–10.

Ahn JS, Ebrahimian S, McDermott S, et al. Association of artificial intelligence–aided chest radiograph interpretation with reader performance and efficiency. JAMA Netw Open. 2022;5(8):e2229289. https://doi.org/10.1001/jamanetworkopen.2022.29289.

Bauer DT, Guerlain SA, Brown PJ. Evaluating the use of flowsheets in pediatric intensive care to inform design. Proc Hum Factors Ergon Soc Annu Meet. 2006;50:1054–8.

Benda NC, Hettinger AZ, Bisantz AM, et al. Communication in the electronic age: an analysis of face-to-face physician-nurse communication in the emergency department. J Healthc Informatics Res. 2017;1:218–30.

Benda NC, Hettinger AZ, Bisantz AM, et al. Communication in the electronic age: an analysis of face-to-face physician-nurse communication in the emergency department. Manuscript Submitting Publication;2016.

Bernstam EV, Hersh WR, Sim I, Eichmann D, Silverstein JC, Smith JW, Becich MJ. Unintended consequences of health information technology: a need for biomedical informatics. J Biomed Inform. 2009.

Biever W, Angell L, Seaman S. Automated driving system collisions: early lessons. Hum Factors. 2020;62(2):249–59.

Bisantz AM, Roth E. Analysis of cognitive work. Ann Rev Hum Factors Ergon. 2008;3:1–43.

Bisantz AM, Pennathur PR, Fairbanks R, Perry SJ, Zwemer FL, Guarrera TK, Wears RL. Emergency department status boards: a case study in information systems transition. J Cogn Eng Decis Mak. 2010a;4:39–68.

Bisantz AM, Pennathur PR, Guarrera TK, Fairbanks RJ, Perry SJ, Zwemer F, Wears RL. Emergency department status boards: a case study in information systems transition. J Cogn Eng Decis Mak. 2010b;4:39–68.

Bisantz A, Roth E, Watts-Englert J. Study and analysis of complex cognitive work. Eval Hum Work Fourth Ed. 2015. https://doi.org/10.1201/B18362.

Braithwaite J, Wears RL, Hollnagel E. Resilient health care: turning patient safety on its head. Int J Qual Heal Care. 2015;27:418–20.

Braithwaite J, Wears R, Hollnagel E. Resilient health care: reconciling work-as-imagined and work-as-done. Resilient Heal Care Reconciling Work. 2017. https://doi.org/10.1201/978131 5366838-1.

Byrne M. Cognitive architecture. In: Sears A, Jacko J, editors. Fundamentals of human-computer interaction. CRC Press; 2009. p. 70–88.

Carayon P. Human factors of complex sociotechnical systems. Appl Ergon. 2006;37:525–35.

Carroll JM, Campbell RL. Artifacts as psychological theories: the case of human-computer interaction. Behav Inf Technol. 1998;8:247–56.

Carroll JM, Rosson MB. Getting around the task-artifact cycle: how to make claims and design by scenario. ACM Trans Inf Syst. 1992;10:181–212.

Casner SM, Hutchins EL, Norman D. The challenges of partially automated driving. Commun ACM. 2016;59:70–7.

Catchpole KR, Hallett E, Curtis S, Mirchi T, Souders CP, Anger JT. Diagnosing barriers to safety and efficiency in robotic surgery. Ergonomics. 2018;61:26–39.

Christian CK, Gustafson ML, Roth EM, Sheridan TB, Gandhi TK, Dwyer K, Zinner MJ, Dierks MM. A prospective study of patient safety in the operating room. Surgery. 2006;139:159–73.

Chung PH, Zhang J, Johnson TR, Patel VL. An extended hierarchical task analysis for error prediction in medical devices. AMIA Ann Symp Proceedings AMIA Symp. 2003;2003:165–9.

Clark LN, Benda NC, Hegde S, et al. Usability evaluation of an emergency department information system prototype designed using cognitive systems engineering techniques. Appl Ergon. 2017;60:356–65.

Cogswell PM, Barakos JA, Barkhof F, Benzinger TS, Jack CR, Poussaint TY, Raji CA, Ramanan VK, Whitlow CT. Amyloid-related imaging abnormalities with emerging Alzheimer disease therapeutics: detection and reporting recommendations for clinical practice. Am J Neuroradiol. 2022;43(9):E19-35.

Crandall B, Klein GA, Hoffman RR. Working minds: a practitioner's guide to cognitive task analysis. The MIT Press;2006.

Crandall B, Getchell-Reiter K. Critical decision method: a technique for eliciting concrete assessment indicators from the intuition of NICU nurses. Adv Nurs Sci. 1993;16:42–51.

Dawber TR, Meadors GF, Moore FE. Epidemiological approaches to heart disease: the Framingham study. Am J Public Heal Nations Heal. 1951;41:279–86.

Department of Homeland Security, Office of Inspector General. "Undercover tests of screener and equipment performance." DHS OIG Report, 2025. https://www.oig.dhs.gov/sites/default/files/assets/Mgmt/OIG_04-37_0904.pdf.

Dierks MM, Christian CK, Roth EM, Member A, Sheridan TB, Fellow L. Healthcare safety: the impact of disabling "Safety" protocols. 2004;34:693–8.

Fairbanks RJ, Guarrera TK, Karn KS, Caplan SH, Shah MN, Wears RL. Interface design characteristics of a popular emergency department information system. In: Proceedings of the human factors and ergonomics society annual meeting, 2008 September, vol. 52, no. 12. Los Angeles, CA: SAGE Publications;2008. pp. 778–82.

Fairbanks RJ, Wears RL, Woods DD, Hollnagel E, Plsek P, Cook RI. Resilience and resilience engineering in health care. Jt Comm J Qual Patient Saf. 2014;376–383

Flanagan JC. The critical incident technique. Psychol Bull. 1954;51:327–58.

Flanagan ME, Saleem JJ, Millitello LG, Russ AL, Doebbeling BN. Paper- and computer-based workarounds to electronic health record use at three benchmark institutions. J Am Med Informatics Assoc. 2013;1–8.

Green RA, Hripcsak G, Salmasian H, Lazar EJ, Bostwick SB, Bakken SR, Vawdrey DK. Intercepting wrong-patient orders in a computerized provider order entry system. Ann Emerg Med. 2015;65:679-86.e1.

Guarrera T, McGeorge N, Clark L, Lavergne D, Hettinger A, Fairbanks R, Bisantz A. Cognitive engineering design of an emergency department information system. Cogn Eng Better Heal Care Syst. 2015.

Gurses AP, Xiao Y, Hu P. User-designed information tools to support communication and care coordination in a trauma hospital. J Biomed Inform. 2009;42:667–77.

Harrer S. Attention is not all you need: the complicated case of ethically using large language models in healthcare and medicine. EBioMedicine. 2023;1:90.

Hegde S, Jackson C. RETIPS revisited: findings from a pilot stage implementation of the resilience engineering tool to improve patient safety. Proc Hum Factors Ergon Soc Ann Meet. 2017;61:648–648.

Hegde S, Wreathall J, Hettinger AZ, Fairbanks RJ, Wears RL, Bisantz AM. Towards the development of a resilience engineering tool to improve patient safety. Proc Hum Factors Ergon Soc Annu Meet. 2014;58:803–7.

Hegde S, Hettinger AZ, Fairbanks RJ, Wreathall J, Wears RL, Bisantz AM. Knowledge elicitation for resilience engineering in health care. Proc Hum Factors Ergon Soc Ann Meet. 2015;59:175–9.

Hettinger A, Fairbanks R, Hegde S, Rackoff AS, Wreathall J, Lewis VR, Bisantz AM, Wears RL. An evidence-based toolkit for the development of effective and sustainable root cause analysis system safety solutions. J Healthc Risk Manag. 2013;33:11–20.

Hettinger AZ, Roth EM, Bisantz AM. Cognitive engineering and health informatics: applications and intersections. J Biomed Inform. 2017;67:21–33.

Hettinger AZ, Ratwani R, Fairbanks RJ. New insights on safety and health IT; 2015. https://psnet.ahrq.gov/perspectives/perspective/181/new-insights-on-safety-and-health-it.

Hollnagel E, Wears R, Braithwaite J. From safety-I to safety-II: a white paper;2015. p. 1–32.

https://www.pewtrusts.org/-/media/assets/2018/08/healthit_safe_use_of_ehrs_report.pdf.

https://www.whitehouse.gov/briefing-room/presidential-actions/2023/10/30/executive-order-on-the-safe-secure-and-trustworthy-development-and-use-of-artificial-intelligence/.

Hu Y-Y, Arriaga AF, Roth EM, et al. Protecting patients from an unsafe system: the etiology and recovery of intraoperative deviations in care. Ann Surg. 2012;256:203–10.

John BE, Kieras DE. Using GOMS for user interface design and evaluation: which technique? ACM Trans Comput Interact. 1996;3:287–319.

Kirwan B, Ainsworth LK. A guide to task analysis. London: Taylor and Francis; 1992.

Klein GA, Calderwood R, MacGregor D. Critical decision method for eliciting knowledge. IEEE Trans Syst Man Cybern. 1989;19:462–72.

Lee J, Kirlik A, Dainoff M. The Oxford handbook of cognitive engineering; 2013.

Lee JD, Wickens CD, Liu Y, Boyle LN. Designing for people: an introduction to human factors engineering. CreateSpace Independent Publishing Platform;2017.

Lowry SZ, Ramaiah M, Patterson ES, Brick D, Gurses AP, Ozok A, Simmons D, Gibbons MC. Integrating electronic health records into clinical workflow. Proc Int Symp Hum Factors Ergon Heal Care. 2014;3:170–7.

McDonald KM, Su G, Lisker S, Patterson ES, Sarkar U. Implementation science for ambulatory care safety: a novel method to develop context-sensitive interventions to reduce quality gaps in monitoring high-risk patients. Implement Sci. 2017;12:79.

Militello LG, Arbuckle NB, Saleem JJ, Patterson E, Flanagan M, Haggstrom D, Doebbeling BN. Sources of variation in primary care clinical workflow: Implications for the design of cognitive support. Health Informatics J. 2014;20:35–49.

Molich R, Nielsen J. Improving a human-computer dialogue. Commun ACM. 1990;33:338–48.

Neilsen J. Usability engineering. Elsevier; 1994.

Nielsen J. 10 usability heuristics for user interface design; 1995. http://www.nngroup.com/articles/ten-usability-heuristics/.

Patterson ES, Rogers ML, Tomolo A, Wears RL, Tsevat J. Comparison of extent of use, information accuracy, and functions for manual and electronic patient status boards. Int J Med Inform. 2010;79:817–23.

Patterson MD, Militello LG, Bunger A, Taylor RG, Wheeler DS, Klein G, Geis GL. Leveraging the critical decision method to develop simulation-based training for early recognition of sepsis. J Cogn Eng Decis Mak. 2016;10:36–56.

Pennathur PR, Bisantz AM, Fairbanks R, Perry SJ, Zwemer FL, Wears RL. Assessing the impact of computerization on work practice: Information technology in emergency departments. In: Proceedings of human factors ergonomics society. 51st Annual Meeting. Baltimore, Maryland;2007. p. 377–81.

Pennathur PR, Cao C, Bisantz AM, Lin L, Fairbanks R, Wears RL, Perry SJ, Guarrera TK, Brown JL. Emergency department patient tracking system evaluation and situation awareness assessment. Int J Ind Erg. 2009.

Ratwani RM, Savage E, Will A, Arnold R, Khairat S, Miller K, Fairbanks RJ, Hodgkins M, Hettinger AZ. A usability and safety analysis of electronic health records: a multi-center study. J Am Med Inform Assoc. 2018;25(9):1197–201.

Roth E, Eggleston R. Forging new evaluation paradigms: beyond statistical generalization. In: Miller JE, Patterson ES, editors. Macrocognition Metrics Scenar. Ashgate; 2010. p. 204–19.

Roth E, Scott R, Deutsch S, Kuper S, Schmidt V, Stilson M, Wampler J. Evolvable work-centred support systems for command and control: creating systems users can adapt to meet changing demands. Ergonomics. 2006;49:688–705.

Roth E, Patterson E. Using observational study as a tool for discovery: uncovering cognitive and collaborative demands and adaptive strategies. In: 5th national decision making conference;2000.

Roth EM, Pritchett AR. Preface to the special issue on advancing models of human–automation interaction. J Cogn Eng Decis Mak. 2018;12:3–6.

Stanton NA. Hierarchical task analysis. In: Karwowski W, editors. International encyclopedia ergonomics human factors. CRC Press, Boca Raton, FL;2001. p. 3183–90.

Stanton N, Salmon P, Rafferty L, Walker G. Human factors methods: a practical guide for engineering and design; 2017.

Thrall JH, Li X, Li Q, Cruz C, Do S, Dreyer K, Brink J. Artificial intelligence and machine learning in radiology: opportunities, challenges, pitfalls, and criteria for success. J Am Coll Radiol. 2018;15(3):504–8.

Tiferes J, Hussein AA, Bisantz A, Kozlowski JD, Sharif MA, Winder NM, Ahmad N, Allers J, Cavuoto L, Guru KA. The loud surgeon behind the console: understanding team activities during robot-assisted surgery. J Surg Educ. 2016;73:504–12.

Tiferes J, Hussein AA, Bisantz A, Higginbotham DJ, Sharif M, Kozlowski J, Ahmad B, O'Hara R, Wawrzyniak N, Guru K. Are gestures worth a thousand words? Verbal and nonverbal communication during robot-assisted surgery. Appl Ergon. 2018; https://doi.org/10.1016/J.APERGO.2018.02.015.

Tolley CL, Forde NE, Coffey KL, Sittig DF, Ash JS, Husband AK, Bates DW, Slight SP. Factors contributing to medication errors made when using computerized order entry in pediatrics: a systematic review. J Am Med Informatics Assoc. 2017. https://doi.org/10.1093/jamia/ocx124.

Truxler R, Roth E, Scott R, Smith S, Wampler J. Designing collaborative automated planners for agile adaptation to dynamic change. Proc Hum Factors Ergon Soc Ann Meet. 2012;56:223–7.

Wears RL. "Just a few seconds of your time…" at least 130 million times a year. Ann Emerg Med. 2015;65:687–9.

Wears RL, Berg M. Computer technology and clinical work: still waiting for Godot. JAMA. 2005;293:1261–3.

Wears RL, Perry SJ, Wilson S, Galliers J, Fone J. Emergency department status boards: user-evolved artefacts for inter- and intra-group coordination. Cogn Technol Work. 2007b;9:163–70.

Wears RL, Fairbanks R, Perry SJ, Bisantz AM, Pennathur P, Zwemer FL. Safety implications of computerizing the ED status board. Am Coll Emerg Physicians Res Forum. 2007a.

Woods DD. Steering the reverberations of technology change on fields of practice: laws that govern cognitive work;2002. p. 14.

Wright A, McCoy AB, Hickman TT, Hilaire DS, Borbolla D, Bowes WA III, Dixon WG, Dorr DA, Krall M, Malholtra S, Bates DW. Problem list completeness in electronic health records: a multi-site study and assessment of success factors. Int J Med Inform. 2015;84(10):784–90.

Xiao Y. Artifacts and collaborative work in healthcare: methodological, theoretical, and technological implications of the tangible. J Biomed Inform. 2005;38:26–33.

Xiao Y, Schenkel S, Faraj S, Mackenzie CF, Moss J. What whiteboards in a trauma center operating suite can teach us about emergency department communication. Ann Emerg Med. 2007;50:387–95.

Xiao T, Sanderson P, Clayton S, Venkatesh B. The ETTO principle and organisational strategies: a field study of ICU bed and staff management. Cogn Technol Work. 2010;12:143–52.

Xiao Y, Fairbanks RJ (Terry), Gurses AP, Nemeth C, Roth E, Wears RL, Gorman DP. User created cognitive artifacts: what can they teach us about design of information technology? Proc Hum Factors Ergon Soc Ann Meet. 2009;53:694–8.

Zahabi M, Kaber DB, Swangnetr M. Usability and safety in electronic medical records interface design: a review of recent literature and guideline formulation. Hum Fact. 2015a;57:805–34.

Zahabi M, Kaber DB, Swangnetr M. Usability and safety in electronic medical records interface design: a review of recent literature and guideline formulation. Hum Factors J Hum Factors Ergon Soc. 2015b. https://doi.org/10.1177/0018720815576827.

Zhou L, Blackley SV, Kowalski L, Doan R, Acker WW, Landman AB, Kontrient E, Mack D, Meteer M, Bates DW, Goss FR. Analysis of errors in dictated clinical documents assisted by speech recognition software and professional transcriptionists. JAMA Netw Open. 2018;1(3):e180530.

Chapter 15
Using Electronic Health Record Metadata to Understand Clinician Work and Behavior

A. Jay Holmgren, Bryan Steitz, Sunny Lou, and Nate Apathy

15.1 Introduction

Electronic health record (EHR) data have become an incredibly valuable resource for researchers, health systems, and policymakers seeking to generate and understand real-world evidence in clinical care delivery. As EHRs have become ubiquitous, Adler-Milstein et al. (2017), Apathy et al. (2021) and clinical work is increasingly centered around the EHR, the use of clinical data to fuel research, operational insights, and health system decision-making has rapidly increased (Weiskopf and Weng 2013). While the utility of clinical data stored in the EHR, ranging from patient vital signs to medication orders and documentation stored in both structured and free-text clinical notes is broadly recognized, another type of data derived from the electronic health record remains under-valued: metadata derived from EHR audit logs.

EHR audit logs, also known as activity or event logs, are metadata: data about data. EHR audit logs are generated as a byproduct of normal EHR use, and keep a granular tracking of every interaction that every user has with the EHR, including details such as what user (e.g., a specific physician, nurse, administrator, medical assistant), what action (e.g., signing a note, ordering a medication, messaging a patient or another member of the care team), what time, for what patient, and more. EHR audit logs

A. Jay Holmgren (✉)
UC San Francisco, San Francisco, CA, USA
e-mail: A.Holmgren@ucsf.edu

B. Steitz
Vanderbilt University, Nashville, TN, USA

S. Lou
Washington University, St. Louis, MO, USA

N. Apathy
University of Maryland, College Park, MD, USA

© The Author(s), under exclusive license to Springer Nature Switzerland AG 2025
K. Zheng et al. (eds.), *Reengineering Clinical Workflow in the Digital and AI Era*,
Cognitive Informatics in Biomedicine and Healthcare,
https://doi.org/10.1007/978-3-031-82971-0_15

have been referred to as a potential "gold mine" for researchers for obvious reasons—they allow accurate, precise measurement of clinical work at scale, a feat that would have been either impossible or prohibitively expensive using standard data collection methodologies such as time-and-motion studies (Adler-Milstein et al. 2020a). While research on EHR audit logs has grown rapidly over the last several years, Rule et al. (2023b) there are a number of important lessons learned, limitations, and best practices for practitioners and researchers as they navigate this new data source. This chapter will outline what audit logs are and how to operationalize them to generate useful insights about clinical work and care delivery, highlight the existing contributions of audit log research, discuss practical considerations of using audit log data for research and operational purposes, and outline future directions for research using EHR audit logs.

15.2   An Introduction to EHR Audit Logs

Why does the EHR audit log exist, what does it look like, and how is it different from other EHR data?

The original purpose of EHR audit logs in the United States, was not to serve as a data source to fuel research or generate operational insights. Rather, audit logs are required as part of the Health Information Technology Certification Program operated by the Office of the National Coordinator for Health Information Technology (ONC) and the Centers for Medicare and Medicaid Services (CMS) to ensure the EHR can meet the requirements for various incentive programs like the Meaningful Use EHR Incentive Program, Promoting Interoperability (PI), and Merit-Based Incentive Payment System (MIPS). The primary goal of the audit log requirement is HIPAA compliant security: to ensure that unauthorized access to protected health information (PHI) can be fully investigated. Knowing the origin of audit logs, and their original use case for security and compliance purposes, is critical to understanding many of the complexities and nuances of working with audit logs: researchers and operational leaders are repurposing the data for a secondary, non-intended use. While audit logs are a rich and valuable data source, they are not without limitations.

While the specific data elements of audit logs vary across EHR systems, they all have several core data elements that all audit logs are required to contain. Put simply, audit logs are time- and user-stamped logs of most, if not all, events that occur within the EHR. User actions that view, modify, or remove data within the EHR are nearly always accompanied by an audit log event due to the EHR certification requirements. Many other log events, not strictly required by the audit log certification criteria, are common across EHR vendor systems. These may include: navigation within the EHR, such as moving between different sections of the user interface; and keystroke actions as users input data, receive and interact with decision support alerts, and more. While often referred to as "event logs", these also fall within the scope of the colloquial use of the term "audit log data." In short, audit logs show a set of discrete user interactions with the EHR over time, often at a very granular level. In practice, audit logs are therefore primarily "user centric:" they begin with the start of the user's EHR session for that day and stop at the end of the session and are often analyzed at the user level. Users are most often a clinician or other employee of the care delivery organization but can also be patients when event log data exists for patient interactions with their EHR-tethered portal.

Given the vast number of activities that a user in the EHR performs each day that generate an audit log event, "raw" audit log data are often messy, complex, and difficult to work with. The majority of audit log analyses therefore aggregates these actions into higher-level categories or measures germane to the project or research question. Common aggregations include time spent in the EHR, and the distribution of that time across clinical functions such as documenting notes, performing chart review, placing orders, or messaging within the electronic inbox. Other common aggregations include measuring discrete tasks, such as the number of orders placed in each encounter or messages sent per day. Because audit logs track how each user interacts with the system, they can also be used to estimate how clinical users collaborate on EHR-based tasks, such as identifying orders placed by a physician that were created and pended by another member of the care team, or inbox messages addressed to clinicians but handled by administrative staff. Much of the work involved in projects using audit log measures for research is therefore in the development and validation of measures that are more interpretable and clinically meaningful than the raw data captured in the audit log.

Equally important to defining audit log data is to define what they are not—specifically, clinical data stored within the EHR. For example, entering data within a structured field would generate an audit log event, and the user, context, and time of that data entry would be data contained within an audit log. The specific content of that data, such as patient vital signs, smoking status, HbA1c level, etc. is *not* part of the audit log, but rather clinical data stored within the EHR. While these data can often be linked, such as studies examining the association between primary care physicians EHR activities and their panel-level quality measures, Rotenstein et al. (2022b) they are conceptually distinct. The user-centricity of audit logs is also in contrast to the majority of clinical data stored in the EHR, which is often centered on a single clinical encounter or a longitudinal set of encounters for a specific patient, rather than the EHR user or clinician. While clinical EHR data represent another important resource for understanding health care delivery at scale, they are outside of the scope of the audit log, which is reserved for user-level metadata tracking EHR actions.

Types of EHR Audit Log Data

Audit log data can take several forms, which vary primarily in their level of granularity and linkability to other sources like clinical EHR data. We describe here three key types of audit log data: active use logs, audit logs, and domain-specific event logs (Rule et al. 2023a). ***Active use logs*** are the least granular and most readily available data. These data capture aggregated measures of user activity over a given period of time, usually a week or a month. This form of audit log data is referred to as "active use log" data because it records measures of "active" EHR system use by a given user over a period of time. These data are compiled by EHR vendors via real-time tracking of keystrokes, mouse movement, and clicks, and uses heuristics and rules to identify "active" vs. "inactive" system use. These tracking methods use a stopwatch-like cumulative time counting function to track and aggregate active time. For example, Epic Systems Corp, a major US EHR vendor, Holmgren and Apathy (2023) starts the stopwatch for a user as soon as they log in, and as long as users register a keystroke or mouse movement or click within 5 s, the stopwatch continues to count. After 5 s of inactivity, the stopwatch is paused until the next keystroke, mouse movement, or click is observed, which resumes the stopwatch. The data capturing keystrokes, mouse movements, and clicks are discarded by vendors after active use time has been measured, because these data are prohibitively large to store, but the aggregated active use time data are preserved and constructed into numerous measures of EHR use.

Active use log data are recorded for all EHR use, but operational leaders are often interested in not only total active time but also active time spent in different domains of the EHR (e.g., in the inbox or writing clinical notes) and at specific times (e.g., after clinic hours or on days off). As a result, active use log data provided by vendors typically divides up activity into common domains of EHR work. For example, Cerner's Advance platform measures overall active use time and divides active time into categories of Notes, Orders, Chart Review, and Other. Epic's Signal platform includes active use time measures for Notes, Orders, Clinical Review (analogous to Chart Review), and InBasket (the clinician inbox), among others. Active use log data sources also often include a measure of "after-hours" EHR use time, usually defined as active time during a fixed window of time (e.g., 7 p.m. to 7 a.m.) or relative to when the clinician is scheduled to work during the day. For example, Epic's Signal counts all active EHR time outside of 30 min prior to a clinician's first scheduled appointment and 30 min after their last appointment as "time outside scheduled hours" (Baxter et al. 2021).

The most readily available active use log data to health care organizations are typically downloadable from vendor-provided analytics platforms like Epic's Signal or Cerner's Advance. These exports provide aggregated measures at the user-month or user-week level, however other more granular exports of active use log are also available from major vendors. These more granular exports aggregate active use log data into much smaller increments of time, in some cases 15-min or one-hour blocks. These data provide a much more precise account of when users were actively using the EHR, and for how long they were active in the system. These tools often also break out active use time by EHR work domain, as noted above. For example, Epic's User Activity Log (UAL) Lite would illustrate for how many minutes a given physician was actively typing clinical notes between 8:00 a.m. and 8:15 a.m. on a specific day. This more granular active use log data are of course far larger than user-week or user-month exports, making it more challenging to manage and analyze and more expensive to store.

A second form of audit log data, and the data at the core of audit log research, is simply called ***audit logs***. This data is distinct from active use log data in that it does not measure the duration of time spent actively using the EHR, but rather audit logs record discrete *events* that occur during the use of EHRs (Rule et al. 2020). Audit logs are—as their name implies—chiefly used for auditing purposes, specifically to ascertain who accessed a given patient chart or performed a given action in a patient chart at what time. This use of audit logs is used to support investigations into things like inappropriate chart access. For example, if a celebrity or head of state is admitted to a hospital, it is important to ensure that no one inappropriately accesses their chart. Audit logs are the source of truth in any such investigations into HIPAA violations like inappropriate chart access; because of this important role, EHR vendors are required to maintain audit logs and preserve them for up to five years.

Audit logs include records for every auditable event that takes place in the EHR, particularly viewing, modifying, or removing any data. EHR system activity generates thousands of auditable events, that can include (but are not limited to) logging in, opening a patient chart, opening a section (e.g., laboratory results) within a chart, responding to a clinical decision alert, recording vital signs, submitting an order, and signing a clinical note. The set of events that are "auditable" is configurable by each organization, and most vendors have a standard set of auditable events that are configured by default. There are two basic components that are required to generate an "auditable event" that appears in audit logs. First, there must be a discrete, observable action that requires user interaction with the EHR (there are system-generated auditable events, but given our focus on user behavior, we focus here on user-generated auditable events). The second component is an "event handler," which is software analogous to a sensor that is configured to recognize and record whenever a given event occurs (Rule et al. 2023a). Importantly, this means that discrete user actions do not appear in audit logs if they do not have event handlers configured to record the action. This leads to a square/rectangle situation: all user-generated events recorded in audit logs represent some type of user action, but not all user actions are recorded in audit logs. Audit logs therefore allow researchers to granularly measure clinician behavior at scale previously impossible, but are not without their own set of limitations that may vary depending on the exact type of audit log data used.

Once all auditable events are compiled into the audit logs, the data resembles the structure in Table 15.1, with each observation representing one auditable event (Rule et al. 2020). Audit logs, at a minimum, will include a timestamp for the time the event was logged, an identifier for the user that performed the action that generated the event, a descriptor or identifier for the specific action that is being logged, and the patient record on which the action was taken (if applicable; many auditable EHR actions take place outside of the context of a single patient's chart, e.g., reviewing a schedule or rooming list). Modern audit logs frequently include far more data than the bare minimum, and often feature additional variables like encounter identifiers, patient room and/or unit information, additional information about the user (e.g., role or specialty), information to link the audit logs to clinical EHR data (e.g., order identifiers for specific orders being placed), and even IP addresses of devices being used.

Finally, ***domain-specific event logs*** are a third form of EHR audit log data that record discrete events much like audit logs, but capture activity that does not get

Table 15.1 EHR audit log example structure

User	Time	Patient record	Action	Location
Physician 1	01/01/2024 04:06:35	16,784,124	View note	Clinic 4 Computer 7
Physician 1	01/01/2024 04:07:31	16,784,124	View problem list	Clinic 4 Computer 7
Physician 1	01/01/2024 04:09:01	17,216,891	View patient summary	Clinic 4 Computer 7
Nurse 1	01/01/2024 05:15:12	17,324,561	View flowsheet	Floor 2 Computer 1
Nurse 1	01/01/2024 05:15:15	17,324,561	Edit flowsheet	Floor 2 Computer 1
Physician 2	01/01/2024 07:26:56	12,354,789	Edit note	Clinic 3 Computer 4
Physician 2	01/01/2024 07:27:01	12,354,789	Sign note	Clinic 3 Computer 4
Physician 2	01/01/2024 07:27:58	24,963,410	View problem list	Clinic 3 Computer 4

recorded in the standard audit log data described above. These data are at a similar level of granularity as audit log data, in that each observation represents a discrete event, but domain-specific event logs often capture events that are not individual user interactions with the EHR. A frequently used example of domain-specific event logs are logs that capture information about the firing and responses to clinical decision support alerts. The type, detail, and granularity of domain-specific event log data captured will vary widely across EHR vendors and individual organizations depending on their specific configuration, in part because these logs are not explicitly required or in any way regulated by ONC and CMS. These types of domain-specific event logs are often created to track a specific operational purpose, such as ensuring that interruptive alerts are not firing too frequently or for the wrong patients.

15.3 Existing Research Using EHR Audit Logs

While audit logs remain a relatively new data source, the number of studies published using audit log data has increased dramatically from fewer than 10 articles per year in 2016 to over 50 in 2021. (Rule et al. 2023b) Rather than a comprehensive literature review, this section provides a high-level overview of published research using audit log data to illustrate common use cases and describe the current state of the field.

Studying Clinician Work with EHR Audit Logs

Given the previously discussed user-centricity of EHR audit logs, and their granular tracking of EHR actions by primarily clinical users, it is unsurprising that the most common use case for audit log data has been the study of clinicians and clinical work. The most obvious use case is studying the amount of time clinicians spend working in the EHR, which has gained particular salience in light of growing concerns over

EHR-driven physician burnout (Adler-Milstein et al. 2020b; Tai-Seale et al. 2023). As a result, a number of studies have quantified the amount of time physicians spend in the EHR across specialties (Overhage and McCallie 2020; Rotenstein et al. 2021), US states (Holmgren et al. 2022b), physician gender (Rotenstein et al. 2022a; Rule et al. 2023c), national health systems (Downing et al. 2018; Holmgren et al. 2020), over time following the onset of the COVID-19 pandemic (Holmgren et al. 2022a; Tsai et al. 2022), and in response to federal reimbursement policy changes (Apathy et al. 2022a; Maisel et al. 2023). Measures often include overall EHR time, EHR time by function, and whether the time was spent during or outside of clinic hours.

Beyond quantifying time spent in the EHR, studies have used audit log data to provide insights into how documentation tools can improve efficiency (Apathy et al. 2022b), the role of organizations in shaping how physicians use the EHR (Cross et al. 2024), the impact of mandatory patient access to clinical notes on physician documentation practices (Holmgren and Apathy 2022), the use of novel EHR features such as secure messaging (Baratta et al. 2023), dashboards to visualize social determinants of health (Wang et al. 2021), or integrated interoperable data exchange (Adler-Milstein and Wang 2020), and to describe differences in EHR use between in-person and virtual telemedicine care (Holmgren et al. 2023b). Due to the granularity of audit log data, it has also been used to identify specific workflows within the EHR (Perros et al. 2020; Chen et al. 2021; Lou et al. 2023b) and to measure the association between these patterns of EHR use and clinician-focused outcomes such as work efficiency (Akbar et al. 2021; Gong et al. 2021). Understanding how clinicians use and interact with the electronic health record is one of the most common use cases for audit log data.

Because so much of clinical work now occurs within the EHR, audit log data has also been used to measure clinical workload more broadly. For example, audit log data has been used to automatically classify work responsibilities for clinicians with multiple roles (Kim et al. 2023), identify work shift boundaries (Dziorny et al. 2019; Moy et al. 2023), track work hours (Shine et al. 2010; Soleimani et al. 2021), and measure the association between work hours and patient outcomes (Ouyang et al. 2016). Patient load has also been measured using audit log data; at the simplest level, this can be approximated using the number of patients with notes or orders (Lou et al. 2022b), but more advanced methods have been developed to handle patient attribution for team-based supervision models (Mai et al. 2020). These measures are particularly useful in the inpatient setting where clinical workload and work hours cannot be easily determined from a clinic schedule like they can in the outpatient setting.

Audit logs have been used to investigate the relationship between EHR use, clinical workload, and a number of outcomes related to clinician wellness, quality, efficiency, and patient safety, and the quality of care. For example, researchers have used audit logs to investigate how different EHR functions are associated with quality of care (Rotenstein et al. 2022b), understand the drivers of the gender pay gap in medicine (Ganguli et al. 2020; Li et al. 2023), measure the relationship between clinical workload and burnout (Adler-Milstein et al. 2020b; Lou et al. 2022c; Tai-Seale et al. 2023) or reimbursement (Lou et al. 2023a) and illustrate how clinician attention resulting from additional EHR burden switching can lead to patient safety errors (Lou et al. 2022a). Other studies have used audit logs to measure concepts outside of the EHR that are otherwise difficult to observe empirically at scale, such as team formation and collaboration (Chen et al. 2019), and the impact of care team experience on health outcomes in clinical settings such as stroke care (Rose et al. 2022). While still a nascent field, EHR audit log research has already made important contributions to clinical, health policy, informatics, and health services research literature.

Understanding Patient Behavior with EHR Audit Logs

Similar to how audit logs detailing health care worker and clinician use of the EHR, patient portals and other consumer-facing health information systems also document audit logs of user interaction. Data detailing access and use of these systems have contributed to a growing literature on how patients and caregivers interact with their health data and remotely with the healthcare system. Patients most commonly access their health data and patient-facing health resources via patient portal, and the sequences of accessed data and resources are captured in the patient portal audit log. Alternatively, a growing number of patients choose to link their portal with third-party applications such as Apple's Health platform (Barker and Richwine 2023). When users access their health data using third-party applications, the portal audit log records when data are accessed or downloaded. However, the specific ways in which users interact with data within third-party applications are not typically captured within the portal audit log. While it is important to understand how patients apply third-party applications to review and interact with their health data, this is a relatively new area of inquiry that is not well covered in the audit log literature.

A breadth of early work has used audit logs to understand how patients and their caregivers access and use the portal to manage their care and interact with the health care system. These studies primarily relied on researcher-derived metrics about access to core portal functionality, such as messaging with the care team, accessing test results, or managing appointments (Steitz et al. 2019). A number of studies have quantified portal use across diverse practice settings and patient populations to understand patterns of adoption and sustained use, including patients managing chronic diseases (Apter et al. 2020; Gleason et al. 2023), children and adolescents (Steitz et al. 2017; Szilagyi et al. 2020), older adults, Gleason et al. (2023) disadvantaged populations (Ancker et al. 2011; Perzynski et al. 2017), and hospitalized patients (Robinson et al. 2017; Fareed et al. 2019). Researchers have used audit logs to study the relationship between portal use and numerous health, utilization, and satisfaction outcomes (Lyles et al. 2016; Graetz et al. 2020; Fareed et al. 2022; Bell et al. 2024).

Recent external factors, including the COVID-19 pandemic and the 21st Century Cures Act, have sparked widespread portal adoption and a new wave of portal-related audit log research. During the COVID-19 pandemic, audit log data were used to evaluate new workflows and approaches to virtual care, including patient use of telehealth (Patel et al. 2020) and self-triage tools (Judson et al. 2020; Lai et al. 2020), while other studies evaluated the impact of the pandemic onset on levels of patient-initiated message volume (Nath et al. 2021; Holmgren et al. 2022a) and how patient messaging behavior changed in response to health systems starting to bill patients for portal messages (Holmgren et al. 2023a). Researchers have also widely applied audit logs to investigate the impact of regulatory decisions on portal use and patient and provider workflows. For example, when health care organizations began releasing electronic health information to the patient portal immediately upon its availability to providers, a number of research studies applied audit logs to investigate the impact of test result availability (Steitz et al. 2021), patient access to visit notes (Sangal et al. 2021), and patient notification settings on patient access to health data (Steitz et al. 2023). Moreover, several studies have incorporated metrics derived from both patient portal audit logs and EHR audit logs to measure how patient access to their health data impacts clinician workload, such as through clinical messages (Steitz et al. 2021; Holmgren and Apathy 2022; Steitz et al. 2023). Combining audit logs across multiple clinical systems offers considerable opportunity to better understand the complex relationship between use of patient-engaging technologies and clinical work. Future research should continue to explore what can be learned from audit log data about how patients navigate the health care system, interact with the patient portal, and consume health care information.

15.4 Practical Considerations for Audit Log Research

EHR audit logs represent an exciting new source of data for researchers and operational leaders to generate new insights into clinician and patient behavior. Due to the relative nascence of the field, however, there are few published guidelines regarding the use of audit log data. In this section, we highlight several common questions and concerns regarding audit log data and provide recommendations for practitioners interested in using EHR audit log data in their own work.

Common Types of Audit Log Data: Investigator and Vendor-Derived Measures

Perhaps the most salient decision for researchers as they begin to consider a project using audit log data is whether to rely on vendor-derived measures, such as Epic's Signal or Cerner's Advance, or build their own custom measures. Each data source has a set of strengths and weaknesses to balance across an array of factors. While this section will not represent a comprehensive discussion of the trade-offs between investigator-derived and vendor-derived audit log data, as the details of each data source will vary across EHR vendors and health systems, we will discuss high-level considerations of each data source in research and operations.

15.4.1 Investigator-Derived Measures

Early EHR audit log research, especially studies published prior to 2019, were conducted almost entirely using what are often called "investigator-derived measures" (Rule et al. 2023b). These measures are constructed from either active use logs, audit logs, and domain-specific logs, or a combination thereof, usually for a specific research question or project. This category also includes measures developed for operational purposes that may be repurposed for research. The defining characteristic of these measures is that they are developed in a bespoke way to address a particular research question or operational purpose, making them distinct from the more "general purpose" vendor-derived measures. The primary strength of investigator-derived measures is that they afford researchers and operational leaders a large degree of freedom and control over how they are constructed, limited only by the availability of data in the user action or audit logs and the investment required to construct the measures. For example, if an investigator is interested in the relationship between telemedicine use and patient portal messaging at the clinician level, they can build a custom dataset that enables them to specify both of those variables in any way they wish—including both video or audio-only visits as telemedicine, measuring patient portal messages both direct to the clinician and to shared pools, adjust the time period of interest (e.g., specifying at the encounter, clinician-day, clinician-week, clinician-month level, etc.), and otherwise exert a large degree of control over the construction of their measures that vendor-derived measures are unable to offer.

However, there are several important limitations to investigator-derived measures that help to explain their relatively low prevalence in published EHR audit log data research following the broad availability of vendor-derived measures (Rule et al. 2023b). First, investigator-derived measures are necessarily much more resource intensive to use. They often require skilled data and software engineers with extensive backgrounds in both database programming and the specific data models used by the EHR product in order to turn complex, messy raw audit logs into a dataset for analysis. Second, beyond the cost of constructing the data, they require investigators to make many decisions regarding the specific definition and construction of each measure, many of which lack published guidance. This makes comparing studies performed at different institutions challenging—even when they examine similar phenomena—due to small differences in how measures are defined. This also limits replicability, especially when the dataset creation code that explicates these design choices is challenging to share publicly because it contains references to EHR vendors proprietary data models. For example, most measures of active use time have a "time-out" period, wherein after a certain amount of time following the last recorded action, time stops counting. Differences in the choice of time-out period have a large impact on overall measures of time (Magon et al. 2024), and decisions about which audit log actions "count" to withhold a time-out are often undocumented or not mentioned in published articles, making it challenging to perfectly replicate the study with only the scientific publication. Finally, investigator-derived measures are challenging to scale. Even institutions using the same EHR vendor platform often have dramatically different site-level customizations (recall the configuration of event handlers from earlier), and some institutions give researchers more access to audit log measures than others, meaning that even two sites using the same EHR vendor may not be able to generate the exact same measures.

15.4.2 Vendor-Derived Measures

Much of the recent growth in EHR audit log research has been driven by the rapid increase in the availability of vendor-derived EHR audit log data (Rule et al. 2023b). These vendor-derived measures are frequently extracted from metadata aggregation platforms provided by the two largest EHR vendors in the United States: Epic's Signal and Cerner's Advance (Holmgren and Apathy 2023). Both Signal and Advance are tools designed primarily for operational purposes and feature interactive, graphical front-end interfaces that allow users to compare their own EHR use measures to national or organizational benchmarks. These systems also allow users to download the raw data, often aggregated to the user-week or user-month level, and frequently store data over time, enabling researchers to analyze data cross-sectionally or longitudinally, and link it to other relevant datasets such as clinical quality, productivity, and others. They are significantly more "ready to use" than investigator-derived measures, which require a significant amount of up-front investment to create an analysis-worthy dataset.

EHR metadata from these platforms have several attractive properties. First, the ease of extracting the data dramatically reduces the cost of EHR audit log research, which allows researchers and operational leaders without external funding or significant organizational commitment to answer important questions quickly and without a large project budget. Second, because the metrics are standardized by the EHR vendor, there are fewer difficult decisions around how to define and construct specific measures (e.g., how much after the last recorded event should pass before a user is no longer considered "actively using" the EHR). Third, because these platforms are broadly available from the largest EHR vendors, using vendor-derived measures greatly streamlines aggregating data from multiple institutions using the same EHR vendor platform. Finally, vendor-derived platforms were developed with significant internal expertise and data access that investigator-derived measures are unable to replicate. For example, Epic Signal's "active use" definition that includes all mouse and keystroke movement, is effectively impossible to replicate using the audit log data available to researchers even when combining data from multiple sources.

However, compared to investigator-derived measures described above, vendor-derived measures also have important limitations. The most salient difference is that the variables included, the details of measurement, and the inclusion and exclusion criteria are constrained by vendor decisions rather than researcher decisions. Epic's Signal platform, for instance, has a 5 s timeout and includes only clinicians with a minimum number of scheduled visits in the reporting period, both of which are non-modifiable design choices. Other metrics may also be limited: for example, Signal only counts patient-initiated medical advice request messages received directly by the focal user, making it difficult to measure the number of messages received in shared inbox pools that were pertinent to the focal user but addressed by another user. Users without scheduled visits are not included in the ambulatory form of Signal at all, making it impossible to measure EHR use for clinicians other than physicians and advance practice providers with scheduled visits. Similarly, Signal and Cerner's Advance have historically been focused on ambulatory care clinicians, especially Epic's Signal platform, with relatively new inpatient platforms that have to-date been limited in their use for research.

15.4.3 Choosing the Right Set of Measures

Both investigator and vendor-derived measures have strengths and weaknesses, as described above. Investigators should carefully consider these as they make decisions on what measures they should use for any given project. Many of these decisions will be constrained by the reality of research design, including the availability of funding, which may limit the ability of investigators to devote time and resources to building their own set of custom measures. Similarly, if a researcher is seeking to understand a component of EHR use that is not present in vendor-derived measures or study a population that is not captured by those vendor platforms, constructing bespoke measures may be a necessity. Another consideration is whether the research is intended to be portable to other sites, and what EHR vendor those sites use. Research or operational projects that rely solely on vendor-derived measures can be rapidly ported to other sites using the same EHR vendor, while collaborations across vendors will likely require significant harmonization of data and analytic code regardless of whether the measures were vendor or investigator-derived. Overall, researchers and operational leaders considering using vendor or investigator-derived measures should carefully weigh the trade-offs between the two data sources for each specific project or research question.

Normalizing Audit Log Measures Across Users

One of the most common challenges that researchers face in using EHR audit log data is how to normalize measures across a diverse set of clinical users with different clinical workloads. Often, researchers or operational leaders will want to compare measures such as time spent in the EHR during or outside of clinic hours, the number of messages received, or time in specific EHR functions across clinicians in their organization. However, comparing non-normalized numbers can be deceiving if clinicians have different levels of clinical effort: 20 h per week in the EHR may be reasonable for a full-time clinician seeing patients for 32 h per week, but unreasonably long for a physician with only 20% clinical effort who only dedicates 8 h per week to seeing patients. This has led many researchers to seek a denominator to normalize EHR use measures across clinicians, the two most common of which are *per encounter* (for ambulatory care clinicians) and *per patient-scheduled time*. The former simply normalizes whatever measure by the number of ambulatory encounters during that time period (e.g., if a user has 1 h of EHR time and 4 encounters in a day, they would have a value of 15 min per encounter), whereas the latter uses scheduled patient care hours, often normalized to 8 patient-scheduled hours to facilitate an interpretation similar to an 8 h work-day (Sinsky et al. 2020). These normalizations enable a "one glance" comparison of EHR use measures across a range of clinical workloads and are likely to be more intuitive and interpretable for non-experts than raw values over a week or month. Other studies forego this normalization in measure construction and instead choose to use multi-variable regression models that include a control variable for clinical workload, either scheduled patient care hours or number of encounters, to facilitate a *ceteris paribus* comparison of EHR use measures across clinicians. While existing studies have made extensive use of these two normalizations, and they have many attractive properties for presenting EHR use data, researchers should carefully consider what normalization—if any—is appropriate for their particular study.

There are several considerations for what normalization to use in any study using EHR audit log data. First, and perhaps most critically, is whether changes in the denominator could confound the parameter of interest. For example, many health systems have employed scribes to assist physicians with documentation and reduce EHR time and may wish to use EHR audit log data to evaluate how effective the program has been. At the same time, many care delivery organizations require physicians to increase their clinical productivity to receive a scribe, thereby increasing the number of encounters over a given period, meaning that the intervention (in this case a scribe) is likely to impact both the numerator (EHR time), and the denominator (number of visits). If a researcher were to normalize by EHR time per visit and perform an evaluation, their results may under-state time savings as both the numerator and denominator change simultaneously. Second, it is important to note that while these normalizations theoretically allow comparisons across clinicians with very different clinical workloads, the normative interpretation of each unit of EHR use may be different across those users. A full-time clinician with a 100% clinical effort may find any EHR time outside of scheduled patient-care hours especially burdensome because that time necessarily cuts into personal time away from work, while a clinician with 20% clinical effort may find that while EHR time outside of their patient scheduled hours eats into their time for research or administration, it does not negatively impact their well-being in the same way. Finally, it may be that the parameter of interest to an investigator is *related* to these differences in clinical effort—many studies of health care find that clinicians who perform a procedure frequently are more efficient and provide better quality of care than clinicians who perform the same procedure less frequently (Joynt et al. 2013). Researchers may be interested in exploring differences in EHR efficiency and use across different clinical workloads, in which case they should carefully consider how they normalize to avoid introducing potential confounders or biasing their results.

Overall, investigators should carefully think through their specific research question, the key outcomes and interventions of interest, and how they may impact both EHR use and any potential denominator before deciding how to normalize their variables. Researchers can avoid these pitfalls by using descriptive statistics: data visualization to assess movement in both the numerator and denominator separately over time is strongly recommended for any longitudinal study to assess where changes in normalized measures result from, as well as evaluating their outcomes non-normalized and with different normalizations to understand whether the decision to normalize impacts the key outcome measures of interest. Given the close relationship between EHR use and clinical volume, especially in ambulatory care delivery, any researcher using audit log data to investigate EHR use should be especially careful in choosing how and when to normalize their data.

15.5   Future Directions in EHR Audit Log Research

Despite the rapid increase in published articles using audit log data since 2019, the field is still in its infancy. As the use of audit log data in research matures, it must continue to develop and grow as it addresses novel questions in new ways. First, audit log data must expand its set of measures. While existing studies have quantified time in the EHR, or specific EHR actions such as messaging, decision support use, or documentation, these only scratch the surface of what we can understand about clinician and patient behavior from audit logs. For example, audit logs can be used to measure and quantify phenomenon such as team formation and stability (Rose et al. 2022), which may enable more rapid cycle, real-time evaluations of team performance. Recent work has also pioneered going beyond the burden of EHR time to measuring clinician cognitive load using audit logs (Bartek et al. 2023), which holds significant promise for identifying when clinicians are tired, burnt out, or exhausted in a way that impairs their decision-making and reduces quality of care. These are just two examples of how using EHR audit log data can enable investigators to quantify and measure critical concepts in health care delivery through the digital footprints of audit logs, and researchers should continue to refine these concepts and develop new measures of theoretically important constructs that are measurable via the audit log.

Beyond building new sets of measures constructed from EHR audit log data, researchers should also expand the set of methods and study designs they employ in their work. Currently, many audit log studies use simple descriptive study designs, or report associations between important measures like EHR time and quality of care. While quantifying and describing EHR use patterns is a critical contribution, and measuring EHR work overtime continues to be a worthwhile and important research agenda, many of the questions researchers wish to answer with audit log data are fundamentally causal, such as the impact of different team structures on clinician productivity and EHR burden, or the relationship between patient-initiated messaging and clinical decision-making and patient outcomes. While these questions are unlikely to be amenable to randomized trials, audit log researchers should employ causal inference research designs developed in statistics and econometrics, such as difference-in-differences, regression discontinuity, or instrumental variables to identify causal effects from observational data (Angrist and Pischke 2008). Further, continued advances in machine learning may also contribute to audit log research for research questions involving prediction, such as understanding when clinicians are most likely to make mistakes given their EHR use behaviors (Mullainathan and Obermeyer 2022). Continuing to incorporate new research designs and state of the art statistical analysis is critical to ensuring audit log research is actionable and robust.

15.6   Conclusion

The digitization of health care delivery through ubiquitous adoption of electronic health records has unlocked a wealth of newly accessible data, including data on EHR use itself recorded in the audit log. While audit log data comes in many forms, and can be challenging and complex to work with, it has enabled investigators to understand clinician and patient behavior at a scale impossible in the paper charting era. Future researchers should incorporate lessons learned from existing work and continue to push the envelope of what we can learn from the digital trails of EHR audit logs.

References

Adler-Milstein J, Wang MD. The impact of transitioning from availability of outside records within electronic health records to integration of local and outside records within electronic health records. J Am Med Inform Assoc. 2020;27(4):606–12. https://doi.org/10.1093/jamia/ocaa006.

Adler-Milstein J, Holmgren AJ, Kralovec P, Worzala C, Searcy T, Patel V. Electronic health record adoption in US hospitals: the emergence of a digital "advanced use" divide. J Am Med Inform Assoc. 2017;24(6):1142–8. https://doi.org/10.1093/jamia/ocx080.

Adler-Milstein J, Adelman JS, Tai-Seale M, Patel VL, Dymek C. EHR audit logs: a new goldmine for health services research? J Biomed Inform. 2020a;101: 103343. https://doi.org/10.1016/j.jbi.2019.103343.

Adler-Milstein J, Zhao W, Willard-Grace R, Knox M, Grumbach K. Electronic health records and burnout: time spent on the electronic health record after hours and message volume associated with exhaustion but not with cynicism among primary care clinicians. J Am Med Inform Assoc. 2020b;27(4):531–8. https://doi.org/10.1093/jamia/ocz220.

Akbar F, Mark G, Warton EM, Reed ME, Prausnitz S, East JA, Moeller MF, Lieu TA. Physicians' electronic inbox work patterns and factors associated with high inbox work duration. J Am Med Inform Assoc. 2021;28(5):923–30. https://doi.org/10.1093/jamia/ocaa229.

Ancker JS, Barrón Y, Rockoff ML, Hauser D, Pichardo M, Szerencsy A, Calman N. Use of an electronic patient portal among disadvantaged populations. J Gen Intern Med. 2011;26(10):1117–23. https://doi.org/10.1007/s11606-011-1749-y.

Angrist JD, Pischke J-S. Mostly harmless econometrics: an empiricist's companion. Princeton University Press; 2008.

Apathy NC, Holmgren AJ, Adler-Milstein J. A decade post-HITECH: critical access hospitals have electronic health records but struggle to keep up with other advanced functions. J Am Med Inform Assoc. 2021;00:8.

Apathy NC, Hare AJ, Fendrich S, Cross DA. Early changes in billing and notes after evaluation and management guideline change. Ann Intern Med. 2022a;M21–4402. https://doi.org/10.7326/M21-4402.

Apathy NC, Rotenstein L, Bates DW, Holmgren AJ. Documentation dynamics: note composition, burden, and physician efficiency. Health Serv Res. 2022b;n/a(n/a). https://doi.org/10.1111/1475-6773.14097.

Apter AJ, Bryant-Stephens T, Perez L, Morales KH, Howell JT, Mullen AN, Han X, Canales M, Rogers M, Klusaritz H, Localio AR. Patient portal usage and outcomes among adult patients with uncontrolled asthma. J Allergy Clin Immunol: In Practice. 2020;8(3):965–970.e4. https://doi.org/10.1016/j.jaip.2019.09.034.

Baratta LR, Harford D, Sinsky CA, Kannampallil T, Lou SS. Characterizing the patterns of electronic health record-integrated secure messaging use: cross-sectional study. J Med Internet Res. 2023;25: e48583. https://doi.org/10.2196/48583.

Barker W, Richwine C. Patient usage of apps to access online medical records. JAMA Netw Open. 2023;6(11): e2343312. https://doi.org/10.1001/jamanetworkopen.2023.43312.

Bartek B, Lou SS, Kannampallil T. Measuring the cognitive effort associated with task switching in routine EHR-based tasks. J Biomed Inform. 2023;141: 104349. https://doi.org/10.1016/j.jbi.2023.104349.

Baxter SL, Apathy NC, Cross DA, Sinsky C, Hribar MR. Measures of electronic health record use in outpatient settings across vendors. J Am Med Inform Assoc. 2021;28(5):955–9. https://doi.org/10.1093/jamia/ocaa266.

Bell SK, Amat MJ, Anderson TS, Aronson MD, Benneyan JC, Fernandez L, Ricci DA, Salant T, Schiff GD, Shafiq U, Singer SJ, Sternberg SB, Zhang C, Phillips RS. Do patients who read visit notes on the patient portal have a higher rate of "loop closure" on diagnostic tests and referrals in primary care? A retrospective cohort study. J Am Med Inform Assoc. 2024;31(3):622–30. https://doi.org/10.1093/jamia/ocad250.

Chen Y, Lehmann CU, Hatch LD, Schremp E, Malin BA, France DJ. Modeling care team structures in the neonatal intensive care unit through network analysis of EHR audit logs. Methods Inf Med. 2019;58(4–05):109–23. https://doi.org/10.1055/s-0040-1702237.

Chen B, Alrifai W, Gao C, Jones B, Novak L, Lorenzi N, France D, Malin B, Chen Y. Mining tasks and task characteristics from electronic health record audit logs with unsupervised machine learning. J Am Med Inform Assoc. 2021;28(6):1168–77. https://doi.org/10.1093/jamia/ocaa338.

Cross DA, Holmgren AJ, Apathy NC. The role of organizations in shaping physician use of electronic health records. Health Serv Res. 2024;59(1): e14203. https://doi.org/10.1111/1475-6773.14203.

Downing NL, Bates DW, Longhurst CA. Physician burnout in the electronic health record era: are we ignoring the real cause? Ann Intern Med. 2018;169(1):50–1.

Dziorny AC, Orenstein EW, Lindell RB, Hames NA, Washington N, Desai B. Automatic detection of front-line clinician hospital shifts: a novel use of electronic health record timestamp data. Appl Clin Inform. 2019;10(1):28–37. https://doi.org/10.1055/s-0038-1676819.

Fareed N, Walker D, Sieck CJ, Taylor R, Scarborough S, Huerta TR, McAlearney AS. Inpatient portal clusters: identifying user groups based on portal features. J Am Med Inform Assoc. 2019;26(1):28–36. https://doi.org/10.1093/jamia/ocy147.

Fareed N, MacEwan SR, Vink S, Jonnalagadda P, McAlearney AS. Relationships between patient portal activation and patient satisfaction scores among CG-CAHPS and HCAHPS respondents. Am J Manag Care. 2022;28(1):25–31. https://doi.org/10.37765/ajmc.2022.88813.

Ganguli I, Sheridan B, Gray J, Chernew M, Rosenthal MB, Neprash H. Physician work hours and the gender pay gap—evidence from primary care. N Engl J Med. 2020;383(14):1349–57. https://doi.org/10.1056/NEJMsa2013804.

Gleason KT, Wu MMJ, Wec A, Powell DS, Zhang T, Gamper MJ, Green AR, Nothelle S, Amjad H, Wolff JL. Use of the patient portal among older adults with diagnosed dementia and their care partners. Alzheimer's & Dementia. 2023;19(12):5663–71. https://doi.org/10.1002/alz.13354.

Gong JJ, Soleimani H, Murray SG, Adler-Milstein J. Characterizing styles of clinical note production and relationship to clinical work hours among first-year residents. J Am Med Inform Assoc. 2021;29(1):120–7. https://doi.org/10.1093/jamia/ocab253.

Graetz I, Huang J, Muelly ER, Fireman B, Hsu J, Reed ME. Association of mobile patient portal access with diabetes medication adherence and glycemic levels among adults with diabetes. JAMA Netw Open. 2020;3(2): e1921429. https://doi.org/10.1001/jamanetworkopen.2019.21429.

Holmgren AJ, Apathy NC. Assessing the impact of patient access to clinical notes on clinician EHR documentation. J Am Med Inform Assoc. 2022;ocac120. https://doi.org/10.1093/jamia/ocac120.

Holmgren AJ, Apathy NC. Trends in US hospital electronic health record vendor market concentration, 2012–2021. J Gen Intern Med. 2023;38(7):1765–7. https://doi.org/10.1007/s11606-022-07917-3.

Holmgren AJ, Downing NL, Tang M, Sharp C, Longhurst C, Huckman RS. Assessing the impact of the COVID-19 pandemic on clinician ambulatory electronic health record use. J Am Med Inform Assoc. 2022a;29(3):453–60. https://doi.org/10.1093/jamia/ocab268.

Holmgren AJ, Byron ME, Grouse CK, Adler-Milstein J. Association between billing patient portal messages as e-visits and patient messaging volume. JAMA. 2023a;329(4):339–42. https://doi.org/10.1001/jama.2022.24710.

Holmgren AJ, Thombley R, Sinsky CA, Adler-Milstein J. Changes in physician electronic health record use with the expansion of telemedicine. JAMA Intern Med. 2023b. https://doi.org/10.1001/jamainternmed.2023.5738.

Holmgren AJ, Downing NL, Bates DW, Shanafelt TD, Milstein A, Sharp CD, Cutler DM, Huckman RS, Schulman KA. Assessment of electronic health record use between US and non-US health systems. JAMA Internal Med. 2020;9.

Holmgren AJ, Rotenstein L, Downing NL, Bates DW, Schulman K. Association between state-level malpractice environment and clinician electronic health record (EHR) time. J Am Med Inform Assoc. 2022b;ocac034. https://doi.org/10.1093/jamia/ocac034.

Joynt KE, Orav EJ, Jha AK. Physician volume, specialty, and outcomes of care for patients with heart failure. Circ: Heart Failure. 2013;6(5):890–7. https://doi.org/10.1161/CIRCHEARTFAILURE.112.000064.

Judson TJ, Odisho AY, Neinstein AB, Chao J, Williams A, Miller C, Moriarty T, Gleason N, Intinarelli G, Gonzales R. Rapid design and implementation of an integrated patient self-triage and self-scheduling tool for COVID-19. J Am Med Inform Assoc. 2020;27(6):860–6. https://doi.org/10.1093/jamia/ocaa051.

Kim S, Lou SS, Baratta LR, Kannampallil T. Classifying clinical work settings using EHR audit logs: a machine learning approach. Am J Manag Care. 2023;29(1):e24–e30. https://doi.org/10.37765/ajmc.2023.89310.

Lai L, Wittbold KA, Dadabhoy FZ, Sato R, Landman AB, Schwamm LH, He S, Patel R, Wei N, Zuccotti G, Lennes IT, Medina D, Sequist TD, Bomba G, Keschner YG, Zhang HM. Digital triage: novel strategies for population health management in response to the COVID-19 pandemic. Healthc (AMST). 2020;8(4): 100493. https://doi.org/10.1016/j.hjdsi.2020.100493.

Li H, Rotenstein L, Jeffery MM, Paek H, Nath B, Williams BL, McLean RM, Goldstein R, Nuckols TK, Hoq L, Melnick ER. Quantifying EHR and policy factors associated with the gender productivity gap in ambulatory, general internal medicine. J Gen Intern Med. 2023. https://doi.org/10.1007/s11606-023-08428-5.

Lou SS, Kim S, Harford D, Warner BC, Payne PRO, Abraham J, Kannampallil T. Effect of clinician attention switching on workload and wrong-patient errors. Br J Anaesth. 2022a;129(1):e22–4. https://doi.org/10.1016/j.bja.2022.04.012.

Lou SS, Lew D, Harford DR, Lu C, Evanoff BA, Duncan JG, Kannampallil T. Temporal associations between EHR-derived workload, burnout, and errors: a prospective cohort study. J Gen Intern Med. 2022b;37(9):2165–72. https://doi.org/10.1007/s11606-022-07620-3.

Lou SS, Liu H, Warner BC, Harford D, Lu C, Kannampallil T. Predicting physician burnout using clinical activity logs: model performance and lessons learned. J Biomed Inform. 2022c;127: 104015. https://doi.org/10.1016/j.jbi.2022.104015.

Lou SS, Baratta LR, Lew D, Harford D, Avidan MS, Kannampallil T. Anesthesia clinical workload estimated from electronic health record documentation vs billed relative value units. JAMA Netw Open. 2023a;6(8): e2328514. https://doi.org/10.1001/jamanetworkopen.2023.28514.

Lou SS, Liu H, Harford D, Lu C, Kannampallil T. Characterizing the macrostructure of electronic health record work using raw audit logs: an unsupervised action embeddings approach. J Am Med Inform Assoc. 2023b;30(3):539–44. https://doi.org/10.1093/jamia/ocac239.

Lyles CR, Sarkar U, Schillinger D, Ralston JD, Allen JY, Nguyen R, Karter AJ. Refilling medications through an online patient portal: consistent improvements in adherence across racial/ethnic groups. J Am Med Inform Assoc. 2016;23(e1):e28-33. https://doi.org/10.1093/jamia/ocv126.

Magon HS, Helkey D, Shanafelt T, Tawfik D. Creating conversion factors from EHR event log data: a comparison of investigator-derived and vendor-derived metrics for primary care physicians. AMIA Annu Symp Proc. 2024;2023:1115–24.

Mai MV, Orenstein EW, Manning JD, Luberti AA, Dziorny AC. Attributing patients to pediatric residents using electronic health record features augmented with audit logs. Appl Clin Inform. 2020;11(3):442–51. https://doi.org/10.1055/s-0040-1713133.

Maisel N, Thombley R, Overhage JM, Blake K, Sinsky CA, Adler-Milstein J. Physician electronic health record use after changes in us centers for medicare & medicaid services documentation requirements. JAMA Health Forum. 2023;4(5): e230984. https://doi.org/10.1001/jamahealthforum.2023.0984.

Moy AJ, Cato KD, Withall J, Kim EY, Tatonetti N, Rossetti SC. Using time series clustering to segment and infer emergency department nursing shifts from electronic health record log files. AMIA Annu Symp Proc. 2023;2022:805–14.

Mullainathan S, Obermeyer Z. Diagnosing physician error: a machine learning approach to low-value health care. Q J Econ. 2022;137(2):679–727. https://doi.org/10.1093/qje/qjab046.

Nath B, Williams B, Jeffery MM, O'Connell R, Goldstein R, Sinsky CA, Melnick ER. Trends in electronic health record inbox messaging during the COVID-19 pandemic in an ambulatory practice network in New England. JAMA Netw Open. 2021;4(10): e2131490. https://doi.org/10.1001/jamanetworkopen.2021.31490.

Ouyang D, Chen JH, Krishnan G, Hom J, Witteles R, Chi J. Patient outcomes when housestaff exceed 80 hours per week. Am J Med. 2016;129(9):993-9.e1. https://doi.org/10.1016/j.amjmed.2016.03.023.

Overhage JM, McCallie D. Physician time spent using the electronic health record during outpatient encounters: a descriptive study. Ann Intern Med. 2020. https://doi.org/10.7326/M18-3684.

Patel PD, Cobb J, Wright D, Turer RW, Jordan T, Humphrey A, Kepner AL, Smith G, Rosenbloom ST. Rapid development of telehealth capabilities within pediatric patient portal infrastructure for COVID-19 care: barriers, solutions, results. J Am Med Inform Assoc. 2020;27(7):1116–20. https://doi.org/10.1093/jamia/ocaa065.

Perros I, Yan X, Jones JB, Sun J, Stewart WF. Using the PARAFAC2 tensor factorization on EHR audit data to understand PCP desktop work. J Biomed Inform. 2020;101: 103312. https://doi.org/10.1016/j.jbi.2019.103312.

Perzynski AT, Roach MJ, Shick S, Callahan B, Gunzler D, Cebul R, Kaelber DC, Huml A, Thornton JD, Einstadter D. Patient portals and broadband internet inequality. J Am Med Inform Assoc. 2017;24(5):927–32. https://doi.org/10.1093/jamia/ocx020.

Robinson JR, Davis SE, Cronin RM, Jackson GP. Use of a patient portal during hospital admissions to surgical services. AMIA Annu Symp Proc. 2017;2016:1967–76.

Rose C, Thombley R, Noshad M, Lu Y, Clancy HA, Schlessinger D, Li RC, Liu VX, Chen JH, Adler-Milstein J. Team is brain: leveraging EHR audit log data for new insights into acute care processes. J Am Med Inform Assoc. 2022;ocac201. https://doi.org/10.1093/jamia/ocac201.

Rotenstein LS, Holmgren AJ, Downing NL, Bates DW. Differences in total and after-hours electronic health record time across ambulatory specialties. JAMA Intern Med. 2021. https://doi.org/10.1001/jamainternmed.2021.0256.

Rotenstein LS, Fong AS, Jeffery MM, Sinsky CA, Goldstein R, Williams B, Melnick ER. Gender differences in time spent on documentation and the electronic health record in a large ambulatory network. JAMA Netw Open. 2022a;5(3): e223935. https://doi.org/10.1001/jamanetworkopen.2022.3935.

Rotenstein LS, Holmgren AJ, Healey MJ, Horn DM, Ting DY, Lipsitz S, Salmasian H, Gitomer R, Bates DW. Association between electronic health record time and quality of care metrics in primary care. JAMA Netw Open. 2022b;5(10): e2237086. https://doi.org/10.1001/jamanetworkopen.2022.37086.

Rule A, Chiang MF, Hribar MR. Using electronic health record audit logs to study clinical activity: a systematic review of aims, measures, and methods. J Am Med Inform Assoc. 2020;27(3):480–90. https://doi.org/10.1093/jamia/ocz196.

Rule A, Melnick ER, Apathy NC. Using event logs to observe interactions with electronic health records: an updated scoping review shows increasing use of vendor-derived measures. J Am Med Inform Assoc. 2023b;30(1):144–54. https://doi.org/10.1093/jamia/ocac177.

Rule A, Shafer CM, Micek MA, Baltus JJ, Sinsky CA, Arndt BG. Gender differences in primary care physicians' electronic health record use over time: an observational study. J Gen Intern Med. 2023c;38(6):1570–2. https://doi.org/10.1007/s11606-022-07837-2.

Rule A, Kannampallil T, Hribar MR, Dziorny AC, Thombley R, Apathy NC, Adler-Milstein J. Guidance for reporting analyses of metadata on electronic health record use. J Am Med Inform Assoc. 2023a;ocad254. https://doi.org/10.1093/jamia/ocad254

Sangal RB, Powers E, Rothenberg C, Ndumele C, Ulrich A, Hsiao A, Venkatesh AK. Disparities in accessing and reading open notes in the emergency department upon implementation of the 21st century CURES act. Ann Emerg Med. 2021;78(5):593–8. https://doi.org/10.1016/j.annemergmed.2021.06.014.

Shine D, Pearlman E, Watkins B. Measuring resident hours by tracking interactions with the computerized record. Am J Med. 2010;123(3):286–90. https://doi.org/10.1016/j.amjmed.2009.10.009.

Sinsky CA, Rule A, Cohen G, Arndt BG, Shanafelt TD, Sharp CD, Baxter SL, Tai-Seale M, Yan S, Chen Y, Adler-Milstein J, Hribar M. Metrics for assessing physician activity using electronic health record log data. J Am Med Inform Assoc. 2020;27(4):639–43. https://doi.org/10.1093/jamia/ocz223.

Soleimani H, Adler-Milstein J, Cucina RJ, Murray SG. Automating measurement of trainee work hours. J Hosp Med. 2021;16(7):404–8. https://doi.org/10.12788/jhm.3607.

Steitz BD, Cronin RM, Davis SE, Yan E, Jackson GP. Long-term patterns of patient portal use for pediatric patients at an academic medical center. Appl Clin Inform. 2017;8(3):779–93. https://doi.org/10.4338/ACI-2017-01-RA-0005.

Steitz BD, Wong JIS, Cobb JG, Carlson B, Smith G, Rosenbloom ST. Policies and procedures governing patient portal use at an Academic Medical Center. JAMIA Open. 2019;2(4):479–88. https://doi.org/10.1093/jamiaopen/ooz039.

Steitz BD, Sulieman L, Wright A, Rosenbloom ST. Association of immediate release of test results to patients with implications for clinical workflow. JAMA Netw Open. 2021;4(10): e2129553. https://doi.org/10.1001/jamanetworkopen.2021.29553.

Steitz BD, Padi-Adjirackor NA, Griffith KN, Reese TJ, Rosenbloom ST, Ancker JS. Impact of notification policy on patient-before-clinician review of immediately released test results. J Am Med Inform Assoc. 2023;ocad126. https://doi.org/10.1093/jamia/ocad126.

Szilagyi PG, Valderrama R, Vangala S, Albertin C, Okikawa D, Sloyan M, Lopez N, Lerner CF. Pediatric patient portal use in one health system. J Am Med Inform Assoc. 2020;27(3):444–8. https://doi.org/10.1093/jamia/ocz203.

Tai-Seale M, Baxter S, Millen M, Cheung M, Zisook S, Çelebi J, Polston G, Sun B, Gross E, Helsten T, Rosen R, Clay B, Sinsky C, Ziedonis DM, Longhurst CA, Savides TJ. Association of physician burnout with perceived EHR work stress and potentially actionable factors. J Am Med Inform Assoc. 2023;ocad136. https://doi.org/10.1093/jamia/ocad136.

Tsai T, Boazak M, Hinz ERM. Increased clinician time using electronic health records during COVID-19 pandemic. AMIA Annu Symp Proc. 2022;2021:1159–68.

Wang M, Pantell MS, Gottlieb LM, Adler-Milstein J. Documentation and review of social determinants of health data in the EHR: measures and associated insights. J Am Med Inform Assoc. 2021;28(12):2608–16. https://doi.org/10.1093/jamia/ocab194.

Weiskopf NG, Weng C. Methods and dimensions of electronic health record data quality assessment: enabling reuse for clinical research. J Am Med Inform Assoc. 2013;20(1):144–51.

Chapter 16
Automated Location Tracking in Clinical Environments: A Review of Systems and Impact on Workflow Analysis

Akshay Vankipuram and Vimla L. Patel

Abstract The ability to track and detect the activities and process that constitute clinical workflow for performance analysis and error detection has been enhanced with the inclusion of modern technological interventions in clinical environments. One such important intervention is automated location tracking which is a system that detects the movement of clinically relevant entities (physicians, nurses, patients, and equipment). In this chapter, we elucidate the technologies associated with automated location tracking focusing on the two most widely used: Radio-Frequency Identification (RFID) and Bluetooth. We describe specific systems of each type to give readers a general model of the technological requirements for similar setups in clinical environments. Our goal in writing this chapter is the provide readers with an overview of the state-of-the-art technologies and analytic methods. This can hopefully serve as a guide for similar setups in other medical organizations and clinical sites. The process of using a location tracking system to perform novel workflow data analytics is achieved using computational methods whose efficacy has been enhanced by the continuous collection of tracking data that can be potentially collected. Case studies from our own research in the emergency department at the Mayo Clinic, are used as illustration. Finally, we use visualization techniques that can be used to convey workflow related information as well as a proof-of-concept visualization dashboard, which can be used to provide continuous and consistent feedback to clinical target users. This will facilitate self-assessment of workflow and related behaviors and potentially detect bottlenecks and sources of error.

Keywords Clinical workflow · Probabilistic modeling · Visualization · Clinical informatics · Emergency department · Quality improvement · RFID · EHR

A. Vankipuram (✉)
Tempe, Arizona, USA
e-mail: akshay.vankipuram@gmail.com

V. L. Patel
Cognitive Studies in Medicine and Public Health, The New York Academy of Medicine, New York, NY, USA
e-mail: vpatel@nyam.org

K. Zheng et al. (eds.), *Reengineering Clinical Workflow in the Digital and AI Era*,
Cognitive Informatics in Biomedicine and Healthcare,
https://doi.org/10.1007/978-3-031-82971-0_16

16.1 Background and Motivation

The impact of workflow on clinical error and consequently on patient safety has been widely known for some time (Frisby et al. 2017). While it may be convenient to blame human error for the findings presented in the report "To Err is Human," this is not a view shared by a majority of patient safety researchers (Henriksen et al. 2008). A more accepted view is to consider the complexity of a medical environment, where errors are typically caused by failure of one or more aspects of the system, leading to a sequence of further failures, which ultimately impact patient safety. Errors more often result from our lack of understanding of the environment and its bottlenecks than from a specific individual within the environment. To that end, thorough analysis of health care professionals' clinical workflow is essential to build a knowledge base of the areas of potential bottlenecks that may compromise patient safety.

Since the publication of the above report, research in clinical workflow has increased significantly. Ethnography is an essential approach to studying complex environments (Malhotra et al. 2007; Patel et al. 2008; Vankipuram et al. 2011). It pertains to the study of the individuals who make up the environments and how their biases and interactions affect the outcome of that setting. Ethnographic observations combined with surveys, interviews, and questionnaires are all techniques that help piece the puzzle of an environment together. However, each data collection method has its limitations. Specifically, these methods rely heavily on single or multiple human observers processing multiple, and at times parallel, streams of information (Vankipuram et al. 2009). Increasing the number of observers can help in such a situation, but this can also quickly lead to logistical issues as accounts are combined.

In writing this chapter, we aim to summarize a critical modern technological advancement that can help enhance our understanding of the intricacies of clinical environments and processes. We will present an overview of automated location tracking technologies, followed by related research on the efficacy of these technologies. We then look at case-studies from our work to elucidate the potential impact of location-tracking in the medical domain. We break down the case-studies into analytics derived from location tracking data and data visualization techniques which can help present this information to relevant target users (i.e., clinicians and researchers).

16.2 Automated Location Tracking Technologies

Automated tracking of entities in a clinical environment has gained popularity over the past decade, with uses ranging from equipment tracking in clinical environments to research. Automated tracking refers to the use of technological advancements to continuously track clinical personnel, patients, and equipment with minimal human supervision. The methods associated with automated tracking were inspired by those in the field of aviation. Specifically, by considering tracking of processes in a complex medical environment to be comparable to a black box in aircrafts (Vankipuram et al. 2011). In this analogy, the black box continuously monitors various aspects of flight, such as pilot communication, altitude, cabin pressure, and relays this information to the ground or recorded for post-flight analysis and in case of emergencies. Clinical environments can be similarly monitored to reveal underlying process bottlenecks or sources of error.

One of the most popular techniques to achieve automated tracking is the use of sensors. Several examples of such technologies exist, including Radio Frequency Identification (RFID), Bluetooth, ZigBee, and Wi-Fi (Vankipuram et al. 2018). The efficacy of these various methods depends greatly on the nature of the environment itself and the constraints (safety protocols, lead-lined walls, inference from other medical devices) placed on signal transmission in medical environments. As a result of these constraints, RFID and Bluetooth have become the most popular technologies for automated tracking (Vankipuram et al. 2018). Lee and colleagues (Lee et al. 2007) compared the various safety protocols discussed above, and while they determined that the suitability of a protocol was most dependent on its use-case, Bluetooth and ZigBee were the most suited protocols for low data, low battery use applications. Near-Field communication was effective for much shorter distances than would be convenient for tracking. Wi-Fi, while a popular method, was found to interfere with existing hospital networks.

16.3   Radio-Frequency Identification (RFID)

RFID tags are typically carried by the subjects being monitored and they relay their information at regular intervals to a central receiver. Typically, multiple receivers are needed in larger areas. Information, such as proximity of tags to the receiver, is used to determine interactions between subjects. This helps build a model of interaction that can be used to analyze the impact of interventions or general workflow. Figure 16.1 shows an early version of RFID tags provided for clinical tracking purposes. These earlier technologies suffered from a significant amount of interference leading to a loss of data quality. Data collection over wireless networks also posed a challenge and often the data collected was stored at a central location by the vendor and had to be specifically requested as a data file when needed. Obviously, this was a significant barrier to adoption due to the circuitous and time-consuming collection process, but, more importantly, resulting from an inability to restrict ownership of potentially sensitive data, especially when dealing with patient tracking. Therefore, these technologies were rarely, if ever, used on patients. Additionally, the receiver stations shown in the figure were meant to be placed, manually, at the most appropriate locations and since they were ground stations it meant that they had a higher probability of interfering with the normal clinical workflow and could be distracting or concerning for patients and physicians.

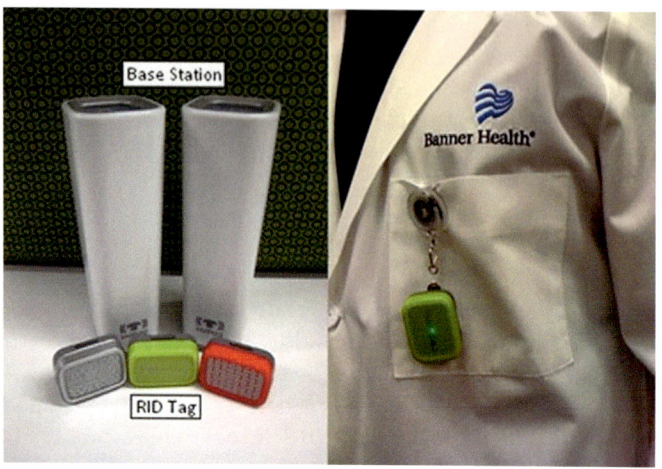

Fig. 16.1 SNiF® RFID tag (Vankipuram et al. 2011)

A modern version of an RFID system is shown in Fig. 16.2 (Versus Technology and Technology 2018). The technologies have been updated to conform with the standards required of medical data including security. In the case of the Versus system, a reduction in the size of the receivers along with an improved tag detection mechanism has allowed the system to improve the efficacy of collected data. While the Versus system is used as an example here, there are several vendors who use variations of similar techniques and achieve similar effectiveness. Additionally, medical organizations have also begun to implement their own solutions because RFID tags and receivers tend to cheap and easily available.

There are two broad classes of RFID technologies that are available:

1. Passive RFID: The tags have no power source and only transmit a signal when they are within range of a receiver. This typically leads to a longer lifespan and passive tags can last up to 10 years. However, due to a lack of onboard power

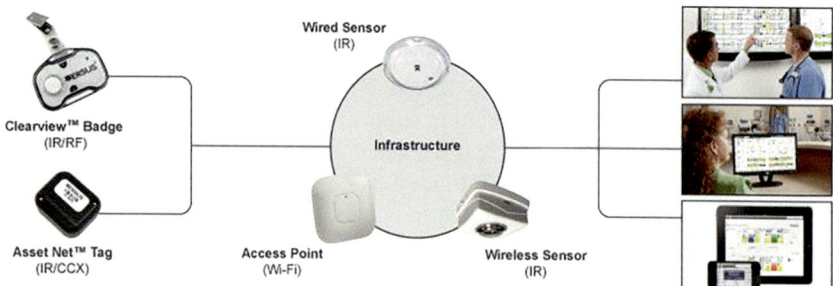

Fig. 16.2 Versus RFID-RTLS system

their detection range is within 40 ft. The receivers are often more expensive than active RFID owing to a need to transmit radio frequency energy.

2. Active RFID: These tags are battery powered and continuously transmit a signal. They have a detection range of over 300ft but have reduced battery lives (3–8 years depending on the range). Receivers are cheaper than their passive counterparts.

Choosing between these technologies is largely based on the characteristics of the medical environment in which they are implemented as well as organizational concerns, such as safety and cost.

16.4 Efficacy of RFID: A Research Perspective

Clinical workflow analyses are especially important when attempting to assess the impact of an intervention or other modifications to everyday processes. An example of such an intervention, and potentially the most relevant to modern medicine, is the introduction of technology into typical clinical workflows. Zheng and colleagues (Zheng et al. 2010) assessed the impact of health information technology implementations (specifically for Computerized Physician Entry (CPOE) forms) on clinical workflows. They introduced a set of new analytics for assessment of impact and demonstrated a means to use data visualization to make complex data more decipherable and useful for quicker assessments. Drawing from this work, Vankipuram and colleagues (Vankipuram et al. 2009) introduced a Hidden Markov Model based approach to capture and analyze interactions using RFID tag-based data.

Fry and Lenert (Fry and Lenert 2005) implemented a system called MASCAL that used RFID technology to track personnel, patients, and equipment in mass casualty events such as natural disasters and other catastrophes. MASCAL involved the use of RFID tags in combination with receivers set around the hospital to track the various resources in real-time at times of emergency. There are two different kinds of RFID tags, active and passive. Active tags constantly broadcast a signal and passive tags wait until they are near a receiver. Ohashi et al. (Ohashi et al. 2008) compared different RFID systems typically employed by hospitals and found that in general both passive and active were affected by the environment. Active tags are battery powered and therefore have a set lifespan whereas passive tags need to have a local receiver to be used.

A study by Elnahrawy and colleagues (Elnahrawy and Martin 2004) compared localization algorithms for tracking precision and found that the uncertainty associated with tracking was likely fundamental and any approach (i.e., Wi-Fi, RFID, Bluetooth, etc.) would suffer from the same issues. Frisby and colleagues (Frisby et al. 2017) implemented a similar system using a beacon to track physicians in the emergency room at the Mayo Clinic hospital, using Raspberry Pi as a receiver. In this study, six receivers and fourteen beacons were used in the hospital.

Fig. 16.3 Estimote®
bluetooth beacons

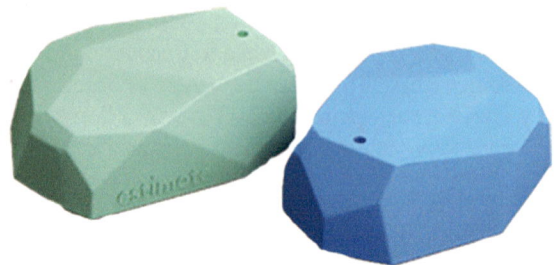

16.5   Bluetooth

Bluetooth based tracking solutions are a more modern approach to clinical tracking. The technique was originally introduced, and is most often used, in non-medical settings (e.g., keyless entry for houses) (Andersson 2014). Bluetooth offers certain advantages over RFID, especially in terms of cost and battery life (Frisby et al. 2017).

The Bluetooth tracking setup is similar to RFID and relies on receivers and tags on tracked entities/personnel. An additional advantage of this technology is its increased compatibility (compared to RFID) with mobile devices and PCs (i.e., most devices can receive and process Bluetooth signals without purchase of a specialized receiver). Bluetooth tracking setups can therefore be more cost effective than the equivalent RFID systems. However, to maximize the efficiency of data collection and minimize the cost, a higher level of technical knowledge is required for setup and maintenance of ad hoc solutions. Bluetooth technologies are classified by their versions. The latest version of Bluetooth, released in 2016, was Bluetooth 5.0. Each subsequent revision of the Bluetooth standard has led to an increase in communication range and a reduction of power/cost. In version 4.0, an associated technology called Bluetooth Low Energy (BLE) was released. This version greatly reduced power consumption of Bluetooth devices while having a comparable communication range. Figure 16.3 shows an example of the Bluetooth tag (beacon) by Estimote (Estimote and Inc. 2018), which is an example of a BLE device. The Estimote tags and similar BLE sensors were estimated to have an increased battery life, making them more efficacious for automated tracking solutions.

As mentioned earlier, Bluetooth signals can be received by a range of commonly found devices, such as mobile phones and laptops. Raspberry Pi (low-cost processors used in mobile devices and computers) have also been used as receivers (Frisby et al. 2017).

16.6   Case Studies: Emergency Room (ER)

In this section, we present our work using location tracking data, specifically, RFID data, in deriving workflow-related analytics in an ER.

16.7 Automated Location Tracking for Clinical Performance Analysis

Positional tracking can be used to derive additional metrics that may function to benchmark emergency room performance. The Center for Medicaid and Medicare Services (CMS) enacted several performance measures that needed to be enacted beginning in 2012 (Blumenthal and Tavenner 2010).

The measures that can be analyzed using location tracking data include:

- Door to Diagnostic Evaluation by a Qualified Medical Professional
- Median Time from ED Arrival to ED Departure for Discharged ED Patients
- Median Time from ED Arrival to ED Departure for Admitted ED Patients
- Admit Decision Time to ED Departure Time for Admitted Patients

Welch and colleagues (Welch et al. 2011) elucidated, in detail, the performance measures for emergency rooms and the salient timestamp or time-interval measures were as follows:

- Treatment space time: Time taken to acquire a bed or room
- Provider contact time
- Arrival to provider time (door-to-doc)
- Arrival to treatment space time
- Length of stay: Arrival to departure

Continuous tracking of these attributes can provide emergency rooms with the ability to continuously monitor and improve their processes.

16.8 Location Tracking Data Collection

To understand the implementation of techniques to analyze clinical workflow and processes using location tracking, we need to understand the structure of tracking data. Most commonly, tracking data is stored in a tabular format. When tracking tags are within the range of a receiver, a single data point is written into the table which may be a locally stored or network relational database. An additional concept to understand is that most effective tracking systems require a high level of coverage (i.e., receivers placed in the environment to achieve a reasonable level of granularity of location data). The data table, therefore, typically has low dimensionality (i.e., few columns, but is usually large since data is recorded per instance of tag detection and this can happen several times a minute per tag that is within the receiver range). It is not uncommon to collect several gigabytes worth of data in a year for a sufficiently large system, such as the one we are describing in this case study. It is therefore incumbent on organizations attempting to implement similar systems to understand their baseline technical requirements and to plan for the growing needs with each year of the system's operation.

Table 16.1 Structure of location tracking data for a single clinician in the ED (Vankipuram et al. 2018). Reprinted with permission from A. Vankipuram, S. Traub, V.L. Patel, A method for the analysis and visualization of clinical workflow in dynamic environments, J. Biomed. Inform. (2018). doi: https://doi.org/10.1016/j.jbi.2018.01.007

Location	Start	End	Duration
Office	11/20/2016 12:04:09AM	11/20/2016 12:06:44AM	0:02:35
Physician workspace	11/20/2016 12:06:47AM	11/20/2016 12:12:11AM	0:05:24

Table 16.1 shows two rows of the RFID data collection for a single tracked clinician in the ED. The columns of the recorded data are as follows:

- Location: The location of the ceiling mounted receiver.
- Start: First instant of time when the tag is within range of the receiver
- End: Instant of time when the tag moves outside the range of the receiver
- Duration: Time spent within range of the receiver

Additionally, each RFID tag was associated with a unique ID which was stored by the receiver, once per row (Table 16.1). The ID could be, therefore, used to identify each tracked clinician. It is worth noting that while this case study deals with RFID data, Bluetooth data will likely need to be similarly structured.

16.9   Data Analytics

Having understood the type of data being collected we can now consider the types of analytics that can be performed on the data. The value of automated techniques over manual observations can best be described by considering methods that require large and higher fidelity datasets, such as the ones we can create using an automated system with good coverage.

16.10   Entropy (Degree of Randomness)

A valuable goal of tracking tasks and movement in a fast-paced, concurrent environment like the ED is to be able to map the inherent structure or lack thereof of the various processes that make up clinical workflow. To that end, we can use the location data to compute the entropy or degree of predictability of processes. Structured processes should have a lower level of entropy or unpredictability since they are, by nature, a series of repeating patterns of movement or behavior. Computing entropy can allow researchers and clinicians a birds-eye view of workflow in an environment like the ED. The entropy of a sequence of movements that underlie a process can be compared to a baseline of truly random movement to get a relative degree of predictability. The associated methods are described in detail in our previous work in the Mayo clinic ED (Vankipuram et al. 2018).

16.11   Discrete Event Simulations (DES)

Demonstrating clinical utility of location tracking data is incumbent on deriving meaningful metrics and relevant ways to present those metrics to the relevant target clinical users. Location tracking data has been used in the creation of new workflow metrics for the ED from RFID data (Vankipuram et al. 2018). As part of this, the clinical environment was modeled using movement transition probabilities to capture its underlying uncertainty. This type of probabilistic model may be visualized to derive specific workflow-related insight, but it can also be used to simulate parameters of interest in the system (Rutberg et al. 2013; Asamoah et al. 2016). These system simulations can be used to assess impact of specific processes or as a predictive model to assess trends.

DES is a technique used to model complex systems by simulating it in action to estimate or predict parameters and outcomes of interest (Rutberg et al. 2013). Systems are typically represented as a series of states, events, and transitions, each of which have a cost associated with them. The net cost of moving through the system in various scenarios is typically then used to estimate the value of the resource that one is looking to optimize. In the medical domain, examples of this could be queue length or wait times for patients (Vankipuram et al. 2018). Traditionally, the costs associated within the system are set based on clinical expertise. Additionally, the movement through the system in the case of branching (concurrent) processes is determined randomly. While this is reasonable approximation of uncertainty, various medical environments may demonstrate varying levels of uncertainty. It is also possible that uncertainty levels may vary during a shift due to cognitive and physical stress (Patel et al. 2008). Using probabilistic models generated from RFID data, we can represent the uncertainty of the system in a way that better represents the actual workflow. One way to progress through a probabilistic system is to use the Monte-Carlo method which has been shown to work in DES (Rutberg et al. 2013).

The task of estimating the underlying distributions associated with parameters of interest in a medical environment has been researched (Asamoah et al. 2016). With automated tracking, we can enhance our understanding of the underlying structure of the uncertainty.

Figure 16.4 represents a simplified view of a clinical movement probability model. Such a model can be utilized to simulate outcomes of interest. Figure 16.5 shows the results of DES for 3 behaviors in ED (providers tracking). The time computed represents predicted time to exam for a physician over 1000 simulated runs. The transition probabilities were used to pick the next location to move in the simulation. To pick the duration at each location, we compute the skew for each duration and generate a random number from a distribution with the same mean, std, and skew.

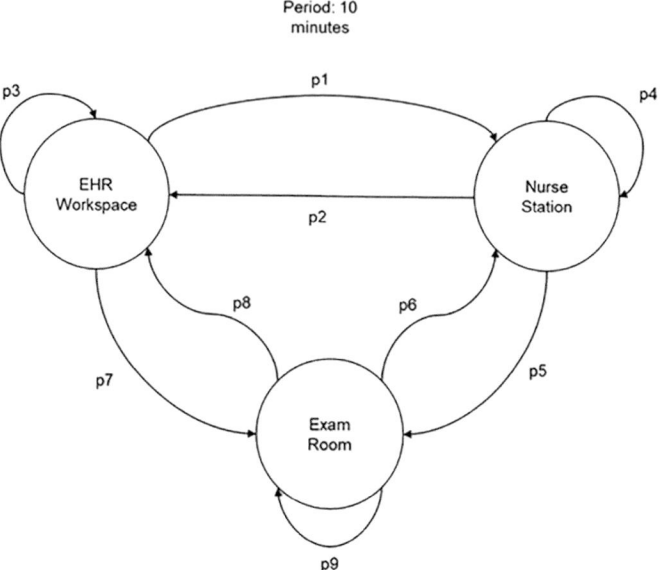

Fig. 16.4 Simplified probability model of the ED (actual model contains all 59 locations)

Figure 16.6 shows the time distributions generated using tracking data that form the underlying models used in this sample simulation.

16.12 Efficient Data Processing at Clinical Scale

Location-based tracking technologies across clinical systems/environments require the ability to process large amounts of data at scale. Modern Bluetooth sensors have data transmission rates of up to 2 Mbps (Park et al. 2020), which is approximately 250 MB per second per sensor. Given that even smaller clinical environments likely require over ten active sensors to collect data at reasonable fidelity, this elevates the importance of having the ability to store large volumes of data. From a data processing perspective, there are likely two types of computing resources required: (i) post-hoc analysis tools that can extract aggregate information about workflows over a larger period, (ii) near real-time event tracking that can serve to power alerting systems where critical problems with workflows that could increase risk of errors can be surfaced and mitigated quickly. The most viable solution that is both scalable and flexible to these requirements is the use of the cloud (Zhai et al. 2023). The use of cloud computing techniques has been stated as being a key factor in moving towards truly smart clinical systems (Singh et al. 2022).

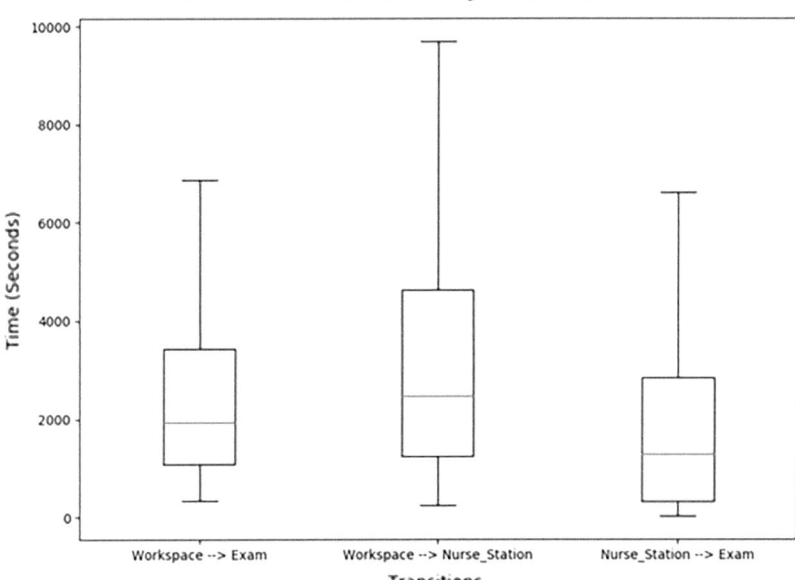

Fig. 16.5 Result of DES for three cases of interest in ED

16.13   Data Visualization

Utility of analytic techniques are the greatest when derived information can be presented to target users in meaningful ways. In the medical domain, users may include clinicians, administrators, or clinical researchers. The theoretical foundations for this space are provided by the science of visual analytics. Visual analytics is the "science of analytical reasoning facilitated by interactive visual interfaces" (Park et al. 2020). Visual analytics can aid in the deeper exploration and insights derived from data and the presentation of this information to specific types of end-users. In this section, we present some examples of visualizations created using the ED location tracking data to illustrate the value further. At the end of the section, we provide a sample workflow dashboard which is used as an example of an ideal-ized outcome of an integrated location tracking analytics system in an ED or similar clinical environment.

16.14   Chord Diagram

Figure 16.7 is a representation of the net duration of interactions between clinicians. Interactions are defined as an event where the clinicians were co-located for a length of time. The practical value of this is its use in process management to provide

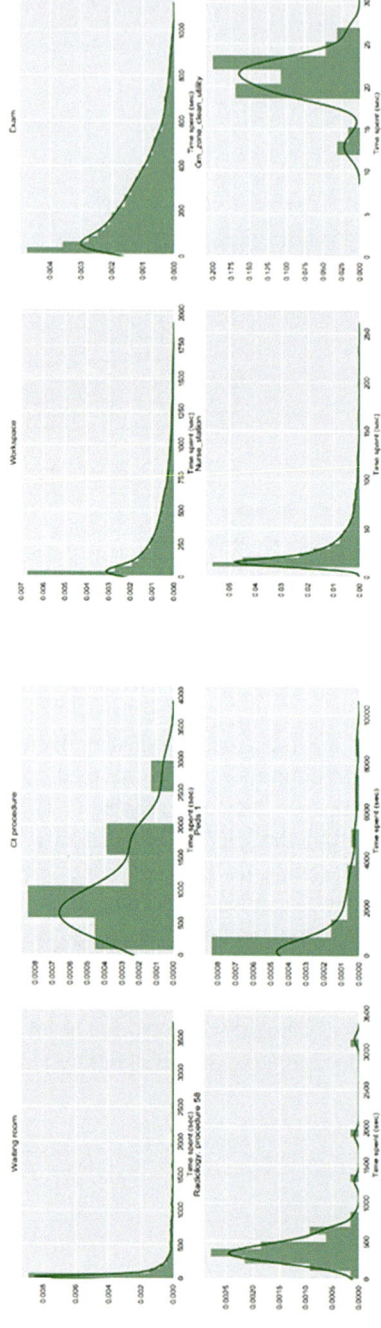

Fig. 16.6 Time distributions for 4 sample locations in two EDs

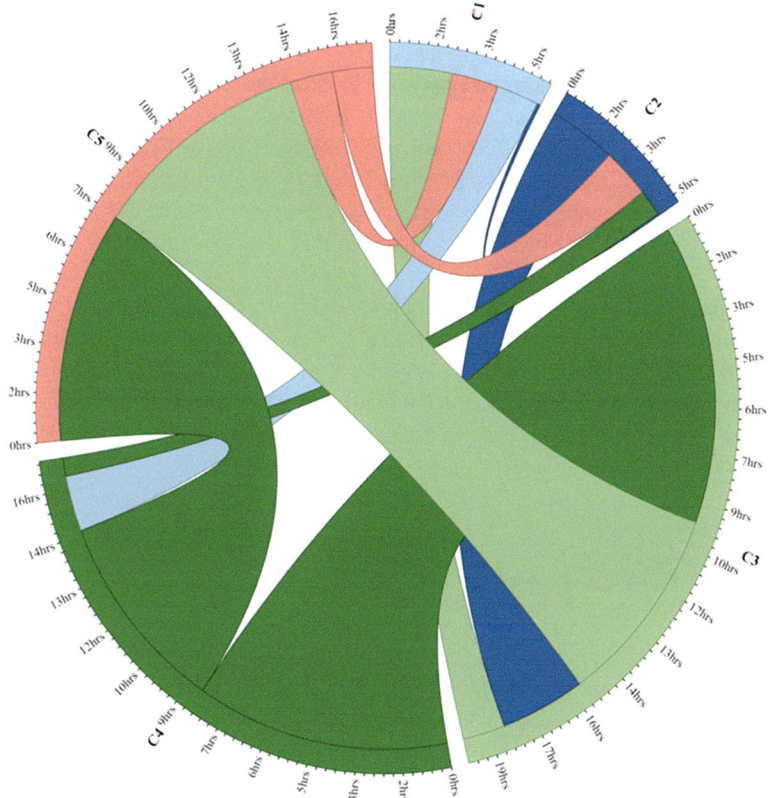

Fig. 16.7 Net duration of interactions between tracked clinicians at mayo clinic

circumstances that maximize interactions and to find pairs of clinicians who are more likely to interact and study them further.

The chord diagram (Fig. 16.7) shows duration of interactions between clinicians. Each colored segment on the boundary represents a different clinician (C1–C5, respectfully). The chords connecting the segments represent a pairwise link and the width of the chord represents the net duration of interaction (the axis of the boundary can be used to estimate the duration).

16.15 Longest Common Subsequence

The longest common subsequence (LCS) is a computational problem that deals with finding the longest common set of sub patterns within two series. An example of this is to find the longest common sequence of nucleotides in two gene sequences. By treating movement data as a series of location sequences, we can compare two sequences of movement, either by time or by tracking personnel, to derive additional insight into behavior.

LCS can be computed for each tracked clinician and visualized as seen for one clinician in Fig. 16.8. This can also be used for process management, but additionally may be used to compare clinicians with varying expertise. The figure shows a movement graph of the most common movements a single tracked clinician makes during a shift. This can be potentially used to compare novices and experts and see if the experts' movement allows them to manage time better or mitigate certain types of error.

The blocks on each axis represent a move within the location (e.g., 'Workspace' to 'Workspace,' with the arrows representing direction of movement). This chart can be compared over lengths of time or between a specific pair of clinicians (e.g., novice vs. expert). It is also possible to use the chart in Fig. 16.8 to view arbitrary length sequences for any clinician, but in this case, we use it to view the LCS of movement across all shifts of a clinician.

16.16   Network Graph-Based Visualization

Relationships and probabilities can be represented as a network graph, as seen in Fig. 16.9, which gives the probability of a clinician's next location. The radius of each colored circle represents the time spent in that location. The strength of the relationship is represented by the number of the links between locations (i.e., more links indicate stronger relationships). These links also show the probability of the physician's next locations from any origin point. This type of graph eliminates any overlapping edges to provide a clearer interpretation of the relationships between locations. Network graphs work well in a dynamic setting, such as an interactive dashboard.

16.17   Radar Chart

A radar plot/chart is a form of visualization that is a good way to represent a single discrete axis. It is a popularly used plot in gamification research, which is the introduction of video-game elements into visualization dashboards to enhance clarity and intuitiveness. Below (Fig. 16.10) we look at an example of a radar plot generated to display the probability of the physician's next location from any origin point.

The radar chart is a useful representation of clinical movement as a Markov process (i.e., when we model the system as a Markov chain where the probability of the clinician being in the current location is only dependent on the immediate previous location). Markov processes are usually a good approximation of complex processes and can be further used in methods like the discrete event and Monte Carlo

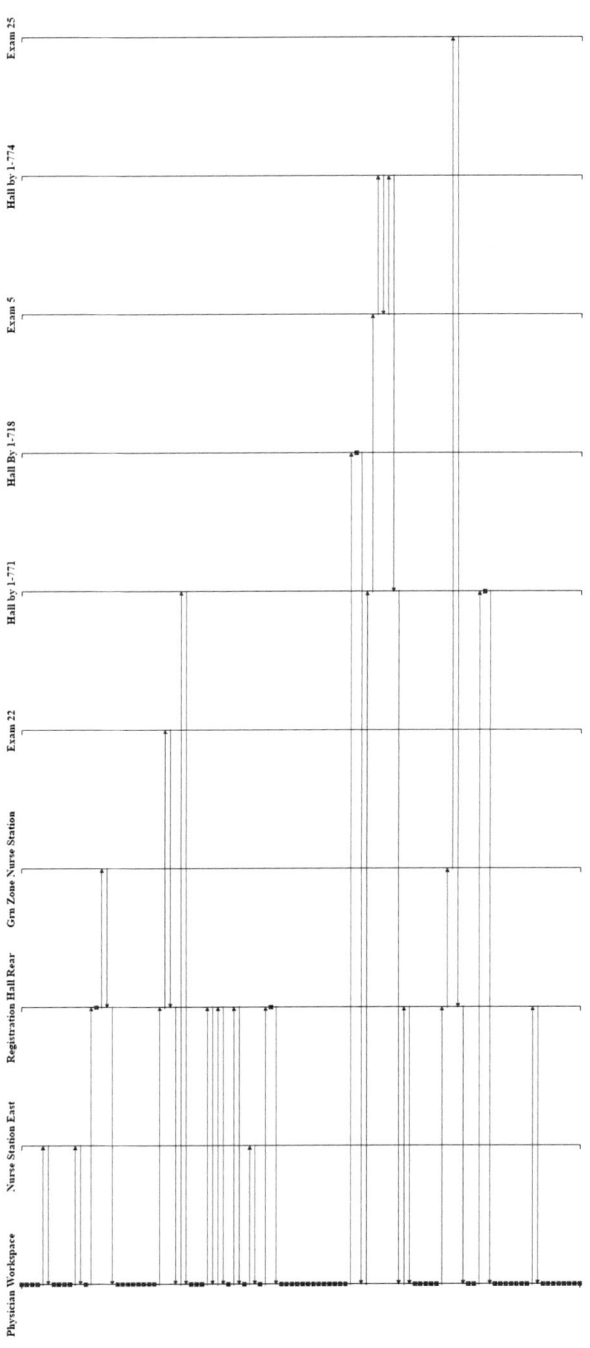

Fig. 16.8 Longest common subsequence for a single clinician over 7 months at mayo clinic

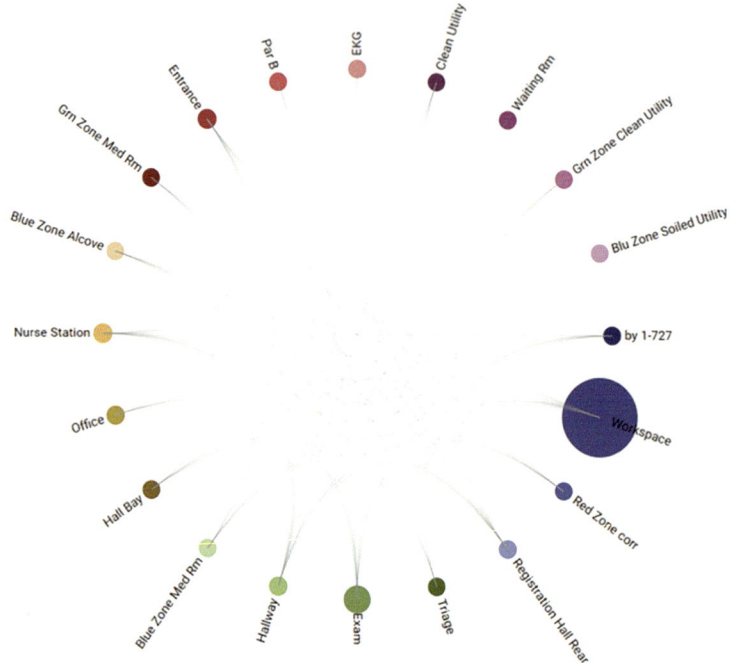

Fig. 16.9 Probability of clinician's next location at mayo clinic

simulations described earlier. Radar charts are an effective way to convey Markov systems.

16.18   Clinical Workflow Dashboard

As mentioned previously, an ideal goal of visual analytics work is to provide a platform for clinicians and researchers to receive feedback on the results of data analysis. Below we present a proof-of-concept dashboard developed using ED location tracking data. Figure 16.11 shows a sample dashboard for a single physician based on measures derided from location tracking. The top row shows instances of direct patient care (movement from workspace to exam room), multiple patient exam room visits, and knowledge transfer (movement from workspace to nurse stations). The plot of the left shows the net count of each of the above metrics per day. The plot on the right shows a single day as selected on the stacked plot (left). This plot is shown per hour of the shift.

The second row shows a set of pie charts representing time spent in various locations within the ED. EHRs have been a disruptive influence on clinical workflow and clinicians are often concerned with time spent with patients compared to other

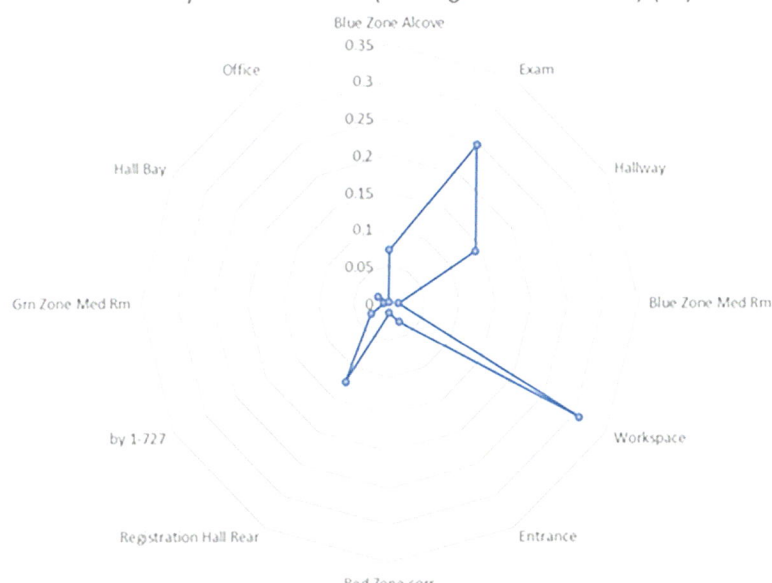

Fig. 16.10 Probability of Next Physician Location, with Nurse's Station Origin. The axis of a radar plot is categorical giving a discrete representation

areas and activities. These plots can convey the proportion of time spent in exam rooms compared to other areas in the ED.

Finally, the transition probabilities described in the radar chart section is represented in the final row. Transition probabilities for a single physician represented as a heatmap (left). The darker squares represent a higher likelihood of movement from location on the column to the location on the row. Useful for presenting net behavior. The radar plot on the right is populated by selecting one of the locations in the heatmap and presents probability values for movement from that location.

Figure 16.11 is an example of an interactive dashboard and can be updated to display measures for any arbitrary length of time. A possible use for such a dashboard could be to observe trends in these measures across time to assess the impact of technological or process interventions.

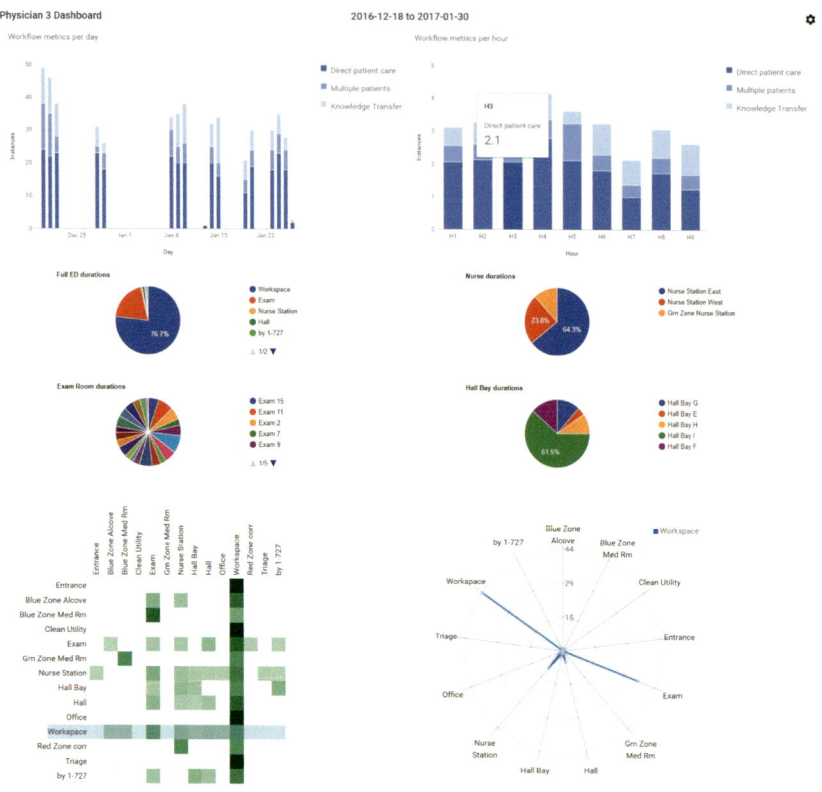

Fig. 16.11 Location tracking analytics visualization dashboard

16.19 Conclusion

In this chapter, we described automated location tracking technologies and associated analytical methods in medical environments. Clinical workflow is inherently complex, and the techniques described above were developed to complement other quantitative methods typically used in the analysis of clinical workflow. Derived measures can assist researchers and clinical stakeholders as they identify bottlenecks which can be further investigated in greater detail using ethnographic techniques. We believe that the most effective way to study workflow is to use a combination of available methods. Our goal in this chapter is to present the utility of, what we believe is, an efficacious modern method to supplement workflow study.

There are also additional sources of data that can be leveraged to create a more holistic picture of clinical processes which we have not included here, but are equally important. Location tracking provides just one dimension of qualitative data. Another example of a valuable data source is EHR trace/usage log files (Adler-Milstein et al. 2020). EHR logs are collected by most mainstream vendors, which includes the use of the system by various authorized personnel. Including this data in clinical workflow analysis can increase the granularity of our view into the medical environment to provide more context to movements and related activities, and thus improve the depth of our automated monitoring capabilities.

Acknowledgements The research in this chapter was supported by grant #R01HS022670 from the Agency for Healthcare Research and Quality (AHRQ). The content is sole responsibility of the authors and does not necessarily represent the official views of the AHRQ.

References

Adler-Milstein J, Adelman JS, Tai-Seale M, Patel VL, Dymek C. EHR audit logs: A new goldmine for health services research? J Biomed Inform. 2020Jan;101: 103343. https://doi.org/10.1016/j.jbi.2019.103343. 2019 Dec 7 PMID: 31821887.

Andersson T. Bluetooth Low Energy and Smartphones for Proximity-Based Automatic Door Locks, 2014. http://www.diva-portal.org/smash/record.jsf?pid=diva2%3A723899&dswid=-8877 (Accessed May 25, 2017).

Asamoah DA, Sharda R, Rude HN, Doran D. RFID-based information visibility for hospital operations: exploring its positive effects using discrete event simulation. Health Care Manag Sci. 2016. https://doi.org/10.1007/s10729-016-9386-y.

Blumenthal D, Tavenner M. The "meaningful use" regulation for electronic health records. N Engl J Med. 2010;363:501–4.

Elnahrawy E, Martin RP. The limits of localization using signal strength: a comparative study, 2004 First Annu. IEEE Commun. Soc. Conf. Sens. Ad Hoc Commun. Networks, 2004. IEEE SECON 2004. (2004). https://doi.org/10.1109/SAHCN.2004.1381942.

Estimote, Estimote, Inc.—indoor location with bluetooth beacons and mesh, (n.d.). https://estimote.com/ (Accessed July 2, 2018).

Frisby J, Smith V, Traub S, Patel VL. Contextual Computing: A Bluetooth based approach for tracking healthcare providers in the emergency room. J Biomed Inform. 2017;65:97–104.

Fry EA, Lenert LA. MASCAL: RFID tracking of patients, staff and equipment to enhance hospital response to mass casualty events. AMIA Annu Symp Proc. 2005;2005:261–5.

Henriksen K, Dayton E, Keyes MA, Carayon P. Chapter 5 . Understanding Adverse Events : A Human Factors Framework Human Factors—What Is It ?, Saf. Qual. An Evidence-Based Handb. Nurses. (2008); 67–86.

Lee JS, Su YW, Shen CC. A comparative study of wireless protocols: Bluetooth, UWB, ZigBee, and Wi-Fi, in: IECON Proc. (Industrial Electron. Conf., 2007. https://doi.org/10.1109/IECON.2007.4460126.

Malhotra S, Jordan D, Shortliffe E, Patel VL. Workflow modeling in critical care: Piecing together your own puzzle. J Biomed Inform. 2007;40:81–92.

Ohashi K, Ota S, Ohno-Machado L, Tanaka H. Comparison of RFID systems for tracking clinical interventions at the bedside., in: AMIA Annu. Symp. Proc., 2008.

Park E, Lee MS, Kim HS, Bahk S. AdaptaBLE: Adaptive control of data rate, transmission power, and connection interval in bluetooth low energy. Comput Netw. 2020;181: 107520.

Patel V, Zhang J, Yoskowitz N, Green R, Sayan O. Translational cognition for decision support in critical care environments: A review. J Biomed Inform. 2008;41:413–31.

Rutberg MH, Wenczel S, Devaney J, Goldlust EJ, Day TE. Incorporating discrete event simulation into quality improvement efforts in health care systems., Am J Med Qual. (2013). https://doi.org/10.1177/1062860613512863.

Singh T, Rastogi P, Pandey UK, Geetha A, Tiwari M, Chakravarthi MK (2022). Systematic health-care smart systems with the integration of the sensor using cloud computing techniques. In 2022 2nd international conference on advance computing and innovative technologies in engineering (ICACITE) (pp. 708–712). IEEE.

Thomas JJ, Cook KA. A visual analytics agenda. IEEE Comput Graph Appl. 2006. https://doi.org/10.1109/MCG.2006.5.

Vankipuram M, Kahol K, Cohen T, Patel VL. Visualization and analysis of activities in critical care environments. AMIA Annu Symp Proc. 2009;2009:662–6.

Vankipuram M, Kahol K, Cohen T, Patel VL. Toward automated workflow analysis and visualization in clinical environments. J Biomed Inform. 2011;44:432–40.

Vankipuram A, Traub S, Patel VL. A method for the analysis and visualization of clinical workflow in dynamic environments. J Biomed Inform. 2018. https://doi.org/10.1016/j.jbi.2018.01.007.

Versus Technology, RTLS Technology. Accurate, Reliable IR-RFID RTLS. Versus RTLS, (n.d.). http://www.versustech.com/rtls-technology/ (Accessed July 2, 2018).

Welch SJ, Asplin BR, Stone-Griffith S, Davidson SJ, Augustine J, Schuur J. Emergency department operational metrics, measures and definitions: Results of the second performance measures and benchmarking summit. Ann Emerg Med. 2011. https://doi.org/10.1016/j.annemergmed.2010.08.040.

Zhai K, Yousef MS, Mohammed S, Al-Dewik NI, Qoronfleh MW. Optimizing clinical workflow using precision medicine and advanced data analytics. Processes. 2023;11(3):939.

Zheng K, Haftel HM, Hirschl RB, O'Reilly M, Hanauer DA. Quantifying the impact of health IT implementations on clinical workflow: a new methodological perspective. J Am Med Informatics Assoc. 2010;17:454–61.

Part IV
Applications and Case Studies

Chapter 17
Examining the Relationship Between Health IT and Ambulatory Care Workflow Redesign

Elizabeth L. Ciemins, Holly J. Lanham, Curt Lindberg, and Kai Zheng

17.1 Introduction

In 2012, the U.S. Agency for Healthcare Research and Quality (AHRQ) launched a research program called "Using Health IT in Practice Redesign: Impact of Health IT on Workflow." The purpose of the program was to fund methodologically rigorous research studies of the implementation of health IT to support practice redesign in ambulatory care settings. The project presented in this chapter was one of the studies funded through this program, entitled "Examining the Relationship Between Health IT and Ambulatory Care Workflow Redesign." This project aimed to (1) employ rigorous and scientifically validated research methods to study the impacts of health IT implementation on healthcare workers' workflow in a diverse set of ambulatory care practices; (2) focus on health IT implementation projects that are initiated to engender or facilitate practice redesign processes; and (3) use multiple complementary methods, with careful results triangulation and member checking, to develop a better understanding of the causal relationship between health IT implementation and ambulatory care workflow.

The empirical study was conducted across six ambulatory care practices from two participating healthcare organizations, Organization West and Organization East,

E. L. Ciemins (✉)
AMGA, Alexandria, VA, USA
e-mail: ECiemins@amga.org

H. J. Lanham
University of Texas Health Science Center, San Antonio, TX, USA

C. Lindberg
Partners in Complexity, Waitsfield, VT, USA

K. Zheng
University of California, Irvine, CA, USA

each serving different patient populations in areas with distinct geographic and socioeconomic profiles. At each organization, a major health IT implementation took place during the project period. The empirical study used a prospective observational design with multiple data collection points before, during, and after these health IT implementations. Data collection methods included ethnographic observations, time and motion observations, log analysis, semi-structured interviews, and member checking focus groups to enrich the insights and triangulate the findings. Through analyzing these data, this project aimed to develop an enhanced understanding of: (1) the causal relationship between health IT implementation and ambulatory care workflow redesign; (2) sociotechnical factors and the role they play in mitigating or augmenting health IT's impacts on workflow processes; and (3) the workflow impacts of health IT magnified through frequently occurring disruptive events such as interruptions and exceptions. In the project, we were particularly interested in studying the workflow dynamics associated with the "team" nature of patient care.

17.2 Methods

17.2.1 Conceptual Models

This study was informed by two conceptual frameworks: the workflow elements model (WEM) and complexity science. The WEM, proposed by Unertl et al. (2010) is grounded in the sociotechnical literature and describes workflow as consisting of five specific elements: *actors* (the people performing actions), *artifacts* (physical or virtual tools), *actions*, *characteristics of actions*, and *outcomes* (the end products of the actions). The model suggests that three pervasive elements apply throughout workflow: *temporality* (scheduling, temporal rhythms, and coordination of events), *aggregation* (the relationship and interaction among different tasks and actors, including elements of coordination, cooperation and conflict), and *context* (physical or virtual workspace and organizational factors). Figure 17.1 displays the mapping of study components to the WEM framework.

Sociotechnical theory, of which the WEM is a part, is a prominent theoretical framework used to study health IT design, implementation and use. Sociotechnical theory seeks understanding and improvement of the fit between the technical and social subsystems that make up an organization (Cherns 1976; Clegg 2000).

Given the rich and contextually nuanced nature of our study data and the limits of the WEM for interpreting such data, we also incorporated complexity science as a theoretical framework to guide our interpretation. Complexity science is the study of systems composed of multiple interacting, interdependent, and heterogeneous agents (Camazine et al. 2001; Holland 1999; Kauffman 1995) Using complexity science as a guiding framework, we conceptualize healthcare delivery organizations

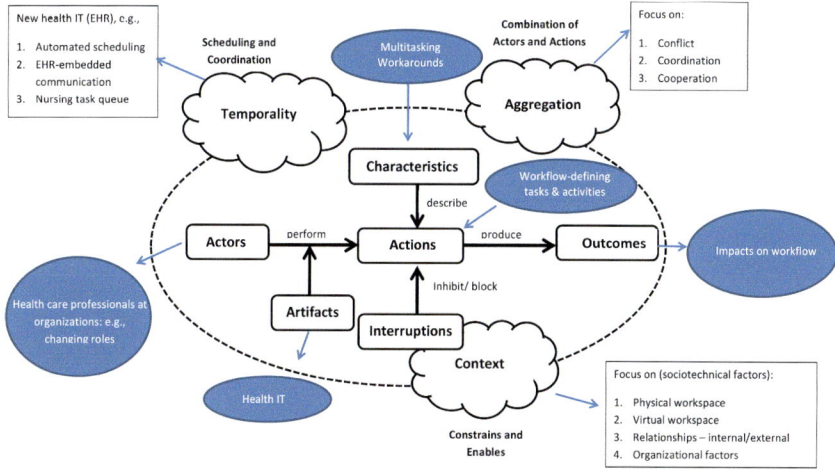

Fig. 17.1 Mapping of study components to workflow elements model (WEM)

as complex adaptive systems characterized by nonlinear interdependencies, self-organization, and irreducible uncertainty (McDaniel et al. 2013; Zimmerman et al. 1998; Kauffman 1995; Cilliers 1998).

17.2.2 Participating Organizations and Study Sites

Organization West is a not-for-profit multispecialty medical group practice serving over 140,000 patients annually, 53% of whom are rural residents, in several western states of the U.S. Its main campus plus two urban branch clinics are located in a medium-size city. Additional regional primary care practices are located in four rural communities within a 200-mile radius. Eighty-seven percent of this rural state's counties have been designated as Health Professional Shortage Areas, Medically Underserved Areas, and/or Physician Scarcity Areas.

Organization East is a non-profit, community-owned health system that serves over 13,000 patients annually at four community health centers and three school-based programs, mostly in rural areas of a U.S. east coast state. Comprehensive preventive and curative primary care services offered including prenatal care, pediatrics, adult chronic and acute care, integrated mental health services, pharmacy, and independent laboratory services. Organization East serves communities with high rates of poverty, behavioral health risks, and chronic diseases.

Three ambulatory care practices participated from each of the two organizations and five of the six practices were primary care clinics. Implementation of patient-centered medical home (PCMH) models of care was underway at both study organizations at the start of the study. Two Organization West sites were rural satellite clinics providing care to patients from resource-poor communities. Organization

Table 17.1 Characteristics of the participating ambulatory care practices

Organization	Study site	Location	Annual patient volume[a]	Number of providers[b]
West	Primary care 1	Rural	19,223	11
	Primary care 2	Rural	17,902	13
	Specialty care	Urban[c]	9,475	7
East	Primary care 1	Rural	3,761	6
	Primary care 2	Rural	4,164	6
	Primary care 3	Rural	4,433	7

[a] Based on data for FY2013
[b] Providers include Medical Doctor (MD), Doctor of Osteopathy (DO), Nurse Practitioner (NP), and Physician Assistant (PA)
[c] "Urban" city population 109,059 (2013 census)

West Specialty Care clinic was included to increase heterogeneity of the study sample and generalizability of research findings. Because specialty clinics may follow different workflow processes and encounter unique challenges in relation to health IT implementation, including a specialty clinic broadened the understanding of the impacts of health IT on workflow practice. Table 17.1 provides basic information on the participating ambulatory care practices.

17.2.3   Health IT Implementations Studied

Table 17.2 summarizes the major health IT implementations that took place at the two participating organizations during the study period. These projects were key to practice redesign, as explained in detail below, and were exemplars of other major practice redesign efforts underway in U.S. healthcare organizations at the time.

Organization West

Organization West had been using a vendor-supplied electronic health records (EHR) system since 2004. During this project, primary care and specialty practices engaged in the clinical advancement project, a major practice redesign effort that included implementation of a series of EHR-based processes to improve ambulatory care, including an electronic patient "homepage," a standardized message center, and enhanced e-prescribing and computerized provider order entry (CPOE).

Table 17.2 Health IT implementations studied

Organization	Health IT	Date	Site affected	Number of providers[a]
West	Clinical advancement project (i.e., electronic homepage; standardized message center; computerized provider order entry; and e-prescribing)	07/16/2013	Primary care 1	11
		08/20/2013	Primary care 2	13
		10/01/2013	Specialty care	7
East	A new, vendor-supplied electronic health record system	9/3/2013	Primary care 1	6
			Primary care 2	6
			Primary care 3	7

[a] Providers include Medical Doctor (MD), Doctor of Osteopathy (DO), Nurse Practitioner (NP), and Physician Assistant (PA)

Organization East

During the project period, Organization East implemented a new EHR system. Some of the functions of the new EHR included automatic patient appointment telephone reminders, documentation of patient medical and social history prior to visit, internal diagnostic test ordering, management of incoming testing and consultation reports, comprehensive patient summaries with updated care plans, automated monitoring and follow-up of no-show patients, monitoring and reporting patient gaps in care, a patient portal, monitoring of team case reviews, and capability of data entry through voice recognition software.

17.2.4 Study Design

The study featured a prospective observational design with multiple data collection points *before*, *during*, and *after* the planned health IT implementations, as shown in Fig. 17.2. The empirical research was conducted using a mixed methods approach consisting of ethnographic observations, time and motion observations, log analysis, semi-structured interviews, and member checking focus groups.

17.2.5 Data Collection Methods

Ethnographic Observations

Based on the work of Agar (1996), and Strauss and Corbin (1998), ethnographic observations helped develop an understanding of the overall characteristics of clinical

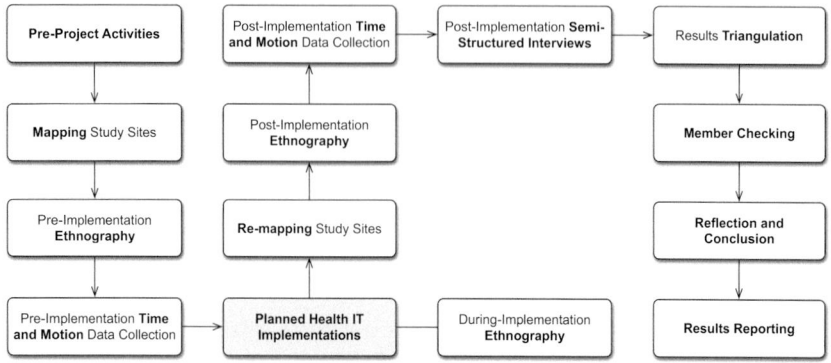

Fig. 17.2 Study design and data collection activities

work at each study practice and inform potential idiosyncrasies of the empirical environments that might affect the conduct of the other study components, data interpretation, and generalizability of findings and conclusions.

Ethnographic observations were conducted across all stages of the planned health IT implementations. At each study practice, the pre-implementation observations focused on: (1) establishing rapport between the investigator team and the clinicians, clinic managers, and other personnel; (2) developing an understanding of the work-flow processes; and (3) mapping the physical practice layout, particularly layout changes after the health IT implementations. Identical ethnographic activities were conducted *during* the planned health IT implementation period to observe distur-bances introduced by health IT implementation; and 3 months *after* the planned health IT implementation to observe healthcare team members performing normal work activities and interacting with the newly implemented health IT systems or products.

Time and Motion Study

A time and motion study involves continuous and independent observations of an individual's work to record data describing each task the individual performs (*what, when, where, for how long*); it is generally regarded as the most reliable method for quantifying work processes and workflow. We conducted a large-scale time and motion study by having two trained research assistants (RAs) shadow clinicians and clinic staff to independently observe their work activities *before* and *after* the planned health IT implementations. Participants were randomly assigned to the two RAs, but the observee-observer pairing stayed the same across the two study stages so that pre-post nuances could be more reliably attributable to true health IT impacts rather than observer biases. The RAs used an iPad-based data recording tool developed by the research team to collect time and motion data. Figure 17.3 is a display of the main screen of the tool.

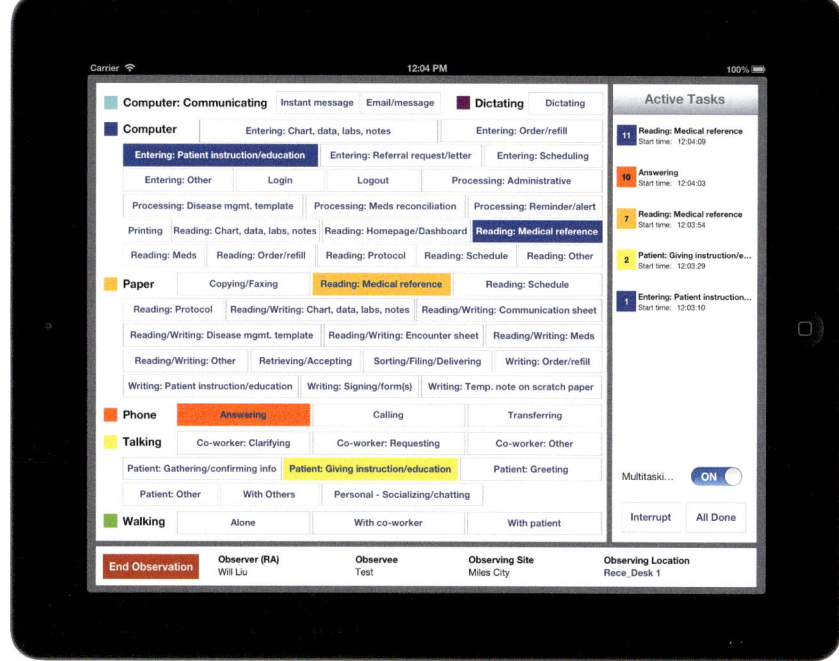

Fig. 17.3 The main screen of the iPad time and motion data recording tool

Log Analysis

For security auditing purposes, all certified EHR systems are required to have the capability of recording and maintaining audit trail logs (CCHIT 2012). These log files contain detailed information regarding end-user interactions with the system such as when a function or a patient document was accessed, and by whom. In this project, we conducted an exploratory log analysis using 5 months of the audit trail logs recorded in the EHR systems at the two participating organizations (2 months before, 1 month during, and 2 months after the health IT implementations). These logs provided us supplemental data to validate and augment the results obtained from time and motion observations, and to analyze clinicians' and clinic staff' off-hours work activities, defined as work conducted outside each clinic's normal business hours.

Semi-structured Interviews

Immediately following the time and motion data collection, we conducted semi-structured interviews to solicit end user beliefs, attitudes, and perceptions about how the health IT implementation altered workflow. Particular attention was paid to sociotechnical integration and how it may mitigate or augment the impacts of health IT on workflow. The interview data also allowed for triangulation with data collected during ethnographic observations, the time and motion study, and from log analysis (Linder et al. 2006).

Member Checking Focus Groups

Individual 60–75 min focus groups were held with staff at each of the six participating study sites. The purpose was to ensure the research findings, as well as the interpretation of the findings, accurately reflected the healthcare teams' practices and experiences with the changes in health IT under study. The focus group sessions were recorded and transcribed for analysis. Management personnel responsible for the study sites recruited the focus group participants who comprised a representative group of six to seven staff members.

17.2.6 Data Analysis

Qualitative Data Analysis

Qualitative data (i.e., ethnographic observation notes and interview and focus group transcripts) were analyzed using a constant comparison approach (Strauss and Corbin 1998) to identify recurring themes related to how the introduction of health IT as part of practice redesign processes affected healthcare teams' workflow. The workflow elements model (WEM) (Unertl et al. 2010) and complexity science informed the qualitative analyses. In addition, the ethnographic observations and semi-structured interviews focused on the flow of clinical work (i.e., patterns in the sequential execution of clinical tasks), interruptions, and exceptions, as described in the *Conceptual Models* section, allowing the research team to attribute changes in workflow to specific elements of health IT implementation and use, or particular features of a health IT system.

Analyses followed three steps: (1) theme formation; (2) theme matching along themes and patterns observed in the data; and (3) theme comparison across practice sites (Yin 2003). Multiple members of the investigator team independently reviewed the data, making methodological memos, theoretical memos, and preliminary interpretations. Individual researcher interpretations were discussed by the research team throughout the project. Themes and patterns were further refined and new themes were co-generated (Crabtree and Miller 1999). All themes were developed through a process of articulating a unifying idea that represented interpretations from multiple data points. Conceptual labels were assigned to organize themes according to a common thread among ideas. In each step, themes were refined whereby similarly labeled ideas were combined into themes and given more general labels. Disagreements were resolved through group discussion until consensus was reached. Iterations of this process provided a platform for comparing the themes within and between the clinics (Eisenhardt 1989). These processes were facilitated by the NVivo qualitative data analysis software (QSR International, Doncaster, Australia).

Quantitative Data Analysis

The quantitative data collected in this project were generated from time and motion observations and computer-recorded audit trail logs. Both data sources captured study participants' work processes and workflow in the form of sequences of time stamped clinical activities, or "event sequences." These event sequences were analyzed using three methods described in Zheng et al. (2010) namely time allocation analysis, workflow fragmentation analysis, and pattern recognition. These methods were designed to quantify how clinicians and clinic staff spend their time on different tasks and to uncover hidden regularities embedded in the flow of their work (Zheng et al. 2010).

Online Workflow Analytical Tool

A majority of quantitative data analyses performed in this project was conducted using a Web-based workflow analytical tool. Figure 17.4 shows a screenshot of its main workspace.

The tool supports interactive data analyses on different measures, using different multitasking calibrating methods and different combinations of clinical roles, study practices, and participating organizations. For example, the *Pre-Post* tab automatically computes the key measures of the project (e.g., time allocation and continuous time spent on a given task) and reports statistics for testing the statistical significance of pre-post differences. The *Multitasking* and *Interruption* tabs provided measures on these two types of events, including their frequency of appearing and common combinations of activities that comprised multitasking or in interrupting/interrupted relationships. The *Interruption* tab further applied network analysis to compute key measures characterizing interrupting/interrupted relationships. The *Pattern Analysis* tab was based on pattern recognition, which discovered frequently occurring sequential patterns representing groups of tasks often carried out together and in a fixed sequential order. This tab also provided transition probabilities among different pairs of tasks based on empirical datasets. Location data and location–task data were analyzed in the tool using similar analytical approaches.

Integrative Analysis of Qualitative and Quantitative Data

Applying the framework of Fetters et al. (2013), a multistage, integrative mixed methods analysis approach was used to determine the impacts of health IT on workflow in the context of ambulatory practice redesign. Integration occurred at the study

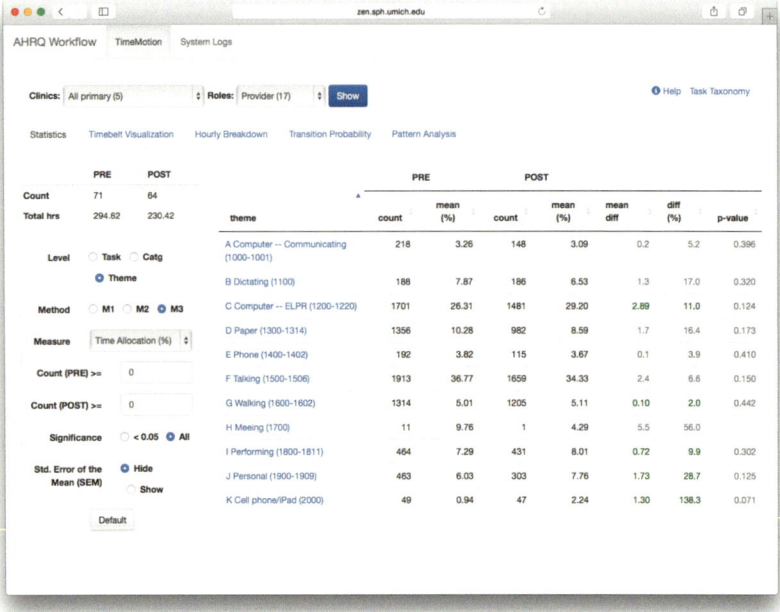

Fig. 17.4 Screenshot of the online workflow analytical tool

design, methods, and interpretation levels. Integration at each level is described. The "fit" of the integration was also assessed.

Integration at the design level. Because a multistage mixed methods framework was employed, combinations of exploratory sequential, explanatory sequential, and convergent approaches were used (Nastasi et al. 2007). Following an *exploratory sequential design*, baseline ethnographic observations and analysis occurred first, in order to inform the development of the task taxonomy and the iPad-based time and motion data collection tool. Qualitative data collection and analysis of the observation data drove changes in the next phase of data collection procedures, the time and motion observation stage. Following an *explanatory sequential design,* the quantitative time and motion observation data were collected first, followed by qualitative interviews, whose content was reflective of the quantitative data collected. The interviews were designed to further explain the findings produced from the ethnographic and time and motion observation data.

Integration at the methods level. Integration of qualitative and quantitative methods occurred through linking the methods of data collection and analysis and by connecting, building, merging, and embedding (Cresswell et al. 2011). Integration occurred through *connecting* when quantitative data were linked with qualitative data through the sampling frame. For example, the interview participants were selected from the population of participants who were followed during the time and motion study phase, as well as those followed during ethnographic observation. Integration through *building* occurred when the initial ethnographic observation informed the design of the time and motion data collection tool. The latter could not have been built without the data collected on tasks performed in the specific participating clinics. Integration through *merging* and *embedding* occurred when quantitative time and motion data was brought together with qualitative observation and interview data for comparison (merging) and then presented (embedded) during the member checking focus groups.

Integration at the interpretation and reporting levels. Integration at the interpretation and reporting levels occurred through narrative. Several approaches were used. A weaving approach was used which involved writing both qualitative and quantitative findings together on a theme-by-theme basis. This approach was used in most of the theme- and concept-based findings. A contiguous approach, or separate reporting of quantitative and qualitative findings, was used for some reporting of quantitative findings where no related qualitative findings existed.

Data integration 'fit'. We found instances of integration to be confirmatory, but not discordant, thus the fit of integration methods was determined to be good. For example, in the log audit data collection phase, the quantitative data confirmed the qualitative data analysis results. During the qualitative interviews, participants reported an increased amount of off-hours work following the health IT implementation. The quantitative log audit data analysis confirmed these findings to be true, with observed significant increases in time spent before and after normal clinic hours.

17.3 Results

17.3.1 Study Sample

At Organization West, a total of 75 clinicians and clinic staff participated in this study, including 17 physicians, 9 advance practitioners (nurse practitioners or physician assistants), 11 medical assistants, 19 nurses, 9 clinical staff members, and 10 other healthcare professionals such as laboratory technicians, physical therapists, registered dietitians, audiologists, and supporting staff members. At Organization East, 53 clinicians and clinic staff participated including 9 physicians, 9 advance practitioners, 18 medical assistants, 17 clinical staff members, and 2 other healthcare professionals.

Description of Qualitative Research Activities

Direct observation involved 122 participants from the six study practices. Interviews involved 39 participants from the six study practices. Focus groups involved 38 participants from the six study practices. Direct observations resulted in approximately 554 single spaced pages of field notes from approximately 366 h of observation. Transcribed interviews resulted in between 3 and 17 pages per interview, with an average of approximately ten pages, of single-spaced text per transcript. Transcribed focus groups resulted in 11–19 pages per focus group, with an average of 15 pages, of single-spaced text per transcript.

Descriptive Analyses of Quantitative Data

The time and motion study involved 29 providers, 16 medical assistants (MAs), six nurses, and six clinic staff (all were receptionists) from the six study practices. Most participated in the study both before and after the health IT implementations, except three providers, one MA, and two nurses who only participated in the pre-implementation phase study, and three staff members who only participated in the post-implementation study phase. A total of 1,173.4 h of data were recorded over 386 sessions. The dataset contained 85,808 distinct records describing the study participants' various clinical tasks or personal activities. The time and motion study in the post-implementation phase had fewer observation hours. This was primarily because several clinicians left the study practices before the post-implementation time and motion data collection began. A total of 66,820 audit trail logs were collected at Organization West and 12,542 were collected at Organization East.

Inter-Observer Validation

After training, the RAs practiced time and motion observation in simulated environments. Then, they paired up to participate in a validation session by simultaneously shadowing the same clinician. The objective was to calibrate the RAs' observations to ensure that the time and motion data collected by different individuals were reasonably consistent.

17.3.2 Findings

Shifting Time Allocation Across Tasks

Using the time and motion data, we examined the amount of time spent on different tasks pre- and post-health IT implementations by clinic role using the time allocation measure, that is, time spent on task as proportion of time spent on all tasks.

Noteworthy and varied changes across the organizations and clinics were seen in: communicating via computer; using computer for entering, processing and reading; paper use; and talking. Table 17.3 presents a summary of these results.

MAs at West Primary Care 2 decreased their time spent communicating using the computer (e.g., email, messaging) by ~5% ($p < 0.05$). Computer entering, login, processing and reading produced mixed results. Significant increases were observed among MAs at West Primary 2 (4.5%) and East Primary 1 (19%) and among providers at East Primary 3 (14.4%), while decreases were observed among clinic staff at West Primary 1 ($p < 0.05$). Use of paper significantly decreased in at least one role at every site. The largest reductions were among MAs at East Primary Care 1 (15.4%) and Staff at West Primary 2 (10%) ($p < 0.05$).

Changes were observed in talking between pre- and post-health IT system implementation. Staff at West Primary Care 1 and nurses at West Primary Care 2 significantly increased their time talking, while providers at East Primary Care 1 demonstrated an eight percent reduction in talking ($p < 0.05$).

Multitasking

A total of 49,961 activities recorded in the time and motion data had overlapping timestamps. After applying the 30-s threshold discussed earlier in the interobserver validation section, excluding likely human observer error, 6,028 activities with overlapping timestamps remained in the dataset.

Table 17.4 shows that except for West Specialty Care, the level of multitasking, both in terms of frequency and average duration, decreased considerably after the health IT implementations, observed as decreases in the All Roles data for all primary care sites ($p < 0.05$). This result is especially prominent among the MAs across all primary care sites and the providers at Organization East.

Workflow Workarounds

Workarounds, behaviors, and processes that circumvent or temporarily fix an evident or perceived workflow problem, occur frequently in care settings undergoing health IT system changes. Using qualitative data, we examined workarounds created in response to health IT implementations, especially those that impacted workflow.

Workflow workarounds were developed at all study sites to address the fear of orders and patients being "lost in the system" or "falling through the cracks." Workarounds for managing this fear usually involved manual or paper-based redundant systems to run alongside or serve as a double check on the newly implemented health IT. This impacted workflow by decreasing efficiency. A provider from West Primary Care 2 described an incident where, in relation to CPOE, "*they didn't have everything in place when they rolled it out.*"

Other workflow workarounds were related to inadequate design of the newly implemented health IT changes. At both organizations, design issues resulted in the health IT's inability to address an exception that occurred during vaccination and medication ordering.

Table 17.3 Selected percent changes in time allocation

Time allocation (%)		West	West	West	West	East	East	East
Theme	Role	Primary 1	Primary 2	Specialty clinic	Primary 1	Primary 2	Primary 3
A. Computer—communicating	MA[a]	6.34	−4.56*	−0.24	0.11	3.36	−0.49
	Staff	0.78	12.44	−	−	−	−0.38
C. Computer—entering, login, processing, reading	Provider	1.19	−0.75	2.55	4.66	−2.62	14.36*
	MA[a]	−2.44	4.50*	0.50	19.05*	5.76	6.05
	Staff	−4.90*	3.38	−	−	−	7.88
D. Paper	Provider	−2.88*	−3.86	−4.11*	−1.71	−4.60*	−3.41*
	MA[a]	−7.07	−6.73*	2.30	−15.40*	−4.92*	−5.22
	Nurse	−	4.20	1.01	−	−	−
	Staff	−3.04	−10.15	−	−	−	−8.34*
F. Talking	Provider	−1.89	3.90	−0.27	−8.33*	−6.25	−2.18
	Nurse	−	10.02*	4.64	−	−	−
	Staff	8.16*	−1.37	−	−	−	−1.80

[a] MA: Medical Assistant
* Significant at the 0.05 level

Table 17.4 Results of multitasking analysis

Measure	Clinical role	Org. west	Org. west	Org. west	Org. west	Org. east	Org. east
		Primary care sites	Primary care sites	Specialty care	Specialty care	All sites	All sites
		Pre	Post	Pre	Post	Pre	Post
Frequency (number of occurrences per hour)	Provider	21.46	18.66	25.47	21.04	29.06	16.59*
	MA[a]	47.49	25.78*	6.24	6.87	24.84	10.87*
	Nurse	12.26	4.23	13.08	9.22	–	–
	Staff	48.12	23.59*	–	–	17.33	13.24
	All Roles	25.62	18.32*	19.97	16.46	26.94	14.04*
Average duration (seconds)	Provider	54.68	47.74	60.86	61.48	61.67	37.25*
	MA[a]	78.18	43.79*	30.02	27.06	54.63	24.89*
	Nurses	36.69	22.77	36.48	29.24	–	–
	Staff	61.16	49.72	–	–	49.83	35.48
	All Roles	53.95	43.89*	50.91	49.49	58.36	32.23*

[a] MA: Medical Assistant (MA)
* Significant at the 0.05 level

Workarounds to improve workflow efficiency were present at all six study sites. At West Primary Care 1 and 2, the computerized vaccination process was "too cumbersome" so a workaround was developed in which the provider gave the nurse written orders, rather than through the EHR queue. This is an example of a paper-based system to circumvent a more structured, computer-based process. In East Primary Care 3 one MA did not use the new EHR post-implementation and instead used paper-based systems combined with the old EHR to perform work tasks.

In summary, workflow workarounds were created in response to the new health IT systems implemented at both organizations. Workarounds were often created in response to an exception the health IT was unable to address. Some decreased efficiency, some reduced quality. Many were implemented because of concerns for patient safety. Several appeared to be temporary while the health IT systems became fully functional. Regardless, the workflow workarounds were disruptive to workflow and the provision of quality patient care.

Impacts of Health IT on Workflow Efficiency

Study participants reported both increased and decreased workflow efficiency following the health IT implementations. For example, benefits of the health IT implementation reported by Specialty Care clinic providers and staff were increased workflow efficiencies related to: the collection of patient data in advance of a patient's visit; the increased detail on radiology orders; short-term follow-up visit scheduling; and message center for provider-nurse communication of non-time sensitive issues.

Another area of increased workflow efficiency was observed at West Primary Care 2 where a "Core Team" model was implemented that was designed to address inefficiencies of wait time for the patient and eliminate redundancies in the provider/nursing workflow process. For Core Team providers, patient encounters increased over a 60-day period and were maintained. At the clinic level, average patients seen per day increased from 70 to 80, with the same level of staffing. The two other Organization West study clinics experienced static or declining use. The Core Teams saw a maximum of 24 patients per day, while the traditional teams saw 18. Not only had providers been able to see more patients per day, but they felt they were providing better care. This also improved efficiency, according to this provider who gets fewer phone messages.

> The other piece is talking amongst the team to get things done because now more people know the story and a secondary benefit of that is, so [the nurse] is in the room with me with the patient, she hears it, so when the patient calls for clarification, [MA] gets the call, [the nurse] can answer most of the questions, so ultimately I get fewer message of people that I have to call.

Another benefit reported by a nurse at West Primary Care 2 was more education for patients:

> The nurse also has done a lot more education with the patient as well…You know, they're able to sit, when the physician is ready to leave, then they can do a little bit of additional education with the patient, so they're getting a lot more education, definitely.

Workflow efficiency improved as patients received needed education at the time of the visit, removing the need for follow up phone calls. Clinicians and clinic staff reported a decreased volume of phone calls following the health IT implementation.

In other clinics, however, the health IT implementation was reported to cause more time on the computer and less time with patients. A provider from West Primary Care 1 said:

> [It is] irritating to me that I have to spend more and more time on the computer and less time with the patient … but I guess it's the way of the future, but I don't like it.

Workarounds resulted in workflow inefficiencies caused by creating paper backup systems or entering double orders to account for EHR system deficiencies during implementation. More computer clicks required more time to complete tasks, increased documentation requirements required more time, and disjointed or fragmented work resulting from systems with more structured documentation requirements led to disjointed and fragmented workflow. Distracted by the computer, staff members reported being less attentive to patients during interactions, which led to patients leaving the clinic with incomplete information and therefore increased phone calls and inquiries back to the clinic at a later time.

Changes in Computer Activities During Off-Hours

Only Organization West had pre/post computer audit logs from the same EHR system. Computer activities conducted before and after normal business hours were quantified through log analysis. The primary measure was the volume of interaction events logged in the EHR systems. Participant perceptions were also solicited in semi-structured interviews and member checking focus groups.

The health IT implementation impacted clinicians' off-hours computer work differently based on their roles. The providers in the Specialty Care clinic were affected most, with a 40% post-implementation increase ($p < 0.05$). MAs in West Primary Care 2 experienced an increase in their off-hours computer activities while other types of clinicians and staff in the same clinic worked less with the computer. Similar patterns were also observed in West Primary Care 1, where the volume of MAs' off-hours computer activities increased while nurses and other staff's off-hours computer activities decreased. Patterns of providers' off-hours computer activities differed by clinic. The reductions in off-hours computer activities among staff at the two West primary care clinics, and the increases in regular clinic hour computer work by providers at Specialty Care clinic, were statistically significant ($p < 0.05$).

A Specialty Clinic surgeon voiced the following during a focus group:

> The continuous dictation I think, for me, I used to try and dictate in between patients and at the end of the day now is when I do all my dictation. I try and do it, but there's just no time, so I end up dictating at 5 o'clock continuously for two hours.

In summary, while all three Organization West clinics experienced increases in off-hours computer work as indicated by the volume of interaction events recorded in the EHR systems, the Specialty clinic was impacted the most, with a considerable increase in computer activities performed outside regular clinic hours.

The Impact of Relationships and Interdependencies on Workflow

Relationships and interdependencies are contextual organizational factors that may constrain or enable workflow according to the WEM (see Fig. 17.1). The number of participant comments gathered in the ethnographic observation and interview data about relationships and interdependencies by site varied. There were many comments about interdependencies and productive interpersonal relationships from all three East sites and from one West site.

Perceptions of what fostered collaboration varied across sites. Staff members at East attributed highly collaborative, helping environment to the organization's culture. Staff member comments frequently included the use of the word "we." The helping seemed informal and pervasive. In the West site that had the most significant collaborative environment, staff comments suggested that the collaboration was primarily a result of a structural intervention—the Core Team model. Staff spoke of high levels of collaboration within teams and the sharing of helpful ideas from team to team by nurses when they filled in on other teams.

Another sociotechnical factor we examined for its mitigating impact on health IT and workflow was team power differentials, a sociotechnical factor highlighted by complexity science and associated with a system's ability to adapt. Differences were observed in this factor across sites. Organization East did not refer to the existence of power differentials. On the contrary, providers often mentioned helping medical assistants as well as nurses and medical assistants helping providers with health IT issues—all evidence of low power differentials across professional disciplines. The situation at West Primary Care 2 seemed similar. Members figured out how best to meet health IT requirements, drawing on expertise within the team.

At the study sites noted for collaboration, in which more references were made to positive relationships and a helping atmosphere, implementation of the planned health IT changes proceeded more smoothly and also with less heterogeneity in patterns of health IT use, according to clinician and clinic staff member comments.

Because staff members knew they could rely on colleagues for support, those at highly collaborative sites generally experienced less frustration and anxiety with the studied health IT changes as reported in ethnographic observations and interviews. Despite a more significant change in health IT at Organization East (entirely new EHR system) than at Organization West (modifications to existing system), the overall level of frustration and anxiety attributed to health IT changes and impact on workflow recorded at Organization East was lower than Organization West.

In the less collaborative sites (Specialty Care and West Primary Care 1) more staff members had to cope with individual decisions made by providers about whether or how to adopt the planned health IT changes, i.e., use of Message Center, CPOE. This led to more heterogeneous, idiosyncratic approaches to practice and workflow in these sites. Multiple different workflows existed side by side and staff had to be aware of these differences and adjust to them.

Impacts Magnified through Interruptions and Exceptions

The time and motion data contained 664 interruptive events. Significant pre-post differences in frequency (number per hour) were found among the providers and MAs at Organization West. These changes were principally driven by the data from West Primary Care 2. As shown in Table 17.5, the providers and MAs from West Primary Care 2 experienced more than a three-fold increase of frequency of interruptions after the health IT implementation.

At Organization East, while there were no significant pre-post differences at the aggregate level, the frequency of interruptions experienced by the providers at Primary Care 3 increased significantly post-implementation.

Across all sites there were two interruptive events that increased significantly and are clinically relevant. These include "Talking to Coworker," which on average increased from 0.31 to 2.53 interruptive events per hour and "Talking to Patient," which on average increased from 0.56 to 5.82 interruptive events per hour.

Observations from the qualitative data provide some context to the struggles that providers, nurses, and clinic staff at both organizations faced as they worked to incorporate the new health IT into their work practices. For example, when an MA at West Primary Care 2 triaged patients, she *didn't know if a person needs their height measured until she is in the exam room going through the screens,*" (the height is only done annually), and that the computer had a hard stop, not allowing her to continue.

Table 17.5 Frequency of interruptive events

Clinical Role	Org. west	Org. west	Org. west	Org. west	Org. west	Org. west	Org. east	Org. east	Org. east	Org. east
	All sites	All sites	Primary care 2	Primary care 2	Special care	Special care	All sites	All sites	Primary care 3	Primary care 3
	Pre	Post	Pre	Post	Pre	Post	Pre	Post	Pre	Post
Provider	0.91	2.18*	0.95	3.25*	1.12	1.33	0.90	0.92	0.39	1.05*
MA[a]	0.77	2.32	0.67	3.20*	1.03	0.28	0.66	1.32	0.29	1.16
Nurse	0.80	0.40*	0.69	0.40	0.73	0.69	–	–	–	–
Staff	0.46	–	0.65	–	–	–	–	0.72	–	0.72
All roles	0.83	1.86*	0.80	2.24*	1.06	1.19	0.79	1.04	0.34	1.05*

[a] MA: Medical Assistants

* Significant at 0.05 level

So if she did not obtain the height before going into the exam room she said she would "*put something in*" and then she "*would have to remember to get the patient's height when they left,*" which our observer noted she forgot to do. A nurse at the same clinic describes several health IT generated interruptions and how they impact her workflow. She says,

> clinical advancement project is not intuitive, and they removed 'no complaint of pain' and put in the scale 0–10, why did they do that? …. Too many clicks and going in and out of screens. I need to go through two different screens to document no prescriptions.

Then as she began printing the growth chart report, that is intended to be shared with families, she continued,

> This is not patient friendly. This report shows the measurements using the metric system. Should use standard for patients to easily understand. I record the standard information next to the metric numbers. Also, It would be helpful if the different formulary names for the same medication could be in here. I need to rely on my knowledge of the various brand names to find the correct one. Why are over the counter medications entered and viewed in a separate location? It would make more sense to be able to view all medications in one area.

The implications for how health IT-generated interruptions impact how individual healthcare professionals approach their work, conceptualize their role in their patients' lives, and make sense of their patients' conditions are perhaps less obvious. For example, a nurse from West Primary Care 1 articulated a concern that "*multitasking combined with phone interruptions during provider order entry could create new medication entry errors.*" In the same clinic, a provider discussed an interruption that presented itself sporadically throughout an entire morning when a biopsy sample was not processed properly. The interruption to workflow in this case was the error, the incorrectly processed biopsy.

Interruptions also seemed to slow workflow and introduce inefficiencies. One provider from West Primary Care 2 said during clinical advancement project implementation that he "*ordered a prescription on the wrong patient, a colonoscopy by the cardiologist, and a vaginal issue with a general surgeon."* He then expressed that he *"feels flustered"* and *"concerned that he isn't giving safe care."*

17.4 Discussion

The results of this project demonstrated that clinical workflow is a complex undertaking that encompasses many facets including discrete work processes, sequential order task execution, task interdependency, communication and interaction patterns, and shared and shifting responsibilities among members of a care team. Clinical workflow is also a dynamic and fragile system impacted by changes introduced into the clinical environment such as implementation of new health IT systems.

The clinical work processes and workflow at the two participating organizations were considerably altered by the new health IT systems implemented as part of ongoing practice redesign initiatives. At one clinic, an entirely new workflow process model (the "Core Team" model) was introduced to enable increased clinical documentation and improved workflow. At other clinics, less skilled positions were phased out during the study period as the newly implemented health IT systems introduced new work task efficiencies and, in some cases, created opportunities for individuals to advance to higher skilled positions. The workflow elements model (WEM) helped organize primary study findings around the key components of clinical workflow. Complexity science as a guiding theoretical framework helped us interpret an extensive amount of rich and contextually nuanced qualitative data to better understand and generate insights into the sociotechnical factors impacting the relationship between health IT implementation and workflow.

17.4.1 The Causal Relationship Between Health IT Implementation and Ambulatory Care Workflow Redesign

Aligned with complex systems theory, health IT had a clear impact on workflow, but it was rare to observe uniform impacts across clinics due to between- and within-clinic heterogeneity in health IT implementation, clinic processes, provider practice patterns, and organizational and clinic-level work environments. For example, the differences observed in time allocation across tasks were heavily influenced at West Primary Care 2 by the simultaneous implementation of a new model of care that specified a shifting of duties for existing clinical roles that was reflected in the time and motion data. For this same clinic, the new model of care itself was designed in such a way to reduce off-hours computer work, therefore partly explaining between-clinic differences.

Another consideration is how providers differentially perceive health IT and how this perception impacts uptake. These perceptions are influenced by how different people process information and react to technology, as well as external influences, such as redesign of clinic processes. For example, in one clinic that had several older providers who did not express a positive relationship with technology, uptake of the new health IT system was limited, with at least half of the providers adopting very few of the new system's features. This impacted workflow in the clinic.

The health IT components themselves had an influence on workflow and on their use and perceived worth. Some health IT features improved workflow, relationships, and communication. Participants at the three Organization West sites noted that internal EHR-based messaging improved inter-professional communication. At most sites, staff members observed that the requirement to gather patient information prior to the provider visit helped build relationships between medical assistants and patients. In several instances it was noted that the "Depart Summary" encouraged greater engagement of patients in their care and productive conversations with staff.

Patient safety concerns played a significant role. Health IT design flaws or insufficiencies led to concerns for patient safety and thus workflow workarounds were developed. Workarounds created to protect patients may have led to a mistrust of the system, leading to even further workarounds. Study participants reported a lack of trust in the new system and the creation of redundant, often paper-based systems, as a reaction to worries that patients would be lost in the new system. Many concerns stemmed from a lack of complete understanding of the new system and may have been mollified by more comprehensive training on the new health IT systems.

Sociotechnical Factors

Sociotechnical factors played a major role in mitigating potentially negative impacts of health IT changes and augmenting favorable impacts of health IT on workflow. One identified factor was the nature of relationships among staff members and the impact of relationships on the work environment. Differences in clinic work environments became apparent through ethnographic observations and interviews. The strong ethic of collaboration and teamwork evident at Organization East seemed to enable their study sites to successfully cope with implementing a new EHR in a very compressed period of time. Helping efforts by staff seemed to be pervasive and an informal part of daily work. Assistance crossed roles and hierarchy. No evidence emerged of self-interested decisions by providers as was seen in some of the West study practices. The collaborative environment in this Organization appeared to enable more learning during the implementation period as well as widespread diffusion of health IT solutions to end users.

In contrast, West Specialty Care staff members mentioned how the differing decisions by providers on how and whether to use new health IT features impacted the workflow of other staff members. Such actions could be viewed as an assertion of decision-making rights by those with more power. This led to more heterogeneous, idiosyncratic approaches to practice and workflow. Differing workflows existed side by side and staff had to be aware of these differences and adjust to them. This may have led to less efficiency in workflow and more differences in use of planned health IT changes. These examples demonstrate how the work environment, in this case the degree of power differentials, can impact health IT implementation and, by association, workflow.

Impacts Magnified Through Interruptions and Exceptions

Little is known about the impact of health IT-related interruptions, and health-IT's response to exceptions, on workflow. We observed health IT-caused interruptions to clinical workflow across all study clinics and work roles. Beyond impacts on workflow efficiency, we observed differences in the quantity of interruptions between the pre- and post-implementation periods by clinic. For example, clinicians and staff at one primary care study clinic experienced a more than three-fold increase in the frequency of interruptions following the health IT implementation, while other clinics experienced no difference. Between-clinic contextual factors may explain some of these differences. For example, more interruptions may be due to a highly collaborative work environment where colleagues actively seek assistance from one another. Patient interruptions are also common when new health IT is introduced because of increased provider documentation requirements and therefore increased time spent on the computer during patient visits. The new health IT may not have been adequately integrated into the workflow design, including the provider-patient interaction. Providers often reported less time to talk to patients during a visit following the health IT implementation. Finally, health IT did not appear to adequately accommodate all care situations, e.g., certain vaccinations, orders, resulting in workarounds. The cause was sometimes the health IT design itself, or the implementation of new design features, which were inadequate in addressing non-typical patients or patient needs.

17.4.2   *Implications and Recommendations*

Key implications and recommendations for implementation of health IT in ambulatory care settings during practice redesign were identified. *Staff engagement* is important in planning changes, making sense of early implementation efforts, and developing thoughtful modifications to health IT features and ongoing implementation efforts. Considering that *different clinics at the same organization may have different implementation plans* is important, recognizing the different work environments and local cultures within a single system. Organizations implementing health IT to support practice redesign efforts need to be alert to the fact that *unexpected developments are likely to occur*, attentive to surprises when they do occur, and capable of making sense of these developments and adjusting plans and systems effectively. Vendors and health IT implementers should consider use of *minimum specifications concept* in health IT feature design and allow variation and flexibility around these core specifications. Consider *reducing staff workload during the health IT implementation period* to provide time for staff to incorporate health IT changes into practice and for staff to help one another. Finally, future research should work to better understand the impact of health IT-generated interruptions on medical professionalism.

17.4.3 Lessons Learned

Several key lessons were learned about studying health IT implementation in ambulatory care practices undergoing practice redesign and the practicalities of applying multiple mixed methods. There are challenges inherent in quantifying workflow. Human observers had limited ability to capture certain tasks performed by clinicians and clinic staff, especially those that occurred rapidly or were not easy to discern such as clinicians' interactions with computer systems. Audit trail logs were also difficult to interpret as they had no signifier for duration, confusing labels, and were overall inconsistent.

Small, rural clinics are challenging to study due to scarcity of resources, including time and staff; low numbers of providers and staff, potentially resulting in scheduling challenges with providers/staff taking vacations, sabbaticals, et cetera; and challenges traveling to distant clinics, especially during the winter. In addition, mistrust by clinic staff of researchers, inherent in small communities, may have hindered studies.

Keeping research plans flexible and being alert for learning opportunities was key. Even when they are part of large health systems, small, rural clinics often act more like independent clinics. This is what occurred at West Primary Care 2 where the Core Team model with scribes was implemented. Because this was topic of national interest at the time, the research team decided to devote more attention to this development, which added richness to the study.

Finally, we learned the two-way value of member checking, i.e., the sites learned as much as we did during this process, and the value of a mixed methods approach. While the quantitative data generated by the project exhibited many prominent pre-post or cross-site differences, these differences carried little meaning without the contextual details rendered by qualitative investigations.

17.4.4 Study Limitations

Limitations included lack of generalizability as the empirical sites included six ambulatory care practices from two participating organizations with unique characteristics that may differ from other ambulatory practices. Second, some study practices were very small only with a handful of participants in each clinical role. A few outliners' behavior could therefore be disproportionally represented in the sample. Third, the vendor-specific idiosyncrasies of the health IT products or systems implemented at each organization could have a strong influence over our study findings. Finally, all study sites had already used EHRs prior to this study. Their experience might thus be very different from those that recently transitioned to health IT from paper-based operations.

17.5 Conclusion

This project used a mixed methods design to study the impacts of health IT on clinical work processes and workflow across six ambulatory care practices at two participating organizations. The results show that health IT supported practice redesign was associated with benefits such as less reliance on paper, increased efficiency, improved referral processes, and, in some cases, more time with patients. However, the results also show that health IT was associated with adverse impacts on workflow. These included more computer activities during both regular hours and off-hours, IT-induced workflow blocks that required circumventing workarounds and caused end-user dissatisfaction. Observed workflow changes were mainly caused by increased documentation requirements and shifted documentation responsibilities, as well as inadequate IT system design. Additional causes included increased complexity in workflow (e.g., for locating information) and fewer face-to-face interactions with co-workers.

The results also show that sociotechnical factors played a significant role in mitigating and augmenting health IT's impacts on workflow. Different study sites developed distinct strategies in response to their new health IT implementation and these strategies relied heavily on the strength of relationships between clinic members, including providers. As a result, the impacts of health IT varied to a considerable degree across the study sites.

Lastly, workflow impacts of health IT were magnified through frequently occurring disruptive events such as interruptions and exceptions. An increased level of interruptions was observed at select clinics and explained by the understanding of influencing sociotechnical factors, such as relationships, and contextual factors, such as local clinic initiatives.

In summary, the impacts of health IT on clinical work processes and workflow are multifaceted and have both beneficial and detrimental effects on many different aspects of patient care delivery and clinic operations. In addition, each ambulatory care practice is unique, and their different work environments and strategies for accommodating health IT could lead to distinctly different results.

References

Agar M. The professional stranger: an informal introduction to ethnography. 2nd ed. San Diego, CA: Emerald Group Publishing; 1996.

Camazine S, Deneuborg J, Franks NR, et al. Self-organization in biological systems. Princeton, NJ: Princeton University Press; 2001.

CCHIT. CCHIT Certified 2011 Ambulatory EHR Certification Criteria 2011 [January 15, 2012.]. http://www.cchit.org/sites/all/files/CCHIT%20Certified%202011%20Ambulatory%20EHR%20Criteria%2020110517.pdf

Cherns A. The principles of sociotechnical design. Hum Relat. 1976;29(8):783–92. https://doi.org/10.1177/001872677602900806.

Cilliers P. Complexity and postmodernism: understanding complex systems. London; New York: Routledge; 1998.

Clegg CW. Sociotechnical principles for system design. Appl Ergon. 2000;31(5):463–77 PMID: 11059460.

Crabtree B, Miller W. Doing qualitative research. Thousand Oaks, CA: Sage; 1999.

Cresswell J, Klassen A, Plano Clark V, et al. Best practices for mixed methods research in the health sciences 2011 [cited 2011 Oct 29, 2013]. http://obssr.od.nih.gov/mixed_methods_research

Eisenhardt K. Building theories from case study research. Acad Manage Rev. 1989;14:532–50.

Fetters MD, Curry LA, Creswell JW. Achieving integration in mixed methods designs-principles and practices. Health Serv Res. 2013;48(6 Pt 2):2134–56. PMID: 24279835. 10.1111.

Holland JH. Emergence: from chaos to order. 1st ed. Cambridge, MA: Perseus Books; 1999.

Kauffman S. At home in the universe: the search for laws of self-organization and complexity. pbk. New York: Oxford University Press; 1995.

Linder JA, Schnipper JL, Tsurikova R, et al. Barriers to electronic health record use during patient visits. AMIA Annu Symp Proc. 2006:499–503. PMID: 17238391. PMCID: 1839290. 86066.

McDaniel RR Jr, Driebe DJ, Lanham HJ. Health care organizations as complex systems: new perspectives on design and management. Adv Health Care Manag. 2013;15:3–26 PMID: 24749211.

Nastasi BK, Hitchcock J, Sarkar S, et al. Mixed methods in intervention research: theory to adaptation. J Mix Methods Res. 2007;1(2):164–82.

Strauss A, Corbin J. Basics of qualitative research: techniques and procedures for developing grounded theory. 2nd ed. Thousand Oaks, CA: Sage Publications, Inc.; 1998.

Unertl KM, Novak LL, Johnson KB, et al. Traversing the many paths of workflow research: developing a conceptual framework of workflow terminology through a systematic literature review. J Am Med Inform Assoc. 2010;17(3):265–73. PMID: 20442143. PMCID: 2995718. 17/3/265.

West B. Where medicine went wrong: rediscovering the path to complexity: World Scientific Publishing Company; 2006.

Yin R. Case study research: design and method. Thousand Oaks, CA: Sage; 2003.

Zheng K, Haftel HM, Hirschl RB, et al. Quantifying the impact of health IT implementations on clinical workflow: a new methodological perspective. J Am Med Inform Assoc. 2010;17(4):454–61. PMID: 20595314. PMCID: 2995654. 17/4/454.

Zimmerman B, Lindberg C, Plsek PE. Edgeware: insights from complexity science for health care leaders. Irving, Texas: VHA Inc.; 1998.

Chapter 18
Health IT-Enabled Care Coordination and Redesign in Ambulatory Care

Jonathan Wald and Laurie Novak

Abstract In this chapter, we present and discuss findings from a study funded by the U.S. Agency for Healthcare Research and Quality (AHRQ) to examine the workflow impact of introducing new technology, My Health Team at Vanderbilt (MHTAV), into primary care clinics to improve care coordination for patients with hypertension and diabetes. The goal of the study was to assess the alignment between health information technology (IT) and clinical workflow during the implementation of MHTAV. Our primary research question was: *what is the workflow impact of implementing health IT-enabled care coordination within six ambulatory primary care clinics?* We approached this question using a human factors and sociotechnical framework. Our aim was to help to fill the evidence gap regarding how health IT adoption impacts workflow, and vice versa.

Keywords Care coordination · Chronic illness · Workflow · Sociotechnical systems · Health IT

18.1 Introduction

Studying workflow and health information technology (IT) adoption is complex because there are many contributing factors and confounders. Research attention to the study of workflow has intensified in the U.S. since the rollout of the meaningful user (MU) program by the Office of the National Coordinator for Health IT (ONC) in 2009. The mounting interest in better understanding clinical workflow in the context of health IT implementation reflects a realization from early pioneer health IT studies—that factors such as site leadership, workflow optimization prior to automation, team communication, and attention to many details of practice and

J. Wald (✉)
SmarterDx, New York City, USA
e-mail: wald.jon@gmail.com

L. Novak
Vanderbilt University Medical Center, Nashville, USA

© The Author(s), under exclusive license to Springer Nature Switzerland AG 2025
K. Zheng et al. (eds.), *Reengineering Clinical Workflow in the Digital and AI Era*,
Cognitive Informatics in Biomedicine and Healthcare,
https://doi.org/10.1007/978-3-031-82971-0_18

367

health IT design and use, can lead to successful adoption of new technology when aligned, or can limit the adoption if gaps are present and remain unaddressed.

The misalignment between workflow and health IT may arise from many contributing factors. These include mismatch between health IT design and the workflow that predated the implementation, insufficient training of users, and inexperienced technical staff responsible for configuring health IT. In addition, health IT often brings together changes in clinical and administrative activities, such as how clinical activities are documented and how the billing process is managed. These, and other sociotechnical challenges, add to the complexity of health IT adoption and implementation research.

Subtle configuration and implementation-related decisions can hurt or help with user experience, such as how users are assigned to system-defined user roles with different levels of access privileges. For example, a mid-level role such as a physician assistant or nurse who functions as a population health manager may perform both clinical and administrative tasks, which doesn't always "fit" the roles pre-defined in health IT systems. Flexible health IT design is therefore needed to accommodate unanticipated task sequences, workflows, and roles. Decisions on how to configure systems for the local context may also introduce usability or workflow challenges, and also may limit the flexibility of the software as clinical redesign takes place.

Many decisions related to user training may also impact health IT adoption. For example, training that uses simulated test environments may not correspond closely to the live environment, although differences may not be apparent until after go-live. During go-live, the more technical users, especially clinicians, may be paired with trainers who lack specific skillsets needed to train certain users. The generic, *one-size-fits-all* design, which is popularly found in today's health IT systems, may be insufficient for supporting complex tasks when there is a significant amount of variation in how they are performed in day-to-day clinical practice. Finally, with increasingly widespread implementation of predictive analytics, consideration must be given to how the users should be trained in the responsible use of these tools. For example, helping users understand the essential elements of an AI algorithm such as training data, type of model, etc., may be an aspect of both design of the clinical decision-support system and mandatory user training.

18.2 Background

18.2.1 Gaps in Prior Research on Workflow

The widespread adoption of health IT to manage electronic patient data and support care delivery has expanded the role that technology plays during work systems redesign in healthcare. However, the anticipated benefits of health IT are difficult to achieve unless implementation and workflow challenges are identified and addressed (Ash et al. 2009; Blumenthal 2011; Dorr et al. 2007; Novak et al. 2012; Holden et al.

2013). Health IT–workflow interactions are often best understood through a human factors and sociotechnical framework (Novak 2010), but large gaps in systematic research of ambulatory care workflow still exist (Carayon et al. 2010).

In 2010, the U.S. Agency for Healthcare Research and Quality (AHRQ) published a comprehensive literature review study that looked into existing research and evidence about the impact of health IT on workflow, its linkage to clinician adoption, and its linkage to the safety, quality, efficiency, and effectiveness of patient care delivery. The study showed evidence of variable quality, little generalizability to non-academic and ambulatory settings, and limited focus on the sociotechnical context of health IT implementation including potentially conflating or mediating factors such as training, technical support, and organizational culture (Carayon et al. 2010). Existing research reviewed in the AHRQ study also did not address redesign of ambulatory care settings, though this is an important aspect of health systems change.

In addition, the AHRQ study identified significant gaps in understanding the interactions between health IT and workflow, and advised that more systematic research was needed, both to establish causal relationships and to produce highly generalizable knowledge in the study of health IT and workflow interactions (Carayon et al. 2010). Accordingly, the study that we describe in this chapter was designed to address two major gaps in the literature:

- **Rigorous research focused on workflow**. This study used a combination of methods (Carayon et al. 2012) specifically designed to understand workflow in the context of a work system implementing new health IT. These adapted methods were implemented by experts in sociotechnical systems research in partnership with clinical subject matter experts in order to provide an understanding of workflow phenomena that are typically ignored or underspecified in prior studies, including: adaptation of health IT, the role of health IT in team-based work, and the coevolution of health IT and workflow.
- **Attention to sociotechnical context**. This study approached workflow as an interactive sociotechnical work system of: (1) people; (2) tools, technologies, and other artifacts; (3) tasks and task characteristics; (4) organizational structures and characteristics; and (5) the surrounding physical, social, and political environment. Data collection and analysis focused on these five factors, alone and in interaction, and how they relate to (for example, constrain or enable) the studied work processes. Attention to the sociotechnical aspects permitted this study to both describe this context and allow comparisons to other contexts. It also permitted the research team to understand what specific contextual factors influenced workflow-related phenomena—for example, the circumstances in which implementing the same health IT system in two or more settings might lead to divergent workflow changes, and why.

18.2.2   Theoretical Framework

The study's theoretical framework was informed by two compatible models that have been applied to workflow research: the adapted SEIPS (Systems Engineering Initiative for Patient Safety) model (Carayon et al. 2006; Karsh et al. 2006; Carayon 2009) and the Workflow Elements Model (WEM) (Carayon et al. 2012; Unertl et al. 2010), depicted in Figs. 18.1 and 18.2. The SEIPS model defines the work system as the interaction of people, tools/technology, tasks, organization, and environment. This work system (structure) shapes workflow (process) that in turn shapes patient and clinician outcomes. The structure-process relationship requires that workflow be studied in the context of the interacting work system. In addition to understanding workflow as process steps or patterns, it must be specified who is involved or not involved (**people**), what artifacts are used or not used (**tools/technologies**), what characteristics such as goals or task demands constrain work (**tasks**), what structures or policies are in place that govern people and processes (**organization**), and where the work takes places (**environment**). This adapted model shown in Fig. 18.1 builds on the SEIPS and related systems models to illustrate workflow as the product of a sociotechnical work system that is transformed by new health IT as well as adaptations over time.

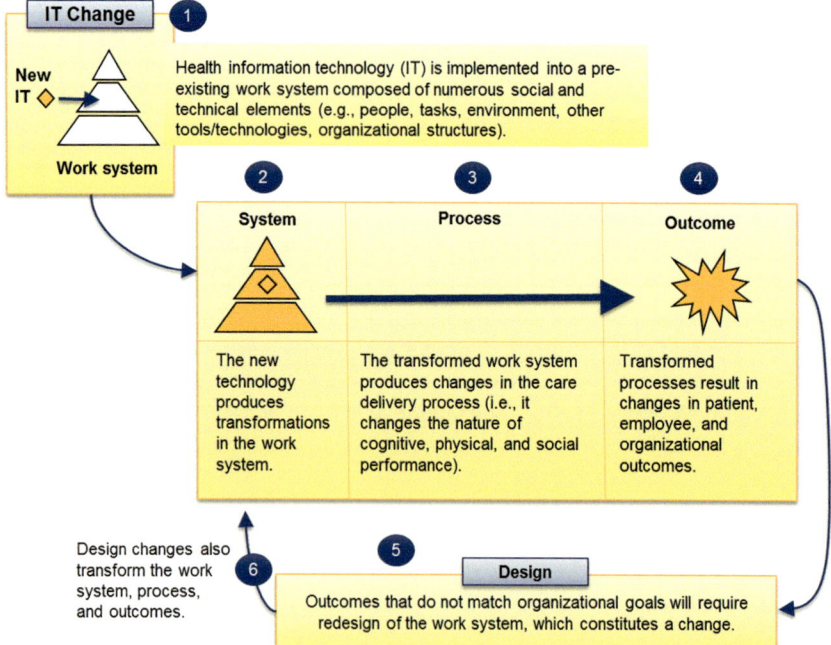

Fig. 18.1   The adapted SEIPS model

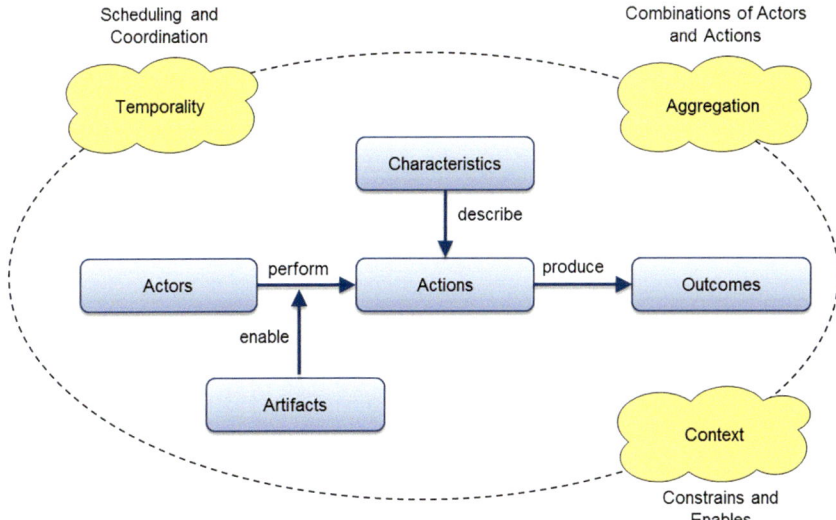

Fig. 18.2 Workflow elements model

Reproduced with modifications from International Journal of Industrial Ergonomics, 41/4, Holden RJ, Brown RL, Alper SJ, Scanlon MC, Patel NR, Karsh BT, That's nice, but what does IT do? Evaluating the impact of bar coded medication administration by measuring changes in the process of care, 371, 2011, with permission from Elsevier (Holden et al. 2011).

Reproduced with modifications from Journal of the American Medical Informatics Association, 17/3, Unertl KM, Novak LL, Johnson KB, Lorenzi NM, Traversing the many paths of workflow research: developing a conceptual framework of workflow terminology through a systematic literature review, 270, 2010, with permission from Oxford Academic (Unertl et al. 2010).

WEM is a broad synthesis of prior workflow research and adds to and refines how one might apply SEIPS generally to the study of workflow (Carayon et al. 2012). WEM specifies three pervasive properties of workflow that shape outcomes or the end products of workflow. First, workflow is dynamic (**temporality**): it occurs across time, changes from moment to moment, depends on a context that may change over time, and often emerges from the activity of individuals and groups working asynchronously in different locations. Second, workflow is collective (**aggregation**): work is carried out by multiple individuals as well as collectives working separately or in concert, synchronously or asynchronously, and toward goals that may converge or diverge. Processes, too, are subject to aggregation and can be delineated into tasks or patterns or seen in combination or as emergent properties of work. Third, workflow occurs in **context**, including work system elements—such as people and technologies—and any other factors that constrain or enable workflow. Examples of contextual factors not explicit in SEIPS include extra-organizational culture, standards, legislation, pressures, and workforce characteristics (Karsh et al. 2006).

The two models in combination guided the data collection of this study in the following ways:

1. Both models promote capturing and analyzing data on sociotechnical system factors (such as people, technologies, and task characteristics) that are relevant to studied processes and steps or patterns.
2. SEIPS specifically promotes capturing and analyzing data on people, tools/ technology, task, organization, and environment factors—as well as interactions between the factors—related to parts of or whole processes.
3. WEM specifically promotes capturing and analyzing data on temporality, aggregation, and contextual properties of parts of or whole processes.
4. Both models promote a focus on processes and related work system factors and pervasive properties that shape key outcomes such as successful, coordinated health and disease management.

18.3 Our Study

18.3.1 Health IT Studied and Empirical Setting

The My Health Team at Vanderbilt (MHTAV) program was initially developed in 2010 by the Vanderbilt Medical Group to be an innovative, ambulatory health care delivery model for a small group of patients with three chronic conditions, diabetes, hypertension, and congestive heart failure, among pilot physicians in one clinic. Vanderbilt received external funding through a U.S. Centers for Medicare & Medicaid Services (CMS) innovations contract in 2012 to greatly expand the program with revised goals: to improve chronic disease management, care coordination, and transition management for all Vanderbilt patients with the three chronic medical conditions.

The expanded MHTAV program was centrally administered and implemented, although the implementation of the program varied somewhat across clinics based on the experience of the care coordinators and the composition of the clinical teams. The MHTAV program included intensified patient engagement and dedicated care coordinators (CCs). CCs were registered nurses who helped coordinate care for patients.

Major IT system components were developed or used in support of care coordination activities, including: (1) the Vanderbilt electronic health record (EHR) system (at the time, StarPanel), (2) cross-patient dashboards for diabetes, hypertension, and congestive heart failure, (3) worklists for use by CCs, (4) a shared view of the patient's plan of care (POC) among clinical staff, (5) alerts and reminders related to care coordination activities, (6) the disease control form, (7) patient portal secure messaging, (8) an interactive voice response (IVR) system, (9) the clinic scheduling system, and (10) online patient education and materials.

A number of health IT components were created or used primarily for MHTAV, including the dashboards, worklists, the POC, and the IVR system, collectively referred to as MHT tools or the MHT system. A key goal of the MHT system was to support structured, bidirectional, and closed-loop communication among members of the care team, including the patient and caregivers. In the context of MHTAV, the providers and clinic nurses provided direct care to patients. CCs managed the MHTAV panel of patients and were supported by MHTAV medical assistants who assisted the CCs with patient education, collection and summaries of patient home monitoring data (blood pressures and blood sugars), and administrative tasks. MHT included a range of information that could be viewed for an individual patient or at the population level. At the patient level, this included demographic information, the patient's condition or disease, and a POC. At the population level, a dashboard showed aggregated statistics for selected indicators. Care coordinator activities were driven by a worklist which showed patients with alerts that were either clinically driven (such as an elevated home blood pressure reading) or process driven (such as a patient who was due for an annual foot exam).

The empirical study involved six study site teams (see Table 18.1). These included a single on-campus medical office (medium-sized; 35 part-time clinicians) and five off-campus primary care offices (small; 2–11 clinicians). All of them are located in Tennessee and staffed with providers (physicians, nurse practitioners), clinic nurses, clinic secretaries, and clinic medical assistants.

Table 18.1 Study sites

Site Team	Attending MDs	Resident MDs	NPs	Setting	MHTAV Adoption**	CC Proximity
1	35	93	0	Urban	April 2010	In separate office, 5 days/week
2	2	0	0	Rural	March 2014	On-site, 2 days/week
3*	4	0	3	Urban	November 2013	On-site, 5 days/week
4	10	0	1	Suburban	October 2012	In office on different floor, 5 days/week
5	11	13	0	Suburban	May 2013	In separate office, 5 days/week
6*	4	0	3	Urban	November 2013	On-site, 5 days/week

MD = physician; NP = nurse practitioner; MHTAV = My Health Team at Vanderbilt; CC = care coordinator. *Two different teams were observed at the same clinic. **At initial observation, MHTAV site teams were already Live at sites 1,4,5; MHTAV-adopting site teams 2,3, and 6 began use of MHTAV after initial study observation

18.3.2 Methods

Study Design

A formal mixed-methods approach was designed, employing direct observation, patient and staff interviews, surveys of staff and patients, artifact and spatial data collection, software use monitoring, and impact on process outcomes for the six site teams at primary care clinics in different phases of adopting MHTAV. Data collection occurred over a 12-month period to capture health IT–workflow interactions over time, and across clinics in various implementation phases.

Care coordinators in this study were licensed as RNs who functioned in the CC role rather than the clinic nurse role, and worked with a care team composed of a provider (i.e., a physician or nurse practitioner), a clinic nurse (i.e., a registered nurse [RN] or licensed practical nurse [LPN]), a medical assistant (MA), and sometimes a scheduler.

Three site teams were already "live" with MHTAV and a CC at the start of the study, and three site teams were introduced to the CC and MHTAV program after the 12-month observation period had begun. Observations and data collection occurred at time zero, after 6 months, and after 12 months for each site team.

CCs in the study were primarily focused on identifying and managing hypertension-associated risks in their panel of patients, and worked to mitigate those risks and help their patients reach blood pressure goals, enabled by health IT. In the last few months of data collection, use of the MHT tools for diabetes-associated risk was added.

Recruitment of the six site teams occurred following approval of the study by both RTI's and Vanderbilt's Institutional Review Boards (IRB).

Data Collection and Analysis

Data collection activities included: (1) project orientation meeting with staff from each clinic site, (2) direct observation of staff work, (3) individual staff interviews, (4) individual patient interviews, (5) staff surveys, and (6) patient surveys. In addition, the Vanderbilt University Medical Center IT department provided utilization data for the MHT system, and diabetes process outcome data were obtained for the providers participating in the study. These data collection methods are summarized in Table 18.2.

Meeting notes and narrative data were entered and analyzed using Dedoose™ through a process of (1) open coding, (2) axial coding, and (3) workflow modeling. Dedoose is a web-based qualitative and mixed-methods data analysis cross-platform application designed to support collaborative data analysis activities. To further support the analysis, we scored staff and patient survey responses and tracked software module use. Quantitative and qualitative data, together, supplemented one another to help us identify complementary themes, resolve conflicting findings, and

Table 18.2 Data collection activities

Data collection activity	Source of data	Data description
1. Staff orientation meeting	Practice staff	Notes of practice staff discussion of practice operations, including health IT support of care coordination issues and challenges
2. Direct observations of care coordination	Care coordinator (if identified); patients; other individuals in the practice responsible for care coordination key workflows including: (a) registering patients, (b) sharing care plan, (c) handling alerts and reminders, (d) compiling and interpreting data from at-home monitoring, and (e) communicating with patients between visits	Field notes of workflow steps, information flow steps, and other information required to create workflow and information flow models; description of health IT components and capabilities relating to care coordination
3. Staff semi-structured interviews	Practice staff participating in direct observations	Responses to interview guide questions gathered from practice staff
4. Patient semi-structured interviews	Patients with diabetes contacted through direct observation or introduced by their physician	Responses to interview questions from patients
5. Staff surveys	Practice staff	Responses to modified Technology Acceptance Model (TAM) survey; (Davis 1989) modification includes responses to additional survey questions focusing specifically on care coordination
6. Patient surveys	Patients	Responses to Patient Activation Measure (PAM) 13-item instrument; (Hibbard et al. 2004) and Summary of Diabetes Self-Care Activities (SDSCA) 10-item instrument

(continued)

Table 18.2 (continued)

Data collection activity	Source of data	Data description
7. Artifact and spatial data collection	Researcher or study participant	Items identified as relevant by researchers during direct observations; examples include: a template of a shared care plan; an appointment reminder postcard, or printed lists used by care coordinators to monitor their work each day
8. Software use monitoring	Data extracts developed for My Health Team (MHT) reporting	Audit logs

provide rich detail to support conclusions about health IT–workflow interactions—in general and across implementation phases.

Coding

During Open coding, data captured after each observation period were reviewed to identify coding elements for "chunks" of textual data, and the coding structure was refined over time as observations were added and higher-level themes were identified.

Next, axial coding was performed to add depth and structure to the constructs (codes) from the open coding phase, synthesizing lower-level constructs into a more integrative theory (Saldaña 2009). During axial coding, all qualitative data were reviewed again and categorized according to the SEIPS model combined with the WEM. The combination of SEIPS and WEM provided the structure for assigning data and codes to the elements shown in Table 18.3.

Applying this framework to hypertension care, primary care providers (actors) perform preventive care and screening procedures (actions) during routine patient care visits, leading to a patient being current on all recommended preventive health care services (outcomes). Health care providers use artifacts in accomplishing their work, including EHRs, paper forms, and paper education materials. Characteristics describing the actions include descriptors such as "routine," "screening," "preventive," and "recurrent." The work of routine preventive care takes place in a specific sequence on a schedule defined by evidence-based guidelines. Routine preventive care work also occurs during days the clinic is open (temporality) and relies on administrative staff and nurses for assistance and information contributions from other health care providers to develop thorough understanding of patient status (aggregation). Permeating all of the workflow processes is the context of the work—the health care organization, the physical space available, the family and support structure for the patient, and the organization's policies and requirements.

Table 18.3 Workflow elements model categories guiding axial coding

Element	Definition	Examples from data
People (actors)	Individuals engaged in work	Care coordinator, medical assistant, physician, clinic nurse, patients
Process (actions)	Steps that actors take to accomplish work	Care coordinator work, medical assistant work, patient work
Outcomes	End results of work	Diabetes adherence, patient education
Tools and technologies (artifacts)	Tools used in work	Message Basket, the EHR, MHT system, Plan of Care Support tab
Tasks (action characteristics)	Descriptions of the work	Patient education, response to alerts/reminders, personal interactions with patients
Temporality	Time-based factors, including scheduling and coordination	Alerts/reminders, patient appointment times, meeting patients in clinic
Aggregation	Collective work across actors and actions, including collaboration	Coordination with multiple providers (including external), coordination with call center, coordination with clinic nurses
Context	Setting for the work, which constrains and enables work activities	Spatial proximity to clinic/providers, technology constraints
Interactions among elements	Phenomena that are the result of interactions among the elements described above	Creation/modification of Plans of Care

Stage 3: Workflow Modeling

The final element of qualitative data analysis involved development of graphical representations of workflow processes, called workflow models. The workflow models were similar to flow charts but contained more detailed documentation of work practices and capture actual work processes as opposed to idealized ones. The modeling process is based on concepts from soft systems methodology (Checkland and Scholes 1999) and hierarchical task analysis (Shepherd 2001). Similar to hierarchical task analysis, during model generation, each larger task is divided into subtasks and each subtask is further divided until a detailed diagram of workflow is generated. For example, the overall work process this project studied is care coordination. Subtasks involved in this overall task may include physicians taking notes in the EHR system, nurses measuring a patient's vital signs, CCs contacting patients directly via phone or e-mail, or many other subtasks. The subtask of CCs contacting patients directly may be further broken down into steps taken to identify patients requiring contact, obtaining contact information, contacting the patient, discussing relevant information with the patient, and documenting the outcomes of the discussion with the patient. All subtasks are captured in the graphical workflow models.

Using the output of earlier data analysis stages, researchers identified the overall flow of CC work and each sub-process involved in CC and manually developed workflow models. Workflow models represent physical space, artifact use, roles, decision points, process variation, organizational policy, and other aspects of workflow related to CC as necessary. For example, the support activity of "Search for Information" was depicted using a diagram that highlighted information flow and artifacts, rather than focusing on physical space, given that most of the activity took place at the CC desk using the computer, notepad, and phone. The modeling process highlights the specific role that health IT plays in CC work and the impact of new health IT functionality on workflow.

Staff Survey Data

Survey data collected from each individual who was interviewed was used to consistently capture additional user information beyond qualitative data such as those obtained through observations and interviews. Responses to the adapted Technology Acceptance Model (TAM) survey were used to evaluate user perceptions and acceptance of technology (Davis 1989). Specifically, the TAM measure includes ease of use and usefulness. Descriptive statistics (for example, mean, standard deviation, and median) were calculated using Microsoft Excel, adding context in interpreting staff perceptions related to health IT.

Patient Survey Data

The patient survey data consistently captured additional information about patient characteristics, such as diabetes self-monitoring measures and levels of patient activation. These measures were analyzed in SPSS to produce descriptive data about the patients surveyed at each site (for example, mean, standard deviation, and median) in order to understand participant differences across the various clinic sites. Quantitative analysis beyond simple descriptive statistics was not performed because of the small number of patients surveyed and the primary qualitative approach.

Data Synthesis

Data synthesis compared and contrasted all health IT and workflow-related data gathered across six sites during two or three (depending on the site) observation periods over 12 months. As detailed earlier, data collection spanned clinic groups in different phases of MHTAV program implementation (already using MHTAV or in the process of adopting MHTAV). Findings gathered from multiple sources with qualitative and quantitative methods were therefore used to examine the strength of support for the

Table 18.4 Description of research product(s) for each analysis activity

Analysis activity	Source of data	Product
A. Workflow diagramming to identify and describe workflows	Semi-structured staff discussion	Set of workflows and workflow elements
	Direct observations	
	Staff interviews	
	Patient interviews	
B. Identification of health IT design elements used in support of care coordination activities	Semi-structured staff discussion	Set of health IT design elements
	Direct observations	
	Staff interviews	
	Patient interviews	
	Staff surveys	
	Usage data	
	Diabetes outcome data	
C. Identification of interactions between workflow and health IT design elements	Analysis activities A and B	Set of interactions, health IT barriers and facilitators to care coordination workflows
	Underlying source data	
D. Analysis of interactions across implementation stage (MHTAV, MHTAV-adopting) and time	Analysis activities A, B, and C	Interaction results by implementation stage
	Underlying data	

identified themes, conflicts in the findings, and the development of final conclusions. Table 18.4 describes the research products that address the research question. Three categories of research products were identified and described: (1) workflows, (2) health IT design elements, and (3) interactions between the workflows and health IT elements.

Interactions Between Health IT and Workflow

The data analyses described above would help us derive a "technology matrix" to capture clinical workflows that comprise care coordination; and the health IT features or components that either support, create barriers for, or have a neutral impact on the workflows. "Good alignment" describes a positive interaction between health IT and workflow. "Neutral alignment" is neither positive nor negative. "Poor alignment" describes a negative interaction. The overall "fit" of a health IT feature in supporting or impeding workflow can be then assessed by looking at the alignment of the feature with individual workflows of a work activity.

18.3.3 Findings

Health IT Impact on Workflow in Key Work Domains

Our study identified seven domains of activity central to the work of care coordination, and around which the study results are organized. Five of these activity areas addressed the primary work of the CCs:

1. Establishing and maintaining relationships with patients
2. Establishing and maintaining a POC
3. Collecting and analyzing home monitoring data
4. Educating and coaching patients
5. Coordinating with other clinicians and patients

The remaining two *supported* the primary work of CCs:

6. Searching for information to support decision making and action
7. Prioritizing tasks and planning work

In this section, we present the findings from two of these seven work domains, namely "establishing and maintaining relationships with patients" and "coordinating with other clinicians and patients." For each of them, we include a *description,* a *workflow diagram* of activities observed and/or discussed in interviews, a *technology matrix* that depicts the level of alignment of health IT features with the workflow, and a summary of findings. We chose to provide a detailed report on only two domains in order to fully explain the methodology we used to analyze and depict the data. We direct readers interested in the additional findings to the final report of the study published by the AHRQ, accessible at https://healthit.ahrq.gov/sites/default/files/docs/citation/hit-enabled-care-coordination-and-redesign-in-tn-final-report.pdf.

Establishing and Maintaining Relationships with Patients

Initial engagement of the patient in the care coordination program. As the MHTAV program was initiated in each clinic, potential patients were displayed on the MHT system worklist, based on dynamic registries using existing EHR data, behind the scenes. The registries used a risk stratification schema that represented two dimensions: a) disease control and stability (for diabetes patients, "level 1" criteria were: documented HbA1c less than 8, fewer than 3 medications for diabetes, no complications OR mild stable complications AND followed by a subspecialist, without severe or frequent hypoglycemia or hypoglycemic unawareness); and b) complexity of primary disease and related comorbid conditions. Initially, the registries were used to populate a worklist of patients that CCs needed to enroll manually into the program, with a face-to-face meeting in the next provider visit. Later, to accelerate enrollment, the decision was made to move to an auto-enrollment model, whereby patients whose records were identified by the registry were automatically enrolled into the MHTAV program and placed on the CC worklist. With this change, face-to-face meetings in the clinic became uncommon, as CCs moved to telephone-based outreach to meet and set up the place of care (POC) for each patient.

In the early phases of the program, a clinician initiated the patient enrollment meeting with the CC, which typically took place face-to-face in the clinic during a scheduled clinic visit. One CC noted that 10 to 11 patients per day were enrolled at first; then after the first few months the number dropped substantially to approximately 7 per week since the majority of eligible patients were already enrolled. At a later point in the MHTAV program, an auto-enrollment process was implemented through which patients who met certain clinical thresholds (for example, HbA1c > 8) automatically became part of the MHTAV program population. CCs were then expected to create a POC for each patient who was auto-enrolled, even without a face-to-face meeting. A CC who described this process pointed out the impact on establishing and maintaining the relationship with the patient: "I can see that it's made a difference. I feel like they, you know… you build that rapport so they trust you and they, they try to… do what you're asking them to do and you know I have a lot of them, [who] take their readings and do, and keep, record that stuff regularly."

Ongoing engagement. The CCs reported that engaging the patients in an ongoing way over time was an important aspect of their work. Developing and maintaining strong relationships with patients helped with obtaining home readings (blood pressure and blood glucose), following up on medication effects, identifying hospital admissions, and monitoring other clinical events. Fostering a friendly and collegial relationship was especially important because CCs could learn about patients' jobs and families, explore with patients what made adherence to clinical recommendations difficult, and share experiences with patients (such as a shared joke), all of which helped establish rapport and trust. For example, one CC could not reach one of her patients for approximately one year, but once the patient met with the CC face-to-face during a clinic visit, she began communicating with the CC regularly about her medical care. Another CC described how the care team was able to keep a patient out of the hospital through education, medication, and diet management. She mentioned the face-to-face communication as key during this process, as both the CC and the patient were able to see and discuss the positive changes as they occurred.

Care coordinators maintained contact with patients through calling on the telephone, messaging through the patient portal, and meeting face-to-face in the clinic. CCs used the clinic schedule to determine if one of the patients they were following would be visiting that day.

However, advances in technology did not always support maintaining patient relationships. For example, when auto-enrollment replaced the need for a face-to-face enrollment meeting with the patient, the CCs felt that their ability to initially engage the patient, and maintain strong engagement, suffered. They stated that the ability to see patient face to face on a regular basis is helpful for maintaining engagement. One CC suggested that Skype or FaceTime may be an alternative strategy for communicating with patients. CCs also noted variation in communication preferences based on a patient's age. They commented there appears to be a cohort of patients (aged approximately 40–50) who prefer to use the messaging function through My Health at Vanderbilt rather than the telephone. The CCs speculated that these patients are employed full time and have more constraints on their time, making online communications easier to accomplish.

Relationship-building activities. The CCs used several strategies to build relationships with patients. These strategies included setting reminders to see patients while they were in the clinic; making notes in the POC Support tab for future reference (memory cues); and providing educational materials to patients. CCs mentioned that having patients visit with them in-person in the clinic helped to create and maintain rapport. For patients who were difficult to engage, CCs described introducing themselves again when the patient came in for an appointment, offering them information and log sheets, and any other assistance to try to reconnect with them.

During our observations, CCs mentioned that reduced in-person contact with patients, either because CCs visited multiple clinics or because their office was outside the clinic building, changed the nature and strength of their relationships with patients. As mentioned previously, CCs also felt that auto-enrollment may be a barrier to establishing strong relationships with each patient.

Figure 18.3 and Table 18.5 present the workflow diagram and technology matrix for establishing and maintaining relationships with patients. Figure 18.3 illustrates the change over time that occurred before, during MHTAV, and later in data collection. As technology was introduced to identify, enroll, and later, contact the patients, direct CC initial contact with many of the patients decreased.

The middle section of the diagram in Fig. 18.3 illustrates the two ways in which relationships are established and maintained within the MHTAV program. Technology-driven refers to the MHT system itself, including algorithms used to trigger alerts and set the status of patients in the MHTAV program. Role-driven refers to ways in which CCs engage patients and establish relationships on a more

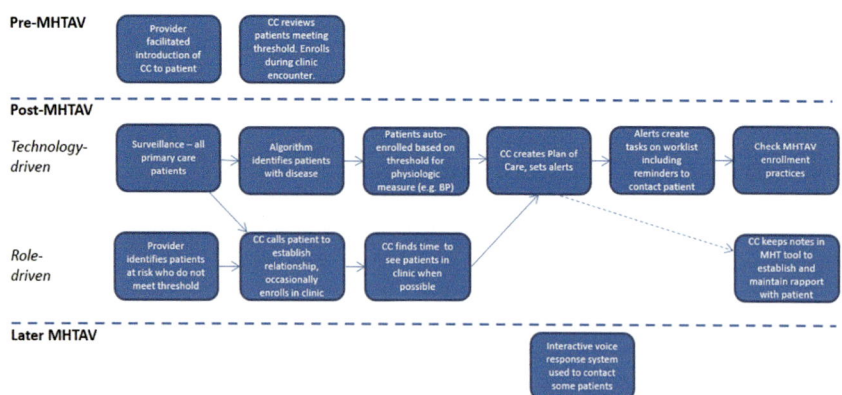

Fig. 18.3 Workflow diagram: establishing and maintaining relationships with patients. CC = care coordinator; BP = blood pressure; MHT = My Health Team; MHAV = My Health Team At Vanderbilt

Table 18.5 Technology matrix: establishing and maintaining relationships with patients

Relevant IT resources or attributes	Workflow: establishing and maintaining relationships with patients	
	Activity: enrollment/ auto-enrollment	Activity: building rapport with patients
Alerts and reminders populate the CC worklist	Reminders are used to connect with patients during clinic appointments. This can assist in educational goals, as well as supporting the patient by providing monitoring equipment, validation of monitoring equipment. **Good alignment**	Reminders to call/message patients or connect with them in clinic. Opportunity for CC to build rapport via face-to-face communication. **Good alignment**
Auto-enrollment	Patients are automatically added to CC's panel based on collected vitals and stratified according to the protocol. **Good alignment**	
Disease Control Form (DCF)	Displays information about patient, including the next appointment. **Good alignment**	DCF shows status of patient and allows CC to update status based on information received from communications with patient. **Good alignment**
POC Support tab	Records activities involving initial patient contact, and assists in establishing the POC for the patient. **Good alignment**	Enables ongoing communication with patient, as well as input of possible pertinent information about the patient home environment ("Red Flags": Activity, Diet, Foot care, Emotion coping skills, Disease monitoring, Unable to reach patient, Physical activity, Medication adherence, Medication reconciliation, Tobacco cessation, and Other categories). **Good alignment**
POC Support tab (continued)		"CC Actions" are entered here, and a history is maintained in the "POC Support Hx." CC Actions contain information about education/coaching given to patient, and also monitoring equipment status (that is, validation of existing equipment or providing one to patient). These serve as memory cues to establish and build rapport with patients. **Good alignment**
Auto-enrollment process was implemented in later stages of MHTAV	Patients enrolled without meeting the CC in the clinic, minimizing CC work. **Good alignment**	CCs reported face-to-face meetings with patients were important to rapport-building. **Poor alignment**

CC = care coordinator; DCF = disease control form; POC = plan of care; Hx = history; MHTAV = My Health Team at Vanderbilt personal level. Before MHT tools were introduced, CCs were introduced to patients by a provider or clinical team member. This continued, though reduced, after the MHT tools were introduced.

Coordinating with Other Clinicians and Patients

As the MHTAV program was implemented, it took time for the clinic teams to embrace the CCs as key members. Initially, a team member sometimes inadvertently duplicated the effort of another team member (for example, LPNs sent messages to the provider and/or patient not realizing the CC also called and/or sent messages about the same topic). Over time, other team members (providers and clinic nurses) learned about the CCs' capabilities and role and learned how the CCs could significantly contribute and efficiently function on the team. However, CCs who were off-site or part-time with the clinical team lacked daily contact with providers, who were in turn less aware of the various tasks and activities that CCs performed. Some CCs reported having to actively promote their abilities, such as assisting with patient education, reviewing home measurement techniques, and spending time responding to patient questions, especially those who relied on electronic communications and telephones to reach physicians/NPs and clinic nurses they did not interact with face-to-face.

The care team often wanted the CC to meet with patients immediately before or after a patient saw his/her provider at a visit, requiring communication. This was challenging when a patient was newly identified for inclusion in MHT, for example in the cases of new patients whose diabetes was not known by the clinic until the initial visit, new laboratory results that indicate diabetic status shortly before or during visit, a patient who shows low adherence and the need for further education, or cases in which a patient requests more information or education regarding the self-management of their chronic illness. However, it was not easy for the CC to figure out which patient needed to be seen, to know when a patient was actually done seeing a provider, or to receive a provider message that they should see the patient, despite multiple communication technologies. The EHR message basket (or email) could be helpful if the CC was at her computer; the online schedule helped the CC prepare for the patients visiting each day; and the online whiteboard assisted the CC in knowing when a patient arrived and checked in. However, messages were not always used to notify the CC, up-to-date information was often missing from the schedule, and the whiteboard often lacked accurate information about when the patient was actually being seen by a provider, making it difficult for CCs and providers to coordinate a face-to-face meeting for the patient with the CC. As a result, CCs often learned later that they needed to schedule a separate appointment to meet with the patient.

MHT worklist alerts, whether system triggered or created by the CC, provided valuable information to the CC in monitoring and acting on "to do's" for each patient. There were a lot of activities to manage, such as requesting and following up on laboratory tests, checking on the patient experience using a new or changed medication, and following up on teaching. CCs reported good alignment between these tools and their work coordinating future activities for patients.

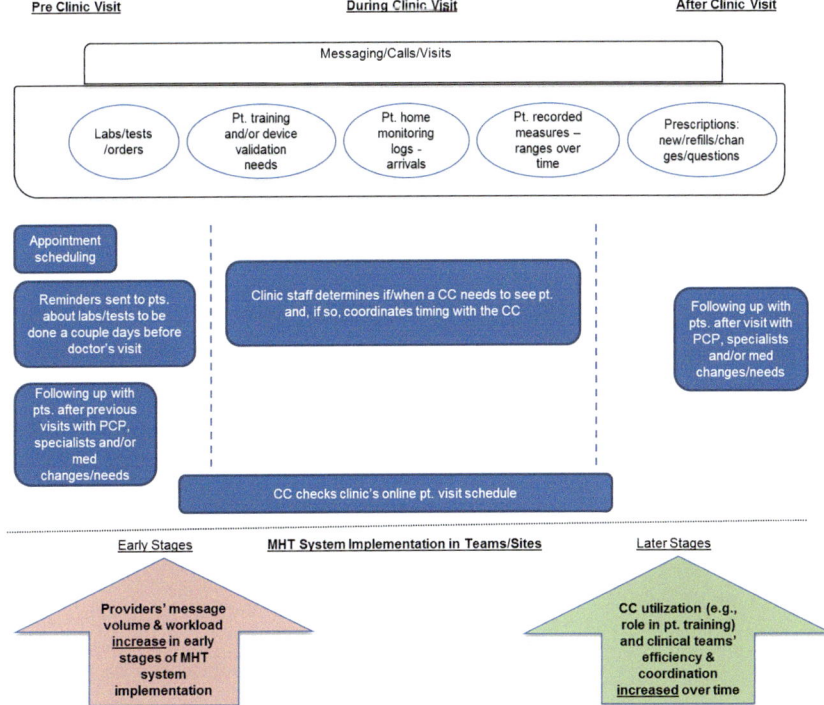

Fig. 18.4 Workflow Diagram: Coordinating with Other Clinicians and Patients

Coordination activities were also observed to vary among teams from urban, suburban, and rural areas. The rural clinic CC interacted with a variety of non-Vanderbilt affiliated hospitals and clinicians, frequently exchanging information via fax. In contrast, CCs in the suburban and urban clinics more often only interacted with Vanderbilt-affiliated hospitals and providers, reflecting real variation in the information ecologies within which the teams worked [22].

Figure 18.4 and Table 18.6 present the workflow diagram and technology matrix for coordinating with other clinicians and patients.

18.4   Discussion

18.4.1   Lessons and Insights

The rigorous, mixed methods study of six site teams at various stages of adoption of health IT to support new care coordination team-based care generated a large amount of data and was itself a complex undertaking. To assess the interaction between

Table 18.6 Technology matrix: coordinating with other clinicians and patients

Relevant IT resources or attributes	Workflow: coordinating with other clinicians (nurses & PCPs)		
	Activity: messaging	Activity: medication changes and refills	Activity: prompts to CCs and patients
MHT worklist alerts and reminders		Notify CCs (or IVR system) to follow-up with patients about new or changed medications on a certain date **Good alignment**	Reminders are used to notify patients to come in for a lab/test a few days before their doctor's appointment **Good alignment**
			Alerts and reminders notify CCs when a patient's status (readmitted to hospital) has changed, a medical appointment has or will soon occur, and/or CCs need to follow up with the patient to see how they are doing and/or how an appointment went. **Good alignment**
Electronic communications: In-basket/MHAV messages	Convenient method for CCs to notify clinicians when they need to act (such as to review a patient's BP or blood glucose data, or that a patient needs training or a monitoring device validated). **Good alignment**	Prescription requests and/or information and questions about medications can be e-mailed among CCs and the clinicians. **Good alignment**	Electronic messaging (MHAV and/or e-mail) has helped CCs when scheduling appointments with patients. **Good alignment**
	Clinicians having a large number of messages sent by the CCs can feel overwhelmed and wish the technology helped to alleviate this **Poor alignment**		
	Messages sent/received to coordinate the best time for the CC to see the patient are often not received in time. *Poor alignment*		

(continued)

Table 18.6 (continued)

Relevant IT resources or attributes	Workflow: coordinating with other clinicians (nurses & PCPs)		
	Activity: messaging	Activity: medication changes and refills	Activity: prompts to CCs and patients
Clinic schedule for viewing by CCs			The online schedule is unreliable due to delays, early arrivals, cancellations, and/or no-shows. CCs often must schedule another appointment to see the Pt at a different time. **Poor alignment**
Interactive voice response (IVR) system asks patients, about new or changed medications (if patient has consented)		IVR system only asks generic and broad questions that often lack specific and contextual information. **Poor alignment**	Since the IVR system is not always reliable, the CC doesn't get sufficient or reliable information and must call the Pt to ask about their new/changed med. **Poor alignment**
CCs schedule or availability status is not accessible remotely/ electronically			Clinic staff are unable to easily and quickly coordinate a face-to-face encounter between a patient and the CC. Instead, staff go to the CC's office or call her, if they have time. **Poor alignment**

BP = blood pressure; CC = care coordinator; HR = heart rate; IVR = interactive voice response; MHAV = MyHealthAtVanderbilt; MHT = My Health Team; Pt = patient

technology and the work system for care coordination, with its multiple workflows, actors, tasks, and multidirectional influences between technology and workflow, we identified and examined seven broad areas of work. Those seven areas included the routine use of technologies by the care coordinator, clinical teams, and patients. Many more use cases were partially addressed or not addressed in this research study, in part due to time and budget limitations. The research team observed that other factors such as cultural, physical, policy, and social environments played an important role in the health IT–workflow interactions we observed, making it important to situate our specific questions about health IT and workflow within the broader context of healthcare and health IT adoption.

18.4.2 Health IT Design

Our main finding, that the overall impact of health IT on workflow was mixed, was not surprising. It made sense that multiple work activities, roles, and technologies interacting in the real-world environment of primary care practices would surface many examples in which workflow was supported by, as well as at odds with, health IT.

The observed differences in alignment of health IT and workflow at different practice sites, and over time, were a strong reminder that technology redesign and practice redesign are both ongoing. Whether technology changes are secondary, made in response to other changes such as new staffing roles, new workflows, or patient direct use of technology, or primary, such as a new dashboard for monitoring population health, our findings suggest that plan-do-study-act (PDSA) steps to observe the actual effects of changes in health IT on workflow are important. Redesign work is best performed by a team of individuals combining their expertise in health IT, workflow, and clinical care. It is not unusual for redesign work to progress through a series of iterations to introduce new features and test their impact. This is especially useful when adapting complex systems where changes in multiple areas are common.

Recently emerging generative artificial intelligence (AI) that uses large language models could significantly improve the alignment of health IT and workflow by impacting many elements of the WEM model simultaneously (Wachter and Brynjolfsson 2024). Through untrained natural language interactions with users and widespread access, these tools are positioned to offer users greater interface adaptability and accelerate innovation that improves workflows, tools, training, communication, timing, and team relationships. Adapting health IT and workflows to take advantage of generative AI is anticipated to accelerate the pace of innovation in healthcare and health IT, as well as generate new knowledge about biomedical and social systems.

18.5 Conclusion

In this mixed methods study assessing the workflow impact of implementing health IT-enabled care coordination in six ambulatory primary care clinics over a 12-month period, we used a human factors and sociotechnical framework that identified five areas of primary work and two areas of supporting work. This approach revealed a complex picture with multiple workflows and varied IT systems used alone and in combination to support those workflows.

Our findings support the WEM assertion that context, aggregation, and temporality can impact the alignment of health IT and workflow. Stronger satisfaction with care coordination tools and processes was noted when there were well-defined workflows, tools designed to fit the workflow, adequate training, good team communication, physical co-location of CCs with other care team members, stronger team relationships, and time to allow the new work system to stabilize and for learning to take place. This study shows that the work of care coordination is broad, complex, and varied. It also demonstrates that even when a specific health IT-enabled program is implemented in a consistent IT environment, its impact varies substantially depending on the physical, social, and policy environment. Alignment between health IT and workflow is dynamic rather than fixed because the implementation of care coordination is changing over time from a narrow scope (a primary focus on the introduction of the new CC role and a few conditions) to a much broader one (a greater focus on team-level communication, multiple contributing roles, and more conditions).

Through the study, we also explored the use of the health IT alignment matrix as a tool to communicate to what extent system components aligned with functional and workflow requirements, and "scoring" of the overall alignment for a work system. Future work is needed to improve the way multiple contributors are identified and tracked during health IT adoption and its redesign over time.

References

Ash JS, Sittig DF, Dykstra R et al. The unintended consequences of computerized provider order entry: Findings from a mixed methods exploration. Int J Med Inform. 2009;78 (Suppl 1):S69–76.

Blumenthal D. Implementation of the federal health information technology initiative. N Engl J Med. 2011;365(25):2426–31.

Carayon P, Schoofs Hundt A, Karsh BT, et al. Work system design for patient safety: The SEIPS model. Qual Saf Health Care. 2006;15(Suppl 1):i50–8.

Carayon P, Cartmill R, Hoonakker P, et al. Human factors analysis of workflow in health information technology implementation. In: Carayon P, editor., et al., Handbook of human factors and ergonomics in patient safety. 2nd ed. Mahwah, NJ: Lawrence Erlbaum; 2012. p. 507–21.

Carayon P. The balance theory and the work system model. Twenty years later. Int J Hum Comput Interac 2009;25:313–27.

Carayon P, Karsh BT, Cartmill R. Incorporating health information technology into workflow redesign—Summary report Prepared by the Center for Quality and Productivity Improvement, University of Wisconsin-Madison, under Contract No. HHSA 290–2008–10036C. Rockville, MD: Quality AfHRa; 2010.

Checkland P, Scholes J. Soft systems methodology in action. New York, NY: Wiley; 1999.

Davis FD. Perceived usefulness, perceived ease of use, and user acceptance of information technology. MIS Quart. 1989;13(3):319–40.

Dorr D, Bonner LM, Cohen AN, et al. Informatics systems to promote improved care for chronic illness: A literature review. J Am Med Inform Assoc. 2007;14(2):156–63.

Hibbard JH, Stockard J, Mahoney ER, et al. Development of the Patient Activation Measure (PAM): conceptualizing and measuring activation in patients and consumers. Health Serv Res. 2004;39(4 Pt 1):1005–26 PMID: 15230939.

Holden RJ, Brown RL, Alper SJ, et al. That's nice, but what does IT do? Evaluating the impact of bar coded medication administration by measuring changes in the process of care. Int J Ind Ergon. 2011;41(4):370–9 PMID: 21686318.

Holden RJ, Rivera-Rodriguez AJ, Faye H, et al. Automation and adaptation: Nurses' problem-solving behavior following the implementation of bar coded medication administration technology. Cogn Technol Work. 2013;15(3):283–96.

Karsh B, Holden R, Alper S, et al. A human factors engineering paradigm for patientsafety: designing to support the performance of the healthcare professional. Qual Saf Health Care. 2006;15(Suppl 1):i59-65.

Novak LL. Improving health IT through understanding the cultural production of safety in clinical settings. In: Nohr C, Aarts J, (eds.) Information Technology in Health Care: Sociotechnical Approaches 2010—From Safe Systems to Patient Safety. Amsterdam: IOS Press; 2010.

Novak LL, Anders SH, Gadd CS. et al. Mediation of adoption and use: A key strategy for mitigating unintended consequences of health IT implementation. J Am Med Inform Assoc. 2012;Online: 26 May 2012. https://doi.org/10.1136/amiajnl-2011-000575

Saldaña J. The coding manual for qualitative researchers. Thousand Oaks, CA: Sage Publications; 2009.

Shepherd A. Hierarchical task analysis. London, UK: Taylor and Francis; 2001.

Unertl KM, Novak LL, Johnson KB, et al. Traversing the many paths of workflow research: developing a conceptual framework of workflow terminology through a systematic literature review. J Am Med Inform Assoc 2010 May-Jun;17(3):265–73. PMID: 20442143.

Wachter RM, Brynjolfsson E. Will generative artificial intelligence deliver on its promise in health care? JAMA. 2024;331(1):65–9.

Chapter 19
Turning "Night into Day": Challenges, Strategies, and Effectiveness of Re-engineering the Workflow to Enable Continuous Electronic Intensive Care Unit Collaboration Between Australia and U.S.

Cheryl Hiddleson, Timothy Buchman, and Enrico Coiera

19.1 Introduction

Safe and effective care of critically ill patients requires a team of professionals including specialty physicians (intensivists) and critical care nurses experienced in providing care for patients in the intensive care unit (ICU). While critical illness can strike at any time and demands continuous attention, allocation of scarce staff follows a predictable pattern. The night shift is more likely to have disproportionately newer and thus less experienced nurses, and the experienced nurses on that shift are engaged in providing care to their own set of patients (Claffey 2006; Floyd 2003). At times this leaves them unable to sufficiently supervise the newer staff. There is also evidence of increased risks at night time with higher in-hospital mortality for admissions at night (Coiera et al. 2014).

There is also a maldistribution of intensivists in the United States with the south-eastern region experiencing a greater need, and there are no intensivists present at many hospitals during the overnight hours. This combination leaves most ICUs in

C. Hiddleson (✉) · T. Buchman
Emory University, Atlanta, USA
e-mail: cheryl.hiddleson@emory.edu

T. Buchman
e-mail: TBuchma@emory.edu

E. Coiera
Macquarie University, North Ryde, Australia
e-mail: enrico.coiera@mq.edu.au

our region struggling with less experienced and diminishing numbers of staff at night. There are fewer resources in many departments of the hospital during night-time hours, requiring these staff to be more independent and resourceful in providing vital care. These novice nurses are not yet prepared for autonomy and are less sure of themselves and of where they might turn for advice or counsel.

To mitigate that nighttime challenge, Emory Healthcare (EHC) supports bedside caregivers with remote guidance from senior intensivists and critical care nurses using an efficient telehealth system, "eICU™" (Lilly et al. 2014). This platform allows the remote caregivers to observe, collaborate and prescribe at 11 ICUs in six hospitals from a single clinical operations room (COR) located in Dunwoody, Georgia. The Emory eICU program has data flowing from the electronic medical records and bedside monitors allowing the remote staff to have continuous access to all patients. The novel displays of data and the corresponding alerts driven by Boolean and trending algorithms in the eICU™ system augment situation awareness and allow early detection when a patient veers off of the expected trajectory.

Every eICU nurse (eRN) has a minimum of five years hands on experience at the bedside and each is certified as a critical care nurse (CCRN) by the American Academy of Critical Care Nurses (AACN). They provide the novice night nurses in the ICUs with "just in time" education and support during hours when onsite resources are not readily available. The bedside nurse pushes a button on the wall in a patient's room to access the eRN who comes on camera in about 15 s. The eRNs provide the newer nurses with insight and support that comes from the in-depth knowledge they acquire after years of providing bedside care to critically ill patients.

The physicians in the eICU are Emory faculty, all board-certified intensivists, have acquired additional training in critical care after completing specialty training in their field of choice. The intensivists in the eICU also provide many forms of support to bedside staff that might otherwise be delayed or not occur at all. That support ranges from just in time education about a drug the staff has never previously had prescribed or administered, to providing support to patients and families approaching the end of a prolonged course of illness.

The caregivers in the eICU are challenged to provide outstanding care throughout the night despite the obvious disruption in their normal wake-sleep cycles. Working through the night time hours exposes clinicians to adverse alterations in their phys-ical, emotional and cognitive abilities. Night shift workers have been shown to exhibit detrimental changes in their health and wellbeing, with the WHO even classifying night work as a "probable carcinogen" in 2007 (Gu et al. 2015). Though these detri-ments to health have been widely acknowledged, solutions for mitigating the effect on caregivers have not been sufficiently explored. In an attempt to further innovate and mitigate these deleterious effects on our staff, Emory proposed, piloted, and established a solution: "Turning Night into Day" (https://clinicaltrials.gov/ct2/show/NCT02895997).

Thus, Emory clinicians that provide remote eICU coverage on the night shift were relocated to the opposite side of the world. From the Antipodes, they would deliver their nighttime care to the patients served at the Emory eICU site, but they would do so from daylight in Australia. (The remote monitoring platform used allows for distance communication and connection with ICUs as far away as 250 miles, so repurposing that platform for ultra-remote coverage 12,000 miles away was technically possible). A six-month pilot research study was proposed to explore the effects on clinicians providing the eICU services when they are moved to a different time zone. Could a geographically dispersed clinical team create quality outcomes for patients as well as increase quality of life for those clinicians? The decision was made to focus on an English-speaking country, with a specific initial focus on a destination familiar to Americans. We were able to leverage a personal connection to establish a relationship with Macquarie University (MU) in Sydney Australia. That university is also home to the Australian Institute of Health Innovation, so it was an ideal location to form a partnership for this forward-looking study. Meetings were scheduled with administrative leadership there to assess the feasibility of this project. There was mutual interest in exploring the project, so the planning phase began.

There were three primary areas of focus for developing this new clinical workflow; how to manage the people, how to manage the legal aspects and how to choose the technical solutions to be used.

19.1.1 Managing the People

Study development and design was a cooperative effort between EHC and MU. The Emory eICU clinicians would be the study subjects and an application for an IRB was completed that focused on studying how the change in location and night/day hours would affect them physically, emotionally and cognitively. Study subjects were chosen on a volunteer basis and would travel to MU for a time of six to nine weeks while performing specific physiologic tests and wearing a heart rate monitor and activity monitoring device. The subject travelers also completed surveys on quality of life and mood status in addition to performing validated tasks to measure efficiency.

Once the study design was complete the focus turned to providing what the clinicians would need to perform effectively in the new environment. The decision was made to send two clinicians. Sending Emory clinicians would lend to assuring a shared sense of purpose and understanding of the primary objective for the study and the Emory eICU Center. This laid a foundation for the primary component of building the dispersed teams. Relocating our own clinicians instead of employing services of local Australian clinicians ensured that the possible obstacles of competing goals and objectives by clinicians from different backgrounds and countries would be avoided (Crowley 2005).

The site in Australia was built to echo the site in Atlanta to help increase clinicians' level of comfort working there. Tools to communicate with the team at home in Atlanta in a seamless and timely manner were needed so there would be no delays in patient care. A video conferencing tool was installed in parallel with the patient-centered eICU tool so clinicians could launch a sidebar video call. This sidebar video conferencing system allowed all clinicians to maintain the perception of being physically collocated, yet they were still thousands of miles apart. To further the sense of teamness, a large screen television/monitor was placed in the MU monitoring room that had a live feed of the Australian COR running for the duration of the shift. A reciprocal monitor was also placed in the COR in Atlanta. In all, there were three video channels used by staff: the video channel embedded in the eICU application facilitating communication between eICU staff and the bedside; the sidebar video link so eICU staff could speak with each other; and the full-room continuous video link providing a sense of "looking into the other room" on the other side of the globe.

19.1.2   Legal Aspects

There were many questions related to liability, insurance, professional credentialing, indemnity and more that had to be answered to arrive at a mutually acceptable contract. Agreements would be governed by Australian law so a contract dispute among the parties would be litigated in Australia. For this reason, EHC chose to hire outside legal counsel in Australia to assist with navigating these questions. Making decisions about how operations function in another country involves being as informed as possible to protect traveling clinicians, Emory Healthcare and the patients treated.

The Australian legal team consulted with the NSW medical and nursing boards to determine what the requirement would be for the clinicians while they worked there. We were informed that Emory's physicians and nurses were not required to apply for registration as health practitioners, apply for licensure or fulfill credentialing requirements in Australia during the six (6) month Project. Even if the Emory employees did not have to register, they were required to comply with relevant codes of conduct for Australian practitioners. They could not provide any type of medical services including consultations to Australian patients at all. All clinicians had to adhere to their scope of practice guidelines and codes of conduct for their place of practice, Atlanta Georgia. Emory clinicians had to comply with EHC employment and HR policies and US laws and regulations. As the Emory employees would not have an Australian employer the Australian minimum conditions, such as pay rates, would not apply during their Australian assignments. However, as they are performing duties in Australia relevant U.S. employment laws would apply, including anti-discrimination, harassment and work health and safety (which in turn covers workplace bullying). Emory had to take reasonable steps to ensure that the Australia workplace is safe for the Emory employees.

They determined that Emory employees could apply for standard visitor's visas electronically online instead of any type of work visa. MU sponsorship was not required because Emory individuals would not be employees or contractors of MU. This was determined because the clinicians would remain Emory employees for the length of their work assignment there and not employed by an Australian entity. They also found that EHC would not need to register with the Australian Securities and Investment Commission as a company doing business in Australia because of the temporary nature of the trial and the fact that it would not be hiring Australian employees. General sales tax would also not be paid because the Emory team would not be generating revenue while there.

To ensure uninterrupted insurance for the clinicians, Emory verified their plan for medical, dental and life insurance had global coverage. There are very different limits and restrictions related to malpractice between the U.S. and Australia, so indemnity had to be granted to the Australian parties involved. The malpractice insurance for all participating clinicians from EHC had to be verified and outlined in the legal contract.

Emory privacy guidelines had to be reviewed with each participating employee before deployment to the Australian site. Any visitors to the Australian site had to complete forms for compliance with HIPPA guidelines around patient confidentiality and privacy. After some preliminary investigation the determination was made that an end-to-end connection from Emory to the distant site in Australia would be the best solution for ensuring adherence to HIPPA guidelines and ensure security for protected health information (PHI).

19.1.3 Technical Aspects

Emory needed to have a connection back home that was private, secure and reliable. The IT team made the determination that an end-to-end circuit was the best option to achieve all three. A multiprotocol label switching (MPLS) network was chosen for the circuit type. This type of circuit could be configured to originate in Atlanta at EHC and terminate at MU in Sydney. This circuit is private and does not involve any transfer of information from one site to another. All the patient data remained on the Emory network, eliminating concerns about adherence to HIPPA guidelines or violation of security of patient information. All patient information remained the property of EHC. The telephones placed in the MU site were also internet based on the EHC network. This offered our clinicians in Atlanta and Australia the ability to make the same local calls with the same numbers and dialing protocols thus avoiding confusion.

The circuit is composed of a fiber connection extending from the U.S. to the street outside the MU building the operations room was located in. Once the fiber was installed the line then had to be connected to the building and up to the COR where it would terminate. There were three vendors that had to be employed for the completion of the build of the fiber line. The line was then connected to a router which was connected to a switch. The switch had network jacks that allowed the computers in the room to connect to the Emory network. All phases of this process had to be managed by the specific vendor and checks had to be made to ensure the access was complete and live. It is essential when developing this type of connection that all vendors are engaged early on, so they can partner and make the process as seamless as possible.

The decision was made that the Emory IT team would purchase and configure the CPUs to be used in Australia. Then the units were shipped to the site at MU. This was another step to ensure patient confidentiality and protection of patient information. Once the computers arrived in Australia, the IT team used remote desktop access to log into the computers and ensure functionality. This remote access also allowed the Emory IT team to apply updates and needed changes to the computers in Australia. There was no need to train or depend on staff at MU to perform those functions thus adding to the reliability of the systems' performance. The computers were also configured using local Atlanta time in order to avoid any confusion or error in documentation by the Australia based clinicians. Upon arrival, the computers were set up by an outside party with Emory IT checking functionality remotely.

The MU site was a locked room with access granted only to Emory staff and essential IT and emergency MU staff. Once again reinforcing protection of PHI and the clinicians themselves that worked weekends when other employees were not present. The computers remained powered on but clinicians logged off after each shift. This action not only added a layer of PHI protection but leaving them on and accessible allowed remote changes or trouble shooting by Emory IT to be performed remotely.

The "sidebar" video sessions were performed via a standard commercial video conferencing tool. This tool was loaded on the secondary computer the clinicians use and also had separate speakers to allow the verbal communication needed. When a nurse in Atlanta called the nurse or physician in Australia, they had an open instance of the video tool and made a call. This resulted in an indicator popping up on the receiving clinician's monitor and they could then answer the call. While the network phones were installed and active, this was the primary means for our staff to communicate back and forth with the staff in Australia.

A 42-in. monitor was installed on the wall in the COR in Atlanta and in Sydney. This monitor had a mini-CPU connected to it, and a live video feed from one side of the earth to the other was established. This feed was the best option for allowing the staff at both sites to have the feel of being collocated. When a nurse in Atlanta had a question or task for the physician to follow up on this live feed allowed them to see what the physician was doing. If the physician was involved in a conversation with another clinician, the nurse in Atlanta could communicate with the nurse in Australia to ensure the question would be answered in a timely manner.

As patient populations change there is a need for healthcare to adapt to provide the care needed to those patients. The Emory eICU represents another option for managing the demands of care delivery for this critically ill population. The expertise and knowledge that might not be available locally to some hospitals can be leveraged through this medium, thus providing patients access to the care they need. The Australia approach affords the clinicians delivering that essential care another option for preserving a quality of life that isn't available while working during night time hours. The audio-visual base of the program affords the ability to put novel workflows in place regardless of the distance between the clinicians and patients. As tele medicine models grow in use, these types of options will increase for clinicians.

We also analyzed qualitative data collected from the clinicians that were study subjects. The model allowed clinicians at the remote site to forge friendships and a level of closeness neither of them expected, and they reported that made the work even more rewarding for them. The clinicians felt more awake and alert while being in Australia because they were able to maintain regular sleep/wake cycles instead of trying to rest ahead or make up for sleep missed working at night. One of our clinicians wrote "The communication from Australia to stateside seemed to be a non-issue when it came to the workflow of the eICU. Personally, it was a chance of a lifetime. I was able to complete my shifts on the weekends and during the week, my time was mine to do as I wanted. The most significant aspect for me, was the change from working nights to working days. I felt like I had more time. When working nights, you can either sleep when your get home, or stay up all day and change to a day routine. Either way, your feel tired, and exhausted, especially working 3 or 4 12-h shifts in a row. In Australia, I completed my assigned shifts, went home and slept. The next morning, I was able to accomplish whatever I had planned. I was not exhausted and did not lose a day just to make the transition from nights to days". Emory Healthcare leadership fully supports their staff and makes efforts to ensure the clinicians are cared for as well as the patients. This program allowed those clinicians a once in a lifetime experience in another country while having the security of continuous employment and financial stability.

As the next phase of the project, we are launching an Emory eICU installation in Perth, Western Australia. Perth is the largest city antipodal to Atlanta and offers the advantage of being either 12 or 13 h out of phase with Atlanta (depending on whether Atlanta is on daylight or standard time.) Our initial experience in Perth will be reported in 2019.

The Australia patient care option did move to Perth Australia in May of 2018, and continued sending one nurse and one physician to Perth in eight to twelve-week rotations. The outreach post did close from the middle of March 2020 to September 2022 due to COVID associated impacts on travel. The program continues to provide increases in satisfaction and productivity of Emory staff when working there.

While there have been extensive changes in healthcare and in the world in general over the last three years, this solution to addressing the deleterious physical and mental effects of night time work has remained stable and still proves to be a successful model of care. Patients have also become aware of the staff location, and become very interested in where their clinician is actually working, yet they have not felt any impact on their care (Oliviero 2018).

Multiple healthcare systems have reached out to Emory to learn more about the build and implementation of the program. This has provided Emory with yet another opportunity to share practice and expertise in a novel program.

References

Claffey, C. Out of darkness. In: Nursing spectrum: Florida edition, vol. 16, no. 19;2006. p. 6–8.
Coiera E, Wang Y, Magrabi F, Concha OP, Gallego B, Runciman W. Predicting the cumulative risk of death during hospitalization by modeling weekend, weekday and diurnal mortality risks. BMC Health Serv Res. 2014;14:226.

Crowley E. Managing dispersed teams: new challenges, new solutions. Handb Bus Strat. 2005;6(1):209–12.

Floyd JP. Crit care nurse. How nurse preceptors influence new graduates, 2003;Suppl:26:52, 95.

Gu F, Han J, Laden F, Pan A, Caporaso NE, Stampfer MJ, Kawachi I, Rexrode KM, Willett WC, Hankinson SE, Speizer FE, Schernhammer ES. Total and cause-specific mortality of U.S. nurses working rotating night shifts. Am J Prev Med. 2015;48(3):241–52.

Lilly CM, McLaughlin JM, Zhao H, Baker SP, Cody S, Irwin RS, UMass Memorial Critical Care Operations Group. A multicenter study of ICU telemedicine reengineering of adult critical care. Chest. 2014;145(3):500–7.

Oliviero H. How Emory Healthcare is taking care of patients here from Australia May 18 2018. Atlanta J Const. 2018. https://www.ajc.com/lifestyles/health/how-emory-healthcare-taking-care-patients-here-from-australia/Zuk24rJv3BfPFKUaa9DQRL/

Chapter 20
Encoding Clinical Pathways: The Impact Beyond the Target

Eugene Y. Kim and Edward H. Suh

Abstract Electronic health record (EHR) designs can lead to unintended practical consequences that are chiefly conspicuous to end users (Colicchio et al. 2019). Though some specific domains such as usability (Melnick et al. 2020) and the EHR's effect on workload (Overhage and McCallie 2020) have recently received increased attention, our understanding of how to best address collateral impacts of EHR design is incomplete. With the aim of grounding conversations regarding users' experience with the EHR within a clinical context, we present a case study demonstrating how encoded workflows such as clinical pathways can potentially have unforeseen impacts on patient care.

20.1 Clinical Case

A 79-year-old man is brought to the Emergency Department (ED) by his family. Family members tell the nurse in triage that he has had a few hours of vomiting, abdominal pain, as well as some weakness on the left side. The triage nurse requests an immediate evaluation by a physician as she recognizes that unilateral weakness is a possible sign of a cerebrovascular accident (CVA). The nursing staff has received extensive training focusing on the importance of early identification of these cases. Early identification is essential to meet the standards for stroke care that are part of the neurology department's preferred approach to CVA management and are also subject to regulatory scrutiny. For example, 'door to needle' time is a critical metric tracking how quickly an ischemic stroke patient may receive a 'clot-busting' medication as the medication may not be effective if not given expediently. 'Door to needle' times

E. Y. Kim (✉) · E. H. Suh
Department of Emergency Medicine, Columbia University Irving Medical Center, New York, NY, USA
e-mail: eyk7@cumc.columbia.edu

E. H. Suh
e-mail: ehs2109@cumc.columbia.edu

© The Author(s), under exclusive license to Springer Nature Switzerland AG 2025
K. Zheng et al. (eds.), *Reengineering Clinical Workflow in the Digital and AI Era*,
Cognitive Informatics in Biomedicine and Healthcare,
https://doi.org/10.1007/978-3-031-82971-0_20

399

are recommended to be under an hour and stroke centers doggedly aim to meet this standard.

The hospital is an academic institution with a stroke program that is known for aggressive intervention. Criteria for "stroke protocol" activation are intentionally set as broadly as possible, in order to capture all possible cases of acute stroke. Representatives from the ED, neurology, and the hospital-wide stroke committee, as well as quality, operations, and medical directors worked with EHR analysts to develop order sets, alerts, scoring systems, (e.g. National Institutes of Health Stroke Scale, scales to assess for a large vessel occlusion) and nursing assessment tools to assist with stroke care. Additionally, custom versions of imaging orders and bundled laboratory test panels, both with a defaulted high priority to expedite their processing, were created. In order to closely track compliance to the protocol, new structured data elements were created and embedded within the order set and nursing flowsheets so that salient time points can be easily extracted to a dashboard.

On the initial evaluation by a resident physician, a history of waxing and waning mental status along with left sided weakness is rapidly obtained from the patient's family members. The resident's cursory first examination reveals a patient with unwell appearance, difficulty following commands, and possibly some limb weakness. She requests the patient elevate both arms symmetrically to check for "pronator drift", a sign of unilateral weakness, but the patient is unable to comply with her instructions. It is not clear whether the difficulty was due to global weakness, an alteration of mental status, inattention, or other factors. When the resident asks the family how long these symptoms have been present, they report that they found the patient in this state approximately an hour and a half ago. They also note that the patient had been recently suffering from an apparent dysrhythmia they cannot recall, and they believe that the cardiologist placed a pacemaker. The clinical team is still at the bedside of the patient and due to the time pressure of the situation has not yet been able to consult the EHR to try to verify any information or place orders.

While the resident physician is conducting her exam, the nurse checks the patient's vital signs and obtains a fingerstick blood glucose. These values are found to be normal. The patient has been in the ED for five minutes at this point. The resident identifies that the patient meets the entry criteria for the hospital acute stroke protocol and is also high-risk because of the cardiac and dysrhythmia history. The resident verbally orders the clerk to call the hospital page operator, who sends simultaneous pages activating all members of the stroke team. Another ED resident assists by entering the "stroke protocol" order set in the EHR which allows them to easily enter the relevant orders. After several hard stops including for blood type and COVID testing, the lab tests, monitoring, and neuroimaging are ordered.

A multidisciplinary team assembles at the patient's bedside. The team includes a neurology fellow, resident, research coordinator, and pharmacist. The laboratory supervisor calls in by telephone to announce that the laboratory is standing by to process the bloodwork. The CT technician removes a different patient who was already on the gurney to be scanned in preparation for the possible stroke patient. Labs are drawn and an ECG is obtained. The patient is attached to the cardiac monitor and transported by the team to the CT scanner, which is located in the ED.

The neurology resident performs a focused history and examination while the patient is being wheeled on the stretcher to the scanner. He obtains a similar history of waxing and waning mental status with possible increased weakness on the left side over the past hour and a half. A past medical history of congestive heart failure, chronic obstructive pulmonary disease, hypertension, and hyperlipidemia is also noted. A stat non-contrast CT scan of the head is performed and appears negative for an acute bleed. The team decides to administer tissue plasminogen activator (tPA). tPA is the primary treatment for ischemic stroke and must be given within a few hours to maximize effectiveness and reduce risk. The decision is not taken lightly, as 6.4% percent of these patients may unfortunately develop serious bleeding within the brain (National Institute of Neurological Disorders and Stroke rt-PA Stroke Study Group. Tissue plasminogen activator for acute ischemic stroke 1995). After a verbal order, the pharmacist opens the sealed medications and begins to mix them in preparation for administration.

Twenty minutes have passed since the patient first arrived in the ED. Four patients were in the process of being triaged when the stroke activation was triggered, and an additional six patients have been triaged in the meantime and are waiting to be seen in different districts of the ED. Overall the ED held approximately 150 patients in various stages of evaluation when the stroke patient arrived. Since that time, three more patients have walked into the ED, as well as two arriving via ambulance. One of the patients who had been waiting for triage, a well-appearing 50-year-old woman, is now having vital signs performed by the nursing assistant. The vitals are notable for a fever to 38.2C orally, as well as tachycardia to 120 beats per minute. The oxygen saturation is 95% and the blood pressure is normal. These measurements are automatically uploaded from the machine into the patient's chart.

On the status board display of the EHR, which gives an overview of all the patients currently in the ED, the febrile patient's name begins to flash in purple and yellow due to the patient's vital signs. This flashing is intended to highlight to clinicians patients at risk for sepsis and activates when the systemic inflammatory response in sepsis (SIRS) criteria is met. This trigger was put into place after a review of patients admitted for severe sepsis and septic shock revealed a substantial number of cases in which the treatment and evaluation did not meet state-mandated guidelines. As the state sepsis guidelines were developed in a relatively algorithmic fashion, the hospital quality committee decided to encode the algorithm into the EHR in the form of automated alerts and order sets in addition to focused education. While initially physicians were concerned that the care pathway left little room for autonomy (e.g. when and which tests, what amount of fluids, or which antibiotics to order), measurements of compliance with the state guidelines have improved dramatically in the year since the initiative was rolled out and it was deemed an outstanding success.

The flashing patient name is present on the nursing computer tracking board too and alerts a nurse monitoring patient flow through triage to send an electronic message through the EHR to the senior resident physician who is assigned the responsibility for managing acute cases. The resident received the notification for the "code sepsis" on her mobile device. She initially ignores this message as she is assisting in the administration of tPA to the stroke patient. Once this is completed, she goes to her workstation to order the tPA, but before she completes this action, she notices she was sent a message by the nurse regarding the sepsis patient. She finishes entering the tPA orders on the stroke patient, which only required one click and entry of her password. She switches over to the possibly septic patient's chart. She notes the vital signs and the history obtained in triage of a cough and fever, and furthermore sees that the past medical history field contains the diagnoses of hypertension, diabetes, chronic obstructive pulmonary disease, and chronic renal insufficiency. The tracking board indicates that the patient had been in the ED for forty minutes already. Sensing the need to expedite care given strict time-based metrics which are tracked at both a departmental and hospital level, she opens the sepsis order set and signs off on the routine panel of tests, interventions, and nursing orders before any further investigation or even meeting the patient. She is thankful she can quickly order the necessary components of the 'sepsis bundle' with one order set. Antibiotics are also ordered, though it is not yet clear if the patient is in fact suffering from a bacterial infection as viral infections may have some similar symptoms at times and the triage note is sparse. Antibiotics have side effects and may also induce antibiotic resistance, but consideration of these risks was deferred as the resident prefers to show high compliance in her care of sepsis cases. Before the EHR will finalize the orders, it produces a series of prompts and hard stops that the resident must clear one by one, checking for proper patient identification, asking that the results of a pregnancy test be entered before the radiology examination, and asking for entry of a patient weight to calculate the intravenous fluid volume. An alert for allergies was bypassed as the provider had not yet interacted with the patient.

The patient's status board entry now indicates the patient is a "code sepsis". The orders entered on her automatically rise to the top of the work list for the nurse assigned to the patient. These include drawing blood cultures, blood gas, venous lactate, as well as a general electrolyte and cell count panel. There are also orders automatically included to obtain urine for analysis and urine culture, a chest X-ray, as well as treatment with antipyretic medications, antibiotics, and intravenous fluids.

Meanwhile, the stroke patient's first bolus of intravenous tPA finishes. As the second dose is starting to infuse, he appears acutely uncomfortable. He is retching, attempting to sit up, and confused. The nurse attending to the patient shouts for help and both the emergency medicine and stroke teams arrive at the bedside. One provider notes that the cardiac monitor is demonstrating what appears to be ventricular tachycardia, a potentially deadly dysrhythmia, but it resolves before intervention and the patient's mental status improves. There is discussion between the neurology and emergency medicine teams on whether to suspend or continue the tPA infusion, but after a few minutes the neurology stroke fellow elects to terminate it. There is confusion as to whether a troponin, a blood test which reflects damage to heart muscle, had been sent as the troponin order is included within a stroke lab order panel whose components are not visible from the order entry workspace. An additional redundant troponin test is sent.

The patient remains stable in the ED, but the disposition of the patient is now unclear. The neurology team requests a cardiology consultation and are advocating for admission to the cardiac care unit. When the cardiology fellow arrives, he disagrees with this assessment. The dispute is escalated to the attending physicians of the two consultative services and the patient is ultimately admitted to the neurological intensive care unit for monitoring. Interrogation of the patient's pacemaker would eventually reveal he had been suffering from intermittent episodes of rapid atrial fibrillation as well as occasional episodes of ventricular tachycardia throughout the day. His pacemaker precludes magnetic resonance imaging of his brain, but after stabilization of his dysrhythmia no further focal neurological symptoms were noted.

During this time, the code sepsis patient finishes an infusion of one liter of normal saline and is started on a second liter. The resident physician finds time to obtain a more in-depth history, which includes fever, cough, nasal congestion, sore throat, and wheeze for the past several days. Her examination is notable for diffuse expiratory wheezing, so the physician orders nebulized albuterol and oral prednisone to treat a possible chronic obstructive pulmonary disease (COPD) exacerbation in the setting of an upper respiratory infection. The chest X-ray and most of the bloodwork ultimately return unremarkable with the exception of a moderately elevated venous lactate, which is flagged as a critical result. The lactate plays an important role within the sepsis pathway and is automatically included in the order set, but otherwise may typically be ordered with particular discretion as false positives may result in further treatment and testing. The attending physician is able to evaluate the patient a few hours after arrival. The elevated lactate is noted and the team makes a plan to repeat the test. The patient, however, has symptomatically improved and is concerned about several pet animals that she has left alone at home. She refuses the repeat blood draw for the second lactate and instead is asking for discharge papers. The emergency medicine team, faced with the elevated lactate in a high-risk patient, discharges the patient with significant consternation, though they do note that lactate may be elevated in the setting of albuterol administration. They provide prescriptions for oral antibiotics that cover community acquired pneumonia, as well as oral steroids for COPD. The team caring for this patient later receives an email that they did not meet the necessary metrics for sepsis care for this case since the team did not document a reassessment after fluid administration using specially developed sepsis documentation tools.

It is now five hours after the stroke alert has been activated and five and a half hours since the "code sepsis" patient had arrived. The ED had received over 60 more patients during this time, which is typical considering the time and day of week. Triage processes had returned to normal as soon as documentation on the stroke patient was completed, but the few minutes of delay has led to a queue forming outside of triage. This in turn had led to some unrest among patients waiting to be evaluated, further increasing pressure on the nurses in triage as people began approaching them to ask when they would be seen. By prioritizing the stroke patient for his CT scan, ED flow had been further disrupted as there had already been delays in the normal turn-around time for CT orders because of difficulty coordinating transportation between the clinical areas and radiology for several moderately sick patients. This led to median times between CT order and test performance to stretch to more than 90 min, well above average for the department. The nursing staff working in the ED also had trouble keeping up with the orders being entered on other patients. Although there was some re-distribution of patients to other districts because of the burden of these two acute cases, there was not enough excess capacity in the nursing group to fully 'catch up' with the patients being evaluated by the medical staff. As a result, average time between first evaluation and disposition decision increased significantly on several patients. This led, in turn, to significantly increased crowding in the clinical areas. The conditions continued to negatively affect care until past midnight, when arrivals to the ED finally tapered to the point where the queue of pending work could be completed.

Two days later, the "code sepsis" patient's blood cultures grow gram positive cocci in one of the two bottles. The patient is asked to return for re-evaluation and she reluctantly complies. On her second visit, she is clinically much improved and it is felt the positive culture was likely due to a contaminant rather than true infection. The patient is discharged again with strict return instructions.

20.2   Discussion

The Emergency Department (ED) presents unique challenges to clinical practice, and consequently to the implementation of ED information systems as well. Patient flow and acuity is variable, patients may need to be treated with limited available information, and there is tremendous clinical heterogeneity and diagnostic uncertainty, all the while care must be delivered in the setting of dynamically constrained resources and compressed timescales. In the field of emergency medicine, there has been a particular push to incorporate clinical pathways into the workup and treatment of critical diagnoses such as stroke, acute coronary syndromes, and sepsis. Due to the high acuity of these diagnoses, the pathways developed tend to be labor-intensive and great effort is devoted to their completion, at any cost. Though pathways and protocols may help standardize care and improve quality, they can also counterintuitively negatively impact the treatment of others and at times for these patients themselves.

In a system with a stroke program, the push to adhere to the timed steps in the pathway compete with the clinician's responsibility to perform a thorough evaluation of the patient and may divert time and resources from other patients. When a complex patient presents with multiple complaints or an unclear clinical picture, a clinician may be induced to simplify the case by focusing on the singular sign or symptom that can, for example, justify a stroke activation and place the patient on a predetermined pathway. As illustrated in this case, fixating on the patient's unilateral weakness allowed the clinician to standardize her evaluation and treatment plan at the expense of a fuller understanding of her complaint. The system itself, designed to optimize care for stroke patients, may also lead clinicians down this route and induce premature diagnostic closure, curtailing a patient's evaluation and thereby limiting the likelihood that they would receive the optimal care for their true ailment. Though the outcome was favorable, the patient's evaluation in the ED was prolonged while his disposition was debated between several services and leadership, resulting in admission to an intensive care unit not specialized in the care of cardiac patients. Additionally, though the EHR may assist in recognizing critical cases and standardizing these patients' workflow, EHR interventions can at times result in extra tests ordered, resources utilized to perform these tests, and consequences from atypical EHR workflows (e.g. increased mental effort, user error) utilized in the care of these patients. Thus, though stroke or sepsis may be more expediently diagnosed and treated, this is not without potential risk to the patient (e.g. misdiagnosis, administration of tPA), the clinical staff (e.g. EHR inefficiencies), and the larger health system and ED (e.g. increased crowding, decreased resources, and the management of critically ill patients).

Similarly, a patient with sepsis may indeed derive benefit from a standardized approach when it enforces compliance with established "best practices". Yet at the same time, many tests or interventions that show some evidence of benefit when studied in a specific population may be less advantageous for a particular individual's circumstances. In this case, while strictly speaking the patient may have met recognized criteria for sepsis, both the likely physiological processes as well as the patient's own preferences made the algorithmic approach far less efficacious. The patient was unlikely to be suffering from the distributive vascular dysfunction and poor tissue perfusion that the sepsis protocol was designed in part to address. In addition, a conversation with the patient revealed strong preference on her part to return home as quickly as possible. Without the flashing patient name to pressure the clinician to abide by the standardized treatment plan, she may have otherwise obtained a more detailed history and physical that could have led to a more focused care plan, relieving the patient and the system from the burden of unnecessary testing and treatment.

These sorts of encoded clinical pathways, however, not only place boundaries on the clinician's approach to the individual patient, but also add new burdens and limitations on the local system as well. Every ED has some areas of constraint, and most have reached a form of resource equilibrium that forces them to operate at or near maximum capacity to achieve standard workflow conditions. In this setting, even seemingly minor perturbations can cause significant downstream effects which may extend far beyond the initial inciting event. The delay in CT scan turnaround time caused by one stroke patient or the backing up of orders to be carried out on other patients while a nurse is called to first attend to a possible sepsis emergency, can result in a significant slowdown in the care of other patients, compromising their outcomes. On a broader scale, it can lead to increased ED crowding, which has its own deleterious effects on clinical outcomes.

20.3 Conclusions

Though self-evident, it bears stressing that clinical staff's priority is clinical care; any activity that does not facilitate patient care directly may be seen as burdensome (Hobensack et al. 2022). Despite the many competing interests that may influence

EHR design and use, including regulatory, financial, institutional and regional priorities (Holmgren et al. 2021), any obtrusiveness or impairment of practical functionality of the EHR is magnified to those using it and even more so when the system is strained or there is a medical emergency. Furthermore, such repercussions can be further reaching than those who interact directly with the EHR. Impractical workflows, or even satisfactory workflows that are under sufficient pressures, may be particularly susceptible to nonadherence or 'workarounds' (Collins et al. 2012) in this environment. This may lead to situations where EHR designers may add additional layers to their workflows in an attempt to enhance conformity, without understanding the overall effect they are having on the local system of care.

Ideally, EHR interventions that closely align with patient-centered care and the system within which they are operating, and clinical outcomes and local real-time impacts, must be considered. As technologies emerge that may, intentionally or not, take decision making out of the hands of clinicians (e.g. machine learning), it is of critical importance that there is a broad recognition of potential downsides of this shift and that clinicians' ability to balance factors and needs not anticipated when these tools were designed are supported. Not doing so may invite suboptimal or disrupted workflows, or unintended impacts in regard to clinical care or the care system in which they are implemented.

References

Colicchio TK, Cimino JJ, Del Fiol G. Unintended consequences of nationwide electronic health record adoption: challenges and opportunities in the post-meaningful use Era. J Med Internet Res. 2019;21(6): e13313. https://doi.org/10.2196/13313.

Collins SA, Fred M, Wilcox L, Vawdrey DK. Workarounds used by nurses to overcome design constraints of electronic health records. NI 2012 (2012). 2012;2012:93.

Hobensack M, Levy DR, Cato K, et al. 25 × 5 symposium to reduce documentation burden: report-out and call for action. Appl Clin Inform. 2022;13(2):439–46. https://doi.org/10.1055/s-0042-1746169.

Holmgren AJ, Downing NL, Bates DW, et al. Assessment of electronic health record use between us and non-us health systems. JAMA Intern Med. 2021;181(2):251–9. https://doi.org/10.1001/jamainternmed.2020.7071.

Melnick ER, Dyrbye LN, Sinsky CA, et al. The association between perceived electronic health record usability and professional burnout among US physicians. Mayo Clin Proc. 2020;95(3):476–87. https://doi.org/10.1016/j.mayocp.2019.09.024.

National Institute of Neurological Disorders and Stroke rt-PA Stroke Study Group. Tissue plasminogen activator for acute ischemic stroke. N Engl J Med. 1995;333(24):1581–1587. https://doi.org/10.1056/NEJM199512143332401.

Overhage JM, McCallie D. Physician time spent using the electronic health record during outpatient encounters: A descriptive study. Ann Intern Med. 2020;172(3):169–74. https://doi.org/10.7326/M18-3684.

Chapter 21
Cognitive Disconnect and Information Overload: Electronic Health Record Use for Rounding and Handover Communications in a Pediatric Intensive Care Unit

R. Stanley Hum

Abstract Bedside working rounds can be one of the most cognitively complex situations in clinical medicine. Team members develop a mental model of the patient synthesizing electronic health record (EHR) information and information that is verbally transmitted during shift-to-shift communication. Each provider must synthesize and filter a large amount of information, which can be error prone. Rounds are also prone to interruptions. Despite interruptions, because the EHR allows for each individual provider to interact with the patient chart and there is an expectation that each team member fulfills a different role for the same patient, the team should develop a shared mental model to enable optimal workflow and provide optimal care. In this case study describing the bedside working rounds in a pediatric intensive care unit (PICU), we will explore each of these issues in depth.

21.1 Case Background

When you think about critical care medicine, you think about a team of healthcare providers frantically performing cardiopulmonary resuscitation on a patient whose heart has stopped. While these situations happen, the more common situation is a critical care team participating in a discussion about a complex patient. In medicine, we call these discussions rounds. What a description of patient cases during rounds may fail to convey is the time pressure imposed on providers. In a typical unit with 14 patients, completing rounds within a 3-h period is not uncommon. Hence, a patient presentation from start to finish needs to be in the order of 10–15 min. During this time, the team discusses a single patient, but interruptions are inevitable. Other

R. S. Hum (✉)
McGill University, Montreal, Canada
e-mail: robert.stanley.hum@mcgill.ca

patients may be deteriorating, new patients may be coming in, and stable patients may need to be discharged to maintain patient flow. This time constraint leaves little time for reflection and contemplation even in the absence of interruptions.

21.2 Case Presentation

Fourteen patients ranging from 2 months through 18 years of age are admitted in a 16-bed PICU. Around 9 AM, the healthcare team is starting to see patients. Standing and gathered in front of the patient's room is the PICU attending physician ("the attending"); the PICU fellow physician (the fellow); four resident physicians ("residents"); and the bedside PICU nurse. The patient can easily be seen from the outside and the patient's parents have come out of the room to listen and participate in the discussion.

The attending, working on a workstation on wheels (WOW), is logged into the patient's electronic health record (EHR). The others are waiting for the attending to finish opening a new physician note for this patient. Using a combination of copying and pasting from the note the attending wrote yesterday, acronym expansion and direct data substitution, the attending is finally ready to hear the presentation.

There are three residents on the team today. Each of them is carrying a stack of stapled paper printouts and each is standing in front of a WOW. These printouts were created just before the shift-to-shift communication ("handover") at 7AM and are summaries of their respective assigned patients including the medication orders, last 24-h of laboratory results and fluid status summaries. They received handover from the overnight resident at 7 AM who has left the unit. Each printout also included handwritten notes including "To Do" reminders, corrections and events which the overnight resident did not enter in the handover document. Each resident also carries a mobile internal phone so that they can be contacted individually.

The resident assigned to this patient ("the presenting resident") starts to report the patient's summary and major events of the last 24 h. Simultaneously, the attending is typing the pertinent information into the interval history section of the patient's EHR note. The attending interrupts the resident as some of presented patient events were reported on the previous day. The resident realizes that some of the handover document events had not been updated. Upon completion of the 24-h events, the attending adds an additional event, which the resident was unaware. After the interval events are described, the bedside nurse ("the nurse") starts their report.

The nurse is standing next to the bedside computer with the patient flowsheet. The nurse has a paper-based written handover aid sheet. The sheet has been updated by the overnight nurse. To ensure consistency, the nurse follows the protocol of reading through the handover sheet in the following order: major 24-h events, neurologic status including sedation, analgesic and muscle relaxant infusions and boluses; cardiovascular status including vasoactive infusions; respiratory status including respiratory rate ranges, ventilator settings and the most recent arterial blood gas as it is written on a sheet by the bedside; fluid balance status; and other systems including skin. Some of the information on the sheet is incorrect, and the nurse reports the correct information. There is also some missing data that has not been updated. Some of the information reported contradicts the resident presentation of the events. The attending asks the team to try to clarify the events. There is no one present with firsthand knowledge of the event in question. Using the bedside computer, the nurse checks the flowsheet data or a nursing note in the EHR but there is no further explanation. The resident checks the handover document interface on the patient's record, but no further information is available.

Simultaneously, while the resident and nurse are presenting, several events happen. First, a nurse pulls the fellow aside because of a deteriorating patient. The fellow returns after the completion of the nurse report, and continues to listen. The fellow has their own sheets on all the patients in the unit. The fellow also received handover at 7am from the overnight fellow.

Second, one of the other residents' internal phone rings. It is another patient's nurse. That patient's medication is due to be given and the nurse would like clarification about the order. The resident steps aside and looks up information on their handover sheets. The nurse asks the resident to update the order. The resident changes to the appropriate patient, enters the order and returns to the discussion.

Once the nurse report is completed, the presenting resident continues by describing their findings on physical examination, followed by the laboratory results. The presenting resident's phone rings. The presenting resident passes the phone to a third resident who answers the phone and steps away. It is one of the consulting services regarding another patient. The third resident takes a message and returns to rounds.

Meanwhile, to save time, another resident has pulled up the patient's chest x-ray (CXR) of this morning along with yesterday's CXR while the presenting resident continues. The attending asks about the CXR, and all eyes move to the display which has been turned so the entire team can see the CXR. The endotracheal tube (ETT) is in a little high. The resident measures the exact distance that the ETT needs to be pushed inwards. The attending confirms that the ETT should be advanced inwards by that distance. Both the presenting resident and the nurse take note as this procedure will need to be performed after the rounds.

The presenting resident the discusses their impression and plan of care. Intermittently, as the resident is corrected by the attending, the presenting resident writes down "To Do" reminders on their handover printout. Since there is minimal time, the handover screen will need to be updated later in the day. One of the other residents starts to enter orders on the patient. As part of the order entry system, there is an alert to notify if the resident is accessing the correct patient's chart which forces a brief period of waiting. Fortunately, the resident notices that the wrong patient's chart has been accessed. In fact, it was the patient that the resident was asked for a medication clarification. The order is cancelled, and the resident switches to the patient being discussed, and the order is re-entered. After waiting, the system allows the order to be finalized.

The other resident continues to enter orders as they are being presented. Another resident is modifying a portion of the handover screen in the EHR. This portion of the handover screen is reserved for the daily checklist. The checklist for the previous day's goals is removed and current goals are entered. The parents are asked if they have any questions. They do not, and the team moves to the next patient of the day.

21.3 Analysis of the Case and Discussion

This case illustrates a typical process preparing for and participating in patient rounds. Upon examination of the case, we will discuss a couple of themes: first, the development of a shared mental model including the effect of technology and use of artefacts to overcome constraints imposed by time and the nature of EHRs, and second, the occurrence of interruptions.

21.3.1 Shared Mental Models

In a recent systematic review, there is a significant body of evidence supporting teamwork in the intensive care unit to provide high-quality care (Donovan et al. 2018). In this example, the work during rounds is distributed across multiple providers with each provider having a different role. Lane et al. (Lane et al. 2013) concluded that a successful communication strategy during patient care rounds included standardized rounding structures and processes with explicit roles for healthcare providers. Ideally, each of the providers should maintain a shared mental model of the patient and the goals of care (Page et al. 2016; Weller et al. 2014; Westli et al. 2010; Reader et al. 2009; Haig et al. 2006; Mathieu et al. 2000). In our example, each of the providers receive their initial patient mental model individually from their overnight counterparts who are not present during rounds. The process of rounding serves to synchronize and reconcile conflicting understanding about the patient amongst the providers as well as to make explicit the goals for the day (Lane et al. 2013). Ideally, the entire team, overnight and daytime, would gather on rounds to handover but these have become increasingly difficult because of duty hour restrictions (Philibert et al. 2011; Education ACfGM. 2017).

With the implementation of reduced duty hours and the increased importance of the healthcare team, handovers to provide continuity of care has become essential (Arora et al. 2014). Handovers have become an increasing important topic of study and handover tools have become more common (Hoskote et al. 2017; Cochran 2018; Mardis et al. 2017, 2016; Keebler et al. 2016; Davis et al. 2015; Abraham et al. 2014). During these handovers, the goal is not only to communicate information but a mental model of the patient in question (Reader et al. 2009; Jiang et al. 2017). Discrepancies between a provider's firsthand knowledge and that which is documented in EHR should be reconciled (Davis et al. 2015).

Sources of error in the EHR can lead to discrepancies in the provider's mental models (Collins et al. 2011; Embi et al. 2004). These sources include incorrect original documentation, incorrect interpretation of an event, copy and pasted information which no longer is accurate and missing information. Based on a provider's expertise and familiarity with the patient, these errors can be accommodated. Unfortunately, in the case of electronic handover tools, which can be a combination of summarized prose by providers and automated summaries extracted from observations documented in the EHR, these errors can lead to incorrect summaries, and can create serious misunderstandings in the mental model developed by inexperienced providers or providers that have never cared for the patient (Davis et al. 2015).

Beyond errors, the amount of information stored in the EHR is immense and can lead to information overload (Farri et al. 2012). Inexperienced providers do not necessarily understand which information is significant and which can safely be ignored and as a result they tend to convey all the information which can impede a succinct description of the patient. Rarely are EHR summaries context aware as to filter out unneeded information. While advances in EHR summarization is being investigated (Pivovarov and Elhadad 2015), mostly, the summaries are aggregators and it is up to the provider to interpret the summary (National Research Council Committee on Engaging the Computer Science Research Community in Health Care I. The National Academies Collection: Reports funded by National Institutes of Health 2009). In fact, Varpio et al. (Varpio et al. 2015) found showed differences between paper and EHR data summarizations and cognitive loads with EHR data summarization being detrimental to clinical reasoning.

Despite the promise of EHRs, many providers still use personal (usually paper) artefacts, such as handover sheets to make up for the deficiencies in the electronic reporting (Kelley et al. 2013; Blaz et al. 2016; Collins et al. 2012; Rosenbluth et al. 2015). In the dynamic environment of the intensive care unit, information about a single patient varies from provider to provider leading to diverging mental models throughout the workday (30). Some of the unintended consequences of healthcare technology include workarounds such as deferred data entry by first documenting on personal artefacts and then subsequently transcribed into the EHR if time permits which can negatively impact documentation quality (Kelley et al. 2013; Blaz et al. 2016; Zheng et al. 2016).

In the previous section, we discussed the discrepancies of information content that needs to be effectively reconciled to develop a shared mental model and how these discrepancies can cause incomplete shared mental models which may lead to suboptimal care. In our case, each of the healthcare providers is situated behind a computer so there is potential for a physical divide between team members. The lack of face-to-face communication and physical barriers is thought to negatively impact rounding effectiveness (Lane et al. 2013; Gharaveis et al. 2018; Morrison et al. 2008). Additionally, each provider is interacting with the computer and thus, their attention is divided between the EHR interface and the group discussion.

While each provider has the overarching goal to provide the best care for the patient, each provider has their own set of priorities (Donovan et al. 2018). Effectively, each handover (nursing, resident, fellow, attending) concentrates on specific sets of information and not all are overlapping (Jiang et al. 2017; Collins et al. 2011; Mamykina et al. 2014). There is a distributive nature of the division of work in rounds. Each provider must have a similar understanding about the patient to be able to most effectively perform interrelated tasks (Page et al. 2016; Weller et al. 2014; Westli et al. 2010; Mathieu et al. 2000). Information from each of the providers must be taken into context, information must be evaluated in terms of being most representative of what occurred. Discrepancies must be reconciled so that a shared mental model can be established. Despite this shared mental model, each provider must augment that mental model to suit the needs and requirements of their own priorities.

21.3.2   Interruptions

Smartphones or rather instant access communications (voice or text) are increasingly common in the clinical workplace (Tran et al. 2014; Wu et al. 2010) and have been shown to improve communication efficiency (Ighani et al. 2010). The ability to immediately contact a remote provider is clearly important and helpful but it can also be a source of increased interruptions and potential interprofessional conflicts (Aungst and Belliveau 2015; Wu et al. 2013a, 2013b; Vaisman and Wu xxxx; Quan et al. 2013). If there are differing interpretations of the significance of a clinical event, then the provider who is being interrupted can become frustrated or experience increased stress (Weigl et al. 2014). With a paging system, it is the provider being interrupted who controls the timing of the communication, whereas, with personal mobile communications, a phone call or text message is generally returned immediately (Lo et al. 2012). In addition to increased interruptions, text paging and smartphones can have negative effects on decreased communication quality compared to face-to-face interactions and potentially leading to weakened interprofessional relationships (Wu et al. 2011, 2012, 2014).

These interruptions can be a source of increased cognitive load due to task switching (Li et al. 2012; Skaugset et al. 2016). Interruptions can lead to gaps information flow (Laxmisan et al. 2007). In our case, the face-to-face interruption and the phone call interruptions require task switching. Providers involved in the interruption must change their focus to another patient and they may miss important information that contribute to shared understanding. These external interruptions are a potential source of rounding efficiency (50) and detrimental to team understanding (Laxmisan et al. 2007). However, Rivera-Rodriguez et al. (Rivera-Rodriguez and Karsh 2010) suggests that not all interruptions are should be considered detrimental. For example, when a presenting member is interrupted by others to clarify information then the mental model remains focused on the same patient and discrepancies can be reconciled and contributing to better shared mental models.

In addition to the effect on information flow, interruptions can be a cause of medical errors (Skaugset et al. 2016). In our case, an interruption was the potential cause of a near-miss with ordering. Several authors have suggested the importance of interruption management such as using physical cues or conscious times to delay or reject interruptions to mitigate errors (52, 53) as well as the importance of error recovery (Patel et al. 2015). Unfortunately, a systematic review of interventions to reduce interruptions showed that the evidence that these interventions reduced errors was equivocal and that further study was needed (Raban and Westbrook 2014).

21.4 Conclusions

The time of the individual provider delivering care is past and teamwork is essential to delivering optimal healthcare. Effectively developing a shared mental model is important in teamwork. Rounding in the intensive care unit is a cognitive complex task involving multiple members of the healthcare team. Participation in rounding serves to distribute work and cognitive load as well as to help solidify shared mental models. The development of shared mental models is affected by the handover process, handover tools including those that involve EHR systems, discrepancies in the experiences of individual team members and errors in the EHR systems. In addition, the demands of using EHR systems at the point of rounding can change the physical environment so that team dynamics are sub-optimal for shared mental model creation. Rounding is also affected by interruptions. Technology can also mediate provider-to-provider communication and be a source of interruptions. Personal communication devices have been shown to make care more efficient, but the technology can also lead to increased interruptions and potentially interprofessional conflicts. These interruptions can be a source of medical error. Recovery from these errors and interruptions is an important process.

21.5 Recommendations

Current processes and workflows, particularly involving handover and rounding, need to be re-evaluated in the light of the distributive nature of work and cognition in the intensive care unit. Processes need to optimize development of shared mental models and support effective teamwork. Implementation of technology needs to be reviewed in this context as it can both be a benefit and a hinderance (for example, smartphones can improve unit efficiency but can also contribute to increased external interruptions or EHR use on rounds can be a cause of distraction and worsening shared mental model development).

References

Abraham J, Kannampallil T, Patel VL. A systematic review of the literature on the evaluation of handoff tools: implications for research and practice. J Am Med Inform Assoc: JAMIA. 2014;21(1):154–62.

Anderson CE, Nicksa GA, Stewart L. Distractions during resident handoffs: incidence, sources, and influence on handoff quality and effectiveness. JAMA Surg. 2015;150(5):396–401.

Arora VM, Reed DA, Fletcher KE. Building continuity in handovers with shorter residency duty hours. BMC Med Educ. 2014;14(Suppl 1):S16.

Aungst TD, Belliveau P. Leveraging mobile smart devices to improve interprofessional communications in inpatient practice setting: A literature review. J Interprof Care. 2015;29(6):570–8.

Blaz JW, Doig AK, Cloyes KG, Staggers N. The hidden lives of nurses' cognitive artifacts. Appl Clin Inform. 2016;7(3):832–49.

Cochran A. Standardized Handoffs in the Intensive Care Unit: Hope or Hype for Improving Critical Care? JAMA surgery. 2018.

Coiera E. Technology, cognition and error. BMJ Qual Saf. 2015;24(7):417–22.

Collins SA, Stein DM, Vawdrey DK, Stetson PD, Bakken S. Content overlap in nurse and physician handoff artifacts and the potential role of electronic health records: a systematic review. J Biomed Inform. 2011;44(4):704–12.

Collins SA, Mamykina L, Jordan D, Stein DM, Shine A, Reyfman P, et al. In search of common ground in handoff documentation in an Intensive Care Unit. J Biomed Inform. 2012;45(2):307–15.

Davis J, Riesenberg LA, Mardis M, Donnelly J, Benningfield B, Youngstrom M, et al. Evaluating outcomes of electronic tools supporting physician shift-to-shift handoffs: a systematic review. J Grad Med Educ. 2015;7(2):174–80.

Donovan AL, Aldrich JM, Gross AK, Barchas DM, Thornton KC, Schell-Chaple HM, et al. Interprofessional Care and Teamwork in the ICU. Critical care medicine. 2018.

Education ACfGM. Accreditation Councll for Graduate Medical Education Common Program Requirements: The Learning and Working Environment (Duty Hours). 2017.

Embi PJ, Yackel TR, Logan JR, Bowen JL, Cooney TG, Gorman PN. Impacts of computerized physician documentation in a teaching hospital: perceptions of faculty and resident physicians. J Am Med Inform Assoc: JAMIA. 2004;11(4):300–9.

Farri O, Pieckiewicz DS, Rahman AS, Adam TJ, Pakhomov SV, Melton GB. A qualitative analysis of EHR clinical document synthesis by clinicians. AMIA Annu Symp Proc AMIA Symp. 2012;2012:1211–20.

Gharaveis A, Hamilton DK, Pati D. The impact of environmental design on teamwork and communication in healthcare facilities: a systematic literature review. HERD. 2018;11(1):119–37.

Haig KM, Sutton S, Whittington J. SBAR: a shared mental model for improving communication between clinicians. Jt Comm J Qual Patient Saf. 2006;32(3):167–75.

Hoskote SS, Racedo Africano CJ, Braun AB, O'Horo JC, Sevilla Berrios RA, Loftsgard TO, et al. Improving the quality of handoffs in patient care between critical care providers in the intensive care unit. Am J Med Qual: off J Am CollE Med Qual. 2017;32(4):376–83.

Ighani F, Kapoor KG, Gibran SK, Davis GH, Prager TC, Chuang AZ, et al. A comparison of two-way text versus conventional paging systems in an academic ophthalmology department. J Med Syst. 2010;34(4):677–84.

Jiang SY, Murphy A, Heitkemper EM, Hum RS, Kaufman DR, Mamykina L. Impact of an electronic handoff documentation tool on team shared mental models in pediatric critical care. J Biomed Inform. 2017;69:24–32.

Keebler JR, Lazzara EH, Patzer BS, Palmer EM, Plummer JP, Smith DC, et al. Meta-Analyses of the effects of standardized handoff protocols on patient, provider, and organizational outcomes. Hum Factors. 2016;58(8):1187–205.

Kelley T, Docherty S, Brandon D. Information needed to support knowing the patient. ANS Adv Nurs Sci. 2013;36(4):351–63.

Lane D, Ferri M, Lemaire J, McLaughlin K, Stelfox HT. A systematic review of evidence-informed practices for patient care rounds in the ICU*. Crit Care Med. 2013;41(8):2015–29.

Laxmisan A, Hakimzada F, Sayan OR, Green RA, Zhang J, Patel VL. The multitasking clinician: decision-making and cognitive demand during and after team handoffs in emergency care. Int J Med Informatics. 2007;76(11–12):801–11.

Li SY, Magrabi F, Coiera E. A systematic review of the psychological literature on interruption and its patient safety implications. J Am Med Inform Assoc: JAMIA. 2012;19(1):6–12.

Lo V, Wu RC, Morra D, Lee L, Reeves S. The use of smartphones in general and internal medicine units: a boon or a bane to the promotion of interprofessional collaboration? J Interprof Care. 2012;26(4):276–82.

Mamykina L, Hum RS, Kaufman D. Investigating Shared Mental Models in Critical Care. In: Patel VL, Kaufman D, Cohen T, editors. Cognitive Informatics in Health and Biomedicine: Springer; 2014. p. 291–315.

Mardis T, Mardis M, Davis J, Justice EM, Riley Holdinsky S, Donnelly J, et al. Bedside shift-to-shift handoffs: a systematic review of the literature. J Nurs Care Qual. 2016;31(1):54–60.

Mardis M, Davis J, Benningfield B, Elliott C, Youngstrom M, Nelson B, et al. Shift-to-Shift handoff effects on patient safety and outcomes. Am J Med Qual: off J Am CollE Med Qual. 2017;32(1):34–42.

Mathieu JE, Heffner TS, Goodwin GF, Salas E, Cannon-Bowers JA. The influence of shared mental models on team process and performance. J Appl Psychol. 2000;85(2):273–83.

Morrison C, Jones M, Blackwell A, Vuylsteke A. Electronic patient record use during ward rounds: a qualitative study of interaction between medical staff. Critical Care (London, England). 2008;12(6):R148.

National Research Council Committee on Engaging the Computer Science Research Community in Health Care I. The National Academies Collection: Reports funded by National Institutes of Health. In: Stead WW, Lin HS, editors. Computational Technology for Effective Health Care: Immediate Steps and Strategic Directions. Washington (DC): National Academies Press (US) National Academy of Sciences.; 2009.

Page JS, Lederman L, Kelly J, Barry MM, James TA. Teams and teamwork in cancer care delivery: shared mental models to improve planning for discharge and coordination of follow-up care. J Oncol Pract. 2016;12(11):1053–8.

Patel VL, Kannampallil TG, Shortliffe EH. Role of cognition in generating and mitigating clinical errors. BMJ Qual Saf. 2015;24(7):468–74.

Philibert I, Amis S. The ACGME 2011 Duty Hour Standards: Enhancing Quality of Care, Supervision and Resident Professional Development. In: Education ACfGM, editor. ACGME Task Force on Quality care and Professionalism. Chicago, IL 2011.

Pivovarov R, Elhadad N. Automated methods for the summarization of electronic health records. J Am Med Inform Assoc: JAMIA. 2015;22(5):938–47.

Quan SD, Wu RC, Rossos PG, Arany T, Groe S, Morra D, et al. It's not about pager replacement: an in-depth look at the interprofessional nature of communication in healthcare. J Hosp Med. 2013;8(3):137–43.

Raban MZ, Westbrook JI. Are interventions to reduce interruptions and errors during medication administration effective?: a systematic review. BMJ Qual Saf. 2014;23(5):414–21.

Ratwani RM, Fong A, Puthumana JS, Hettinger AZ. Emergency physician use of cognitive strategies to manage interruptions. Ann Emerg Med. 2017;70(5):683–7.

Reader TW, Flin R, Mearns K, Cuthbertson BH. Developing a team performance framework for the intensive care unit. Crit Care Med. 2009;37(5):1787–93.

Rivera-Rodriguez AJ, Karsh BT. Interruptions and distractions in healthcare: review and reappraisal. Qual Saf Health Care. 2010;19(4):304–12.

Rosenbluth G, Bale JF, Starmer AJ, Spector ND, Srivastava R, West DC, et al. Variation in printed handoff documents: Results and recommendations from a multicenter needs assessment. J Hosp Med. 2015;10(8):517–24.

Skaugset LM, Farrell S, Carney M, Wolff M, Santen SA, Perry M, et al. Can you multitask? evidence and limitations of task switching and multitasking in emergency medicine. Ann Emerg Med. 2016;68(2):189–95.

Tran K, Morra D, Lo V, Quan S, Wu R. The use of smartphones on General Internal Medicine wards: a mixed methods study. Appl Clin Inform. 2014;5(3):814–23.

Vaisman A, Wu RC. Analysis of Smartphone Interruptions on Academic General Internal Medicine Wards. Frequent Interruptions may cause a 'Crisis Mode' Work Climate. Applied clinical informatics. 2017;8(1):1–11.

Varpio L, Day K, Elliot-Miller P, King JW, Kuziemsky C, Parush A, et al. The impact of adopting EHRs: how losing connectivity affects clinical reasoning. Med Educ. 2015;49(5):476–86.

Weigl M, Muller A, Angerer P, Hoffmann F. Workflow interruptions and mental workload in hospital pediatricians: an observational study. BMC Health Serv Res. 2014;14:433.

Weller J, Boyd M, Cumin D. Teams, tribes and patient safety: overcoming barriers to effective teamwork in healthcare. Postgrad Med J. 2014;90(1061):149–54.

Westli HK, Johnsen BH, Eid J, Rasten I, Brattebo G. Teamwork skills, shared mental models, and performance in simulated trauma teams: an independent group design. Scand J Trauma, Resusc Emerg Med. 2010;18:47.

Wu RC, Morra D, Quan S, Lai S, Zanjani S, Abrams H, et al. The use of smartphones for clinical communication on internal medicine wards. J Hosp Med. 2010;5(9):553–9.

Wu R, Rossos P, Quan S, Reeves S, Lo V, Wong B, et al. An evaluation of the use of smartphones to communicate between clinicians: a mixed-methods study. J Med Internet Res. 2011;13(3): e59.

Wu RC, Tran K, Lo V, O'Leary KJ, Morra D, Quan SD, et al. Effects of clinical communication interventions in hospitals: a systematic review of information and communication technology adoptions for improved communication between clinicians. Int J Med Informatics. 2012;81(11):723–32.

Wu RC, Lo V, Morra D, Wong BM, Sargeant R, Locke K, et al. The intended and unintended consequences of communication systems on general internal medicine inpatient care delivery: a prospective observational case study of five teaching hospitals. J Am Med Inform Assoc: JAMIA. 2013a;20(4):766–77.

Wu RC, Tzanetos K, Morra D, Quan S, Lo V, Wong BM. Educational impact of using smartphones for clinical communication on general medicine: more global, less local. J Hosp Med. 2013b;8(7):365–72.

Wu R, Appel L, Morra D, Lo V, Kitto S, Quan S. Short message service or disService: issues with text messaging in a complex medical environment. Int J Med Informatics. 2014;83(4):278–84.

Zheng K, Abraham J, Novak LL, Reynolds TL, Gettinger A. A survey of the literature on unintended consequences associated with health information technology: 2014–2015. Yearb Med Inform. 2016;1:13–29.

Chapter 22
Clinical Workflow: The Past, Present, and Future

Kai Zheng, Johanna Westbrook, and Vimla L. Patel

As evident from the discussions throughout this book, workflow plays a central role in ensuring smooth functioning of all clinical activities—from patient encounter to medication administration to population health management. Any disruption to workflow can result in severe, adverse consequences such as decreased time efficiency and greater patient safety risks. In the past few decades, the most systemic disruption to clinical workflow is associated with the widespread implementation of health IT systems, electronic health records (EHR) in particular, and more recently due to the adoption of artificial intelligence (AI)-based applications.

In the digital and AI era, coordination of clinical workflow increasingly relies on the use computerized systems with sophisticated decision-making capabilities embedded. However, it has been well recognized that current generation health IT systems "appear designed largely to automate tasks or business processes," providing limited support for clinical workflow and the cognitive tasks of clinicians (National Research Council 2009). Disruption to workflow as a result of health IT implementation is thus common, which is a manifestation of a wide range of design and implementation problems including poor software usability, complex intersystem dependencies, and the lack of sociotechnical integration of software systems into their complex use environments.

Understanding the impact of health IT on clinical workflow has been a key focus of the research on health IT-related unintended consequences (Bloomrosen et al. 2011; Zheng et al. 2016). In this body of the literature, there has been a general consensus

K. Zheng (✉)
University of California, Irvine, USA
e-mail: kai.zheng@uci.edu

J. Westbrook
Macquarie University, North Ryde, Australia

V. L. Patel
The New York Academy of Medicine, New York, USA

© The Author(s), under exclusive license to Springer Nature Switzerland AG 2025   417
K. Zheng et al. (eds.), *Reengineering Clinical Workflow in the Digital and AI Era*,
Cognitive Informatics in Biomedicine and Healthcare,
https://doi.org/10.1007/978-3-031-82971-0_22

that the top-down approach in the prevalent health IT design, which predominantly emphasizes administrative efficiency, is responsible for many of the adverse effects observed (National Research Council 2009). Because newly introduced health IT systems often fail to adequately support clinical workflow, clinicians are forced to develop or maintain their own workflow processes deviating from the 'recommended' practice, which as a result could increase workload and introduce new threats to patient safety.

There have been some efforts to address this issue. For example, the U.S. Agency for Healthcare Research and Quality (AHRQ) funded a project to develop a toolkit to help small and medium-sized outpatient practices more effectively manage their workflow (Carayon and Karsh 2010); and subsequently launched a funding program, "Using Health IT in Practice Redesign: Impact of Health IT on Workflow," to specifically support research that studies the causal relationship between health IT and workflow processes (Zheng et al. 2015a; Wald et al. 2015; Carayon et al. 2015). Further, the U.S. National Institute of Standards and Technology (NIST) issued a guideline in 2014 recommending the use of human factors modeling methods to better align EHR design with ambulatory care clinical workflow; and to move away from a billing-centered design to a patient-centered design in order to support better workload management and more flexible flow of patients and tasks (Lowry et al. 2014).

However, as several chapters in this book point out, there remain significant knowledge and methodological gaps in clinical workflow research. Even though disruption to workflow is a topic frequently discussed in the literature, very few studies actually measure workflow changes directly. Instead, most studies speculated that workflow might have been modified because of differences observed in outcomes-oriented measures (e.g., improved guideline adherence and reduced patient safety events) (Carayon and Karsh 2010). Even among studies that have attempted to directly quantify health IT's impact on workflow, many focused on changes in time utilization (e.g., average total time spent in direct patient care activities vs. using the computer), rather than 'flow' of the work (Zheng et al. 2010). This distinction is important because the spirit of workflow lies in the chronological organization of clinical tasks and the temporal (inter)dependencies among them.

In the literature that directly measures workflow, the most commonly used approaches are qualitative methods, such as ethnographic observations, interviews, and focus groups, and quantitative analysis of data collected from self-reported questionnaire surveys. While such approaches provide an important means for studying workflow and understanding the disruptive effects of health IT, they often fall short of measuring the magnitude of the impact; and their results are susceptible to prejudices (e.g., clinicians' negative emotions due to reluctance to change rather than shortcomings of health IT) and biases (e.g., cognitive heuristics, recall errors).

Quantitative studies on workflow that do not rely on self-reported data usually employ a pre-post observational design to assess changes in workflow. Time and motion is the most commonly used approach, which collects workflow data by having human observers observe clinicians for a continuous period of time to record how they perform their clinical tasks (what, when, for how long) (Zheng et al. 2011).

Compared to alternative methods (e.g., work sampling and self-reported questionnaires), the time and motion method is considered the most accurate way to quantify workflow. However, conducting time and motion studies is resource demanding, and their results are subject to many limitations, such as small sample size, observer bias, and the Hawthorne effect (when being observed, clinicians may demonstrate different behavior from their usual practice) (Zheng et al. 2011).

In recent years, several new methods have emerged for studying workflow using data automatically collected through software tools (e.g., screen capture software) or sensor technology such as eye tracking devices, 3D infrared laser projectors (e.g., Microsoft Kinect), and radio-frequency identification (RFID) (Furniss et al. 2017; Calvitti et al. 2017; Kannampallil et al. 2011). These methods, collectively referred to as "computational ethnography," present an automated and less obtrusive means for collecting in situ data reflecting real end users' actual, unaltered behaviors in real-world settings (Zheng et al. 2015b). These methods have the potential to substantially reduce the resource requirement for conducting workflow studies while producing more granular data than what could not be captured by human observers.

Log analysis of security audits, in particular, can be a valuable solution to enabling large-scale workflow studies at a very low cost. In the U.S., mandated by Health Insurance Portability and Accountability Act (HIPAA) and the Meaningful Use criteria, all computerized systems in healthcare must implement security auditing mechanisms for detecting malicious access to, or alteration of, protected health information. These security logs record each and every clinical activity and the associated metadata (when, by whom, the nature of the action, and the IP address or geocode of the device used), providing very rich information on how medical work is conducted. Such data are also highly structured, and can be readily analyzed to reveal insights into workflow through reconstruction of the spatiotemporal distribution of clinical activities. While still limited, workflow researchers have started to tap into this rich data resource. Chapter 16, entitled "Using Electronic Health Record Metadata to Understand Clinician Work and Behavior," is a new chapter included in this second edition of the book that describes recent efforts in using security log data captured in EHR systems to study clinical workflow.

In conclusion, understanding and reducing disruption to clinical workflow as a result of health IT implementation is of vital importance, because of its critical patient safety consequences and the broader concerns about inefficiency and clinician burnout that may result from suboptimal workflow. To develop a systematic solution, it requires a collective effort from multiple stakeholders and an evidence-based approach. This includes regulatory oversight, continued effort by the industry to improve the design of their products, and development of new, patient- and clinician-centered implementation models to better incorporate software systems into clinical workflow. It should also be recognized that there does not exist a *one-size-fits-all* solution, especially considering the complexity of medical work and the variability across specialties and settings. More adaptable software designs are therefore desired, to better respond to the dynamic nature of clinical workflow to allow changes and deviations both during and after system adoption. In addition, clinicians' knowledge of and expectation for health IT also need to be updated to accommodate technological interventions, such as emerging AI-based technologies. Clinicians need to develop a more informed understanding of the new methods of medical work enabled by computerized systems, and the limitations thereof, to better leverage technology in their clinical practice. Through this book, we hope to establish a solid foundation toward these goals by compiling a collection of high-quality scholarly works that seek to provide clarity, consistency, and reproducibility, with a shared view of clinical workflow and its relevance to health IT design, implementation, and evaluation. We also hope that the discussions presented in this book will lead to actionable, pragmatic insights for informatics practitioners in designing, implementing, and evaluating workflow changes to better accommodate the adoption and use of health IT.

References

Bloomrosen M, Starren J, Lorenzi NM, Ash JS, Patel VL, Shortliffe EH. Anticipating and addressing the unintended consequences of health IT and policy: a report from the AMIA 2009 health policy meeting. J Am Med Inform Assoc. 2011;18(1):82–90.

Calvitti A, Hochheiser H, Ashfaq S, Bell K, Chen Y, El Kareh R, Gabuzda MT, Liu L, Mortensen S, Pandey B, Rick S, Street RL Jr, Weibel N, Weir C, Agha Z. Physician activity during outpatient visits and subjective workload. J Biomed Inform. 2017;69:135–49.

Carayon P, Karsh B-T. Incorporating health information technology into workflow redesign—summary report. AHRQ Publication No. 10–0098-EF. Rockville, MD: Agency for Healthcare Research and Quality; 2010.

Carayon P, Hoonakker P, Cartmill R, Hassol A. Patient-reported health information technology and workflow. AHRQ Publication No. 15–0043-EF. Rockville, MD: Agency for Healthcare Research and Quality; 2015.

Furniss SK, Burton MM, Grando A, Larson DW, Kaufman DR. Integrating process mining and cognitive analysis to study EHR workflow. AMIA Annu Symp Proc. 2017;2016:580–9.

Kannampallil T, Li Z, Zhang M, Cohen T, Robinson DJ, Franklin A, Zhang J, Patel VL. Making sense: sensor-based investigation of clinician activities in complex critical care environments. J Biomed Inform. 2011;44(3):441–54.

Lowry SZ, Ramaiah M, Patterson ES, Brick D, Gurses AP, Ozok A, Simmons D, Gibbons MC. Integrating electronic health records into clinical workflow: an application of human factors modeling methods to ambulatory care. NISTIR 7988. Gaithersburg, MD: National Institute of Standards and Technology; 2014.

National Research Council. Computational technology for effective health care: immediate steps and strategic directions. Washington D.C.: National Academies Press; 2009.

Wald JS, Novak LL, Simpson CL, et al. Health IT-enabled care coordination and redesign in Tennessee. AHRQ Publication No. 15–0048-EF. Rockville, MD: Agency for Healthcare Research and Quality; 2015.

Zheng K, Haftel HM, Hirschl RB, O'Reilly M, Hanauer DA. Quantifying the impact of health IT implementations on clinical workflow: a new methodological perspective. J Am Med Inform Assoc. 2010;17(4):454–61.

Zheng K, Guo MH, Hanauer DA. Using the time and motion method to study clinical work processes and workflow: methodological inconsistencies and a call for standardized research. J Am Med Inform Assoc. 2011;18(5):704–10.

Zheng K, Hanauer DA, Weibel N, Agha Z. Computational ethnography: automated and unobtrusive means for collecting data in situ for human–computer interaction evaluation studies. In: Patel VL, Kannampallil TG, Kaufman DR, editors. Cognitive informatics for biomedicine: human computer interaction in healthcare. Cham, Switzerland: Springer International Publishing; 2015b. p. 111–40.

Zheng K, Abraham J, Novak LL, Reynolds TL, Gettinger A. A survey of the literature on unintended consequences associated with health information technology: 2014–2015. Yearb Med Inform. 2016;1:13–29.

Zheng K, Ciemins E, Lanham HJ, Lindberg C. Examining the relationship between health IT and ambulatory care workflow redesign. AHRQ Publication No. 15–0058-EF. Rockville, MD: Agency for Healthcare Research and Quality. 2015.